D. GALVIN

VOCATIONAL REHABILITATION:
PROFESSION AND PROCESS

Publication Number 831

AMERICAN LECTURE SERIES®

A Publication in

The BANNERSTONE DIVISION *of*
AMERICAN LECTURES IN SOCIAL AND REHABILITATION PSYCHOLOGY

Consulting Editors

JOHN G. CULL, Ph.D.
Director, Regional Counselor Training Program
Department of Rehabilitation Counseling
Virginia Commonwealth University
Fishersville, Virginia

and

RICHARD E. HARDY, Ed.D.
Chairman, Department of Rehabilitation Counseling
Virginia Commonwealth University
Richmond, Virginia

The American Lecture Series in Social and Rehabilitation Psychology offers books which are concerned with man's role in his milieu. Emphasis is placed on how this role can be made more effective in a time of social conflict and a deteriorating physical environment. The books are oriented toward descriptions of what future roles should be and are not concerned exclusively with the delineation and definition of contemporary behavior. Contributors are concerned to a considerable extent with prediction through the use of a functional view of man as opposed to a descriptive, anatomical point of view.

Books in this series are written mainly for the professional practitioner; however, academicians will find them of considerable value in both graduate and undergraduate courses in the helping services.

VOCATIONAL REHABILITATION: PROFESSION AND PROCESS

Third Printing

JOHN G. CULL, Ph.D
*Director, Regional Counselor Training Program
Department of Rehabilitation Counseling
Virginia Commonwealth University
Fishersville, Virginia*

and

RICHARD E. HARDY, Ed.D.
*Chairman, Department of Rehabilitation Counseling
Virginia Commonwealth University
Richmond, Virginia*

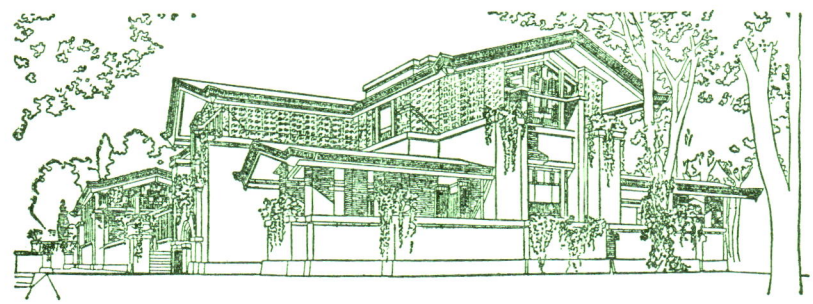

CHARLES C THOMAS • PUBLISHER
Springfield • Illinois • U.S.A.

Published and Distributed Throughout the World by
CHARLES C THOMAS • PUBLISHER
BANNERSTONE HOUSE
301-327 East Lawrence Avenue, Springfield, Illinois, U.S.A.

This book is protected by copyright. No part of it may be reproduced in any manner without written permission from the publisher.

© *1972 by* CHARLES C THOMAS • PUBLISHER
ISBN 0-398-02266-6
Library of Congress Catalog Card Number: 78-172453

First Printing, 1972
Second Printing, 1974
Third Printing, 1977

With THOMAS BOOKS *careful attention is given to all details of manufacturing and design. It is the Publisher's desire to present books that are satisfactory as to their physical qualities and artistic possibilities and appropriate for their particular use.* THOMAS BOOKS *will be true to those laws of quality that assure a good name and good will.*

Printed in the United States of America
N-1

Contributors

Beatrix Cobb, Ph.D.: Director of Counselor Training Program and Horn Professor of Psychology, Texas Tech University. Formerly, Research Fellow, Hogg Foundation for Mental Hygiene; Head, Medical Psychology Section, University of Texas, M. D. Anderson Hospital and Tumor Institute; and Associate Professor University of Texas Post-Graduate School of Medicine. Dr. Cobb has published widely in various professional journals and has been a contributing author to textbooks in rehabilitation.

John M. Cobun, M.A.: Candidate for Ed.D., American University, Washington, D.C.; Supervisor of Staff Development, Maryland Division of Vocational Rehabilitation. Formerly, Counselor with the Maryland Division of Vocational Rehabilitation.

Craig R. Colvin, M.Ed.: Assistant Professor, Regional Counselor Training Program, Department of Rehabilitation Counseling, School of Community Services, Virginia Commonwealth University. Formerly, State Coordinator for the North Carolina Department of Correction; Vocational Rehabilitation Counselor, North Carolina Division of Vocational Rehabilitation; co-author *Contemporary Field Work Practices in Rehabilitation*. Charles C Thomas, Publisher.

William A. Crunk: Associate Regional Commissioner for Rehabilitation and Self-Support Services, Social and Rehabilitation Services, Department of Health, Education and Welfare (Region III). Formerly, Field Representative, Office of Field Coordination, Office of the Secretary, Department of Health, Education and Welfare; Administrator, Central Alabama Rehabilitation Center and Crippled Childrens Clinic; Rehabilitation Supervisor and Counselor, Alabama Division of Vocational Rehabilitation. Special Assignments: Manpower Program Coordination Team, President's Committee on Manpower; Staff Member, Secretary's Task Force on Handicapped Children and Child Development.

John G. Cull, Ph.D.: Director, Regional Counselor Training Program and Professor, Department of Rehabilitation Counseling, School of Community Services, Virginia Commonwealth University; Lecturer, Medical Department Affiliate Program, Woodrow Wilson Rehabilitation Center. Formerly, Rehabilitation Counselor, Texas Commission for the Blind and Texas Division of Vocational Rehabilitation; Director of Research and Program Development, Virginia Department of Vocational Rehabilitation; co-author *Social and Rehabilitation Services for the Blind* and *Contemporary Field Work Practices in Rehabilitation,* Charles C Thomas, Publisher. Dr. Cull has contributed more than fifty publications to the professional literature in psychology and rehabilitation.

Wayne S. Gill, Ph.D.: Rehabilitation Psychologist in independent practice, San Antonio, Texas; Member, Texas State Board of Examiners of Psychologists; Consultant, Texas Rehabilitation Commission, State Commission for the Blind, Goodwill Industries and various school districts; Lecturer, Graduate Program in Rehabilitation, Our Lady of the Lake College. Dr. Gill is the author of twenty articles in various psychology and rehabilitation journals.

Richard E. Hardy, Ed.D.: Chairman, Department of Rehabilitation Counseling, School of Community Services, Virginia Commonwealth University. Formerly, Rehabilitation Counselor in Virginia, Chief Psychologist and Supervisor of Training, South Carolina Department of Vocational Rehabilitation; Rehabilitation Advisor, Rehabilitation Services Administration, Department of Health, Education and Welfare; co-author *Social and Rehabilitation Services for the Blind,* Charles C Thomas, Publisher. Dr. Hardy has contributed more than fifty publications to the professional literature in psychology and rehabilitation.

Paul R. Hoffman, Ed.D.: Chairman, Department of Rehabilitation and Manpower Services and Professor, School of Education, Stout State University; Technical Assistant, Division of Rehabilitation Facilities, Rehabilitation Services Administration, Department of Health, Education and Welfare; First President of Vocational Evaluation and Work Adjustment Association; Developer of first graduate program in work evaluation and initiation of national Materials Development Center in work evaluation and work adjustment; Recipient of Distinguished Service Award from the University of Arizona Alumni Association. Dr. Hoffman is the author of numerous articles in various publications, including national and foreign professional journals.

John D. Hutchinson, IV, M.S.: Assistant Professor and Academic Coordinator, Regional Counselor Training Program, Department of Rehabilitation Counseling, Virginia Commonwealth University. Formerly, Counselor, Administrative Supervisor of Medical Services Department and Supervisor of Evaluation Department at Woodrow Wilson Rehabilitation Center. Prior to accepting his current position, he was supervisor for staff training for the Virginia Department of Vocational Rehabilitation. Mr. Hutchinson was editor of *Vocational Rehabilitation of the Disadvantaged Disabled in the Rural Setting,* published by the U. S. Government Printing Office for the U. S. Department of Health, Education and Welfare.

Contributors

George R. Jarrell, Ph.D.: Coordinator of the Work-Study Program and Associate Professor, Department of Rehabilitation Counseling, Virginia Commonwealth University; Vocational Consultant, Bureau of Hearing and Appeals, Social Security Administration, Washington, D. C.; Training Consultant, Virginia Employment Commission, Richmond, Virginia. Formerly, Rehabilitation Counselor, Mental Health Commission, Columbia, South Carolina.

Robert A. Lassiter, Ph.D.: Chairman, Rehabilitation Counseling Program, School of Education, University of North Carolina at Chapel Hill. Formerly, State Director of Vocational Rehabilitation in North Carolina; Executive Director, North Carolina Society for Crippled Children and Adults; Rehabilitation Counselor and Supervisor in the Florida Vocational Rehabilitation program. Dr. Lassiter is the author of articles in various professional publications.

W. Alfred McCauley, M.A.: Executive Director, National Rehabilitation Counseling Association, Washington, D. C.; Visiting Lecturer, Virginia Commonwealth University and Pennsylvania State University, Rehabilitation Counselor Education. Formerly, Associate Regional Representative, Rehabilitation Services Administration, Department of Health, Education and Welfare, Region III, and Coordinator of Rehabilitation Counselor Training, West Virginia University. Mr. McCauley is the author of *The Blind Person as a College Teacher*, American Foundation for the Blind, and contributor to various rehabilitation publications.

Leslie F. McCoy, M.D.: Regional Medical Coordinator, Social and Rehabilitation Service, Department of Health, Education and Welfare, Region III, Philadelphia. Certified by the American Board of Internal Medicine.

Parnell McLaughlin, Ed.D.: Director, Division of Rehabilitation, Colorado Department of Social Services. Formerly, Rehabilitation Counselor; Consultant, Department of Education; Chief of the Division of Vocational Rehabilitation, Department of Rehabilitation; Director, Department of Rehabilitation. Dr. McLaughlin taught at the University of Denver and was Associate Clinical Professor at the University of Colorado School of Medicine, Physical Medicine and Rehabilitation Department. He served as a member of the Rehabilitation Counselor Training Committee and Chairman of the Personnel Committee, Council of State Administrators.

Leon Meenach, M.A.: Director, Program Planning and Development, Office of Rehabilitation Services, Atlanta, Georgia. Formerly, Director, Rehabilitation Services, Bureau of Rehabilitation, Frankfort, Kentucky. Mr. Meenach served as a counselor and consultant in the area of rehabilitation of the mentally ill and after-care facilities. He is a member of the Advisory Committee of the University of Georgia and Georgia State University Rehabilitation Graduate Training Programs and Chairman of the State of Georgia Coordinating Committee on Mental Disabilities.

Clayton A. Morgan, Ed.D.: Professor of Psychology and Coordinator, Rehabilitation Counselor Training Program, Oklahoma State University. Member of faculty, Creative Problem Solving Institute, State University of New York at Buffalo. Formerly, Vocational Rehabilitation Counselor, Texas Education Agency, Corpus Christi, Texas; secondary school teacher, Ellisville, Mississippi; speaker, resource person, and contributor of numerous publications in various areas of vocational rehabilitation.

Joe C. Morrow, M.A.: Director of Research and Training, North Carolina Division of Vocational Rehabilitation, Department of Public Instruction. Formerly, Director of North Carolina Statewide Comprehensive Planning; Consultant in Rehabilitation Counseling, Mental Retardation Training Institute, University of North Carolina; Counselor, Oklahoma Division of Vocational Rehabilitation.

Edward Newman, Ph.D.: Commissioner, Rehabilitation Services Administration, Social and Rehabilitation Service, U. S. Department of Health, Education and Welfare. Formerly, Assistant for Program Planning and Coordination of the Human Resources Programs Division of the Bureau of the Budget; Executive Director, Vocational Rehabilitation Planning Commission of the Commonwealth of Massachusetts. Dr. Newman is the author of various publications on aspects of planning for social and welfare services.

William R. Phelps, M.S., M.A.: Program Director, Regional Counselor Training Center, Institute, West Virginia. Formerly, Rehabilitation Counselor, State Psychologist, Assistant Administrator and Administrator of the West Virginia Rehabilitation Center. He is a consultant for the Social Security Administration and has published numerous articles in various journals related to mental retardation.

Corbett Reedy, M.A.: Deputy Commissioner, Rehabilitation Services Administration, U. S. Department of Health, Education and Welfare, Washington, D. C. Formerly, Regional Commissioner, Social and Rehabilitation Services Administration, Department of Health, Education and Welfare, Region III, Philadelphia; Director, Virginia Division of Vocational Rehabilitation. Mr. Reedy is Past President, National Rehabilitation Association; teacher, lecturer, writer in diverse subjects in the field of rehabilitation and founder of the short-term training program for rehabilitation counselor trainees at the Woodrow Wilson and West Virginia Rehabilitation Centers.

Edward F. Rose, M.Ed.: Director, Public Policy Employment Programs, United States Civil Service Commission. For his success in this assignment he received the Arthur S. Flemming Award as one of the ten outstanding young men in government for 1968. Formerly, Director of the George Mason Center for Retarded Children in the Arlington County Public

School System; Project Director of an occupational center for the retarded young adult.

Harold F. Shay, M.A.: Director, Division of Manpower Development, Rehabilitation Services Administration, Social and Rehabilitation Services, U. S. Department of Health, Education and Welfare, Washington, D.C. Prior to entering federal service, Mr. Shay held positions in the fields of Rehabilitation and Hospital Administration in Massachusettes and New York.

Harry W. Troop, M.S.: Deputy Director, Facilities Planning and Development, Illinois Division of Vocational Rehabilitation. Formerly, Consultant for Deaf and Hard of Hearing, Chief of Guidance, Training and Placement; Deputy Director, Client Services and Special Programs with the Illinois Division of Vocational Rehabilitation.

James A. West, Ph.D.: Coordinator, RSA Management Training Program, Business and Industrial Services, University of Oklahoma; Mr. West has held positions with Oklahoma Division of Rehabilitation Services from rehabilitation counselor through state director. Some of the several publications he has which resulted from research and demonstration grants include *One Volunteer, Fill the Gap,* 1963; *Mobile Rehabilitation Evaluation Team, Vocational Rehabilitation and the Juvenile Delinquent, Bridging the Gap between School and Employment,* 1964; *A Cooperative Program of Correctional Rehabilitation, Vocational Rehabilitation Services in the State Penitentiary System,* 1967; *Operation Research Program in the Oklahoma Vocational Rehabilitation Agency,* 1970.

Keith C. Wright, M.A.: Professor, Department of Rehabilitation Counseling, School of Community Services, Virginia Commonwealth University. Formerly, Research Analyst, West Virginia Division of Vocational Rehabilitation; Counselor and Research Analyst, United States Public Health Service, Past President Virginia Rehabilitation Association; Past President Virginia Association of Workers for the Blind; Coordinator Short-Term In-Service Training Institutes in Rehabilitation. Mr. Wright is the contributor of numerous articles to the professional literature.

To
Linda

Preface

FOR QUITE some time we, the authors, have felt the need for a basic introductory text in vocational rehabilitation counseling which would serve additionally as a reference for the practicing counselor. While a sizeable body of literature is developing in the area of vocational rehabilitation, there appears to be a paucity of practitioner-oriented material. The purpose of this book is to communicate with the practitioner in the field. It was intended to be limited in the areas of philosophy, theory and academia (the bulk of our professional literature covers these areas). In order to communicate with practitioners we chose contributors who themselves had experience as professional practitioners in the field or who had developed a close relationship with rehabilitation counselors lasting over a number of years.

As the title indicates, this book looks at vocational rehabilitation from two sides in an effort to provide an orientation to the counselor. It describes the counselor as a practitioner in various work settings, as a professional involved in the delivery of services and as a professional interacting with other professionals. Both the papers contained in the book and the contributors were selected after a great deal of planning. Generally, after the selection of the subject of each paper and its contributor, one and, in more critical areas, several extended discussions were held in order to insure each subject complimented the other without unnecessary overlapping and duplication.

The introductory section, Part One, lays the foundation for the book. It traces the history of the rehabilitation concept and considers the place of work in our culture. On this foundation the next two chapters build a prediction of the future through a discussion of changing manpower utilization and other trends developing in rehabilitation.

Part Two is a description of the rehabilitation counselor from two points of view. Chapter 5 describes the counselor by discussing the professional training experiences he should have. There is the common misconception that a professional is an individual filling a professional position. Chapter 5 belies this concept. Chapter 6 continues with a discussion of the professional status of rehabilitation counseling.

Part Three breaks the array of services provided by vocational rehabilitation into five areas. These areas include case finding; evaluation, which includes the most commonly used evaluations—vocational, medical, psychological and social; techniques of counseling (many writings are concerned with the philosophy and theory of counseling but few mention the mechanics or techniques of counseling); the selective training of clients in the rehabilitation process, including all types of training; and finally a chapter by Dr. Hardy which discusses the final phase of the rehabilitation process—placement and follow-up.

Part Four looks at counselor functions in various settings. The chapter on administration concerns in cooperative programs is of concern to counselors in all cooperative programs since it discusses the rationale and development of cooperative programs. Additionally this chapter points out areas of which the counselor should be aware in a cooperative relationship with another service agency. Two chapters are included on the school unit; one of which is oriented administratively, the second is functionally oriented. The remaining chapters treat the specific concerns of specialized counselors in other settings such as psychiatric rehabilitation, correctional rehabilitation and the counselor working with the blind.

In Part Five, Dr. Morgan has prepared an unusual but highly effective chapter for this text to provide insight into some of the characteristics of the client. The next chapter concerns the adjustment process to disability. It covers both adjustment mechanisms and factors which influence the adjustment process. While the aged are not at present eligible for rehabilitation services based on "age" alone, they constitute a large segment of our population and as such merit a discussion of their rehabilitation needs.

The last section of the book, Part Six, is devoted to the other professionals with whom the counselor interacts. Obtaining and using psychological services is an area of some confusion to counselors; therefore, three chapters of this section are devoted to this area. The remaining chapters include working with the physician, the rehabilitation facility and the community.

As with all efforts of this magnitude, there are many who played integral roles in the development of this book. We are indebted to the contributors who wrote such interesting and pertinent chapters. We wish to express our appreciation to them for their patience with us and with our continuing requests, suggestions and, on occasion, proddings. Also we wish to express our appreciation for the assistance we received from the faculty and staff of the Department of Rehabilitation Counseling, Virginia Commonwealth University.

Stuarts Draft, Virginia

JOHN G. CULL
RICHARD E. HARDY

Contents

Contributors v

Preface xiii

PART ONE
INTRODUCTION TO VOCATIONAL REHABILITATION

Chapter   *Page*

1. HISTORY OF THE REHABILITATION MOVEMENT IN AMERICA ... 5
2. PHILOSOPHICAL CONSIDERATIONS IN REHABILITATION AND WORK 59
3. CHANGING REHABILITATION MANPOWER UTILIZATION 66
4. DEVELOPING TRENDS IN REHABILITATION 77

PART TWO
THE REHABILITATION PRACTITIONER

5. THE CHALLENGE OF NEW DIMENSIONS IN REHABILITATION COUNSELOR EDUCATION IN THE SEVENTIES 123
6. THE PROFESSIONAL STATUS OF THE REHABILITATION COUNSELOR 150

PART THREE
THE REHABILITATION PROCESS

7. CASE FINDING 177
8. WORK EVALUATION: AN OVERVIEW 188
9. TECHNIQUES OF COUNSELING IN THE REHABILITATION PROCESS 212

Chapter	Page
10. SELECTIVE TRAINING	227
11. VOCATIONAL PLACEMENT	236

PART FOUR

THE REHABILITATION PRACTITIONER IN A WORK SETTING

12. ORIENTATION OF THE COUNSELOR IN THE GENERAL REHABILITATION PROGRAM	259
13. COOPERATIVE PROGRAMMING	274
14. ADMINISTRATIVE CONCERNS IN COOPERATIVE PROGRAMS	292
15. THE VOCATIONAL REHABILITATION—PUBLIC EDUCATION COOPERATIVE PROGRAM	304
16. THE SCHOOL UNIT COUNSELOR	336
17. THE CORRECTIONAL INSTITUTION AND VOCATIONAL REHABILITATION	351
18. REHABILITATIVE COUNSELING IN CORRECTIONAL SETTINGS	380
19. THE MENTAL HEALTH REHABILITATION COUNSELOR	386
20. PROVIDING COUNSELING SERVICES TO BLIND AND SEVERELY VISUALLY IMPAIRED PERSONS	396

PART FIVE

THE CLIENTS IN THE REHABILITATION PROCESS

21. I, THE CLIENT	409
22. ADJUSTMENT TO DISABILITY	421
23. THE REHABILITATION NEEDS OF THE OLDER ADULT	435

PART SIX

WORKING WITH OTHER PROFESSIONALS IN THE REHABILITATION PROCESS

Chapter	Page
24. Working with the Physician	449
25. The Psychologist and Rehabilitation	470
26. Planning for Psychological Services in Vocational Rehabilitation: A Priority Consideration	484
27. State Rehabilitation Administrators' Views on Psychological Evaluation	498
28. Working with the Rehabilitation Facility	503
29. Working with the Community	526
Index	539

VOCATIONAL REHABILITATION: PROFESSION AND PROCESS

PART ONE

INTRODUCTION TO VOCATIONAL REHABILITATION

History of the Rehabilitation Movement in America
Philosophical Considerations in Rehabilitation and Work
Changing Rehabilitation Manpower Utilization
Developing Trends in Rehabilitation

1

History of the Rehabilitation Movement in America

Robert A. Lassiter

Tyrone: Mary! For God's Sake, forget the past!
Mary: How can I? The past is the present, isn't it? It's the future, too. We all try to lie out of that but life won't let us.
                EUGENE O'NEILL, *Long Day's Journey into Night*, Act II, Scene 2

The Expanding Role of Rehabilitation
Industrialization and the Rehabilitation Movement
Urbanization and the Rehabilitation Movement
Medicine and the Rehabilitation Movement
Development of Workman's Compensation
Psychology and the Rehabilitation Movement
Religion and Rehabilitation
Social Reform and Rehabilitation
The Vocational Education Movement
The Vocational Rehabilitation Act
The Early Role of the Counselor and Rehabilitation
Broadening the Scope of Rehabilitation
The Development and Impact of Public Law 565
Rehabilitation in the 1960's
Summary
References and Notes

THE EXPANDING ROLE OF REHABILITATION

IN RECENT years, the vocational rehabilitation movement has experienced an unprecedented period of growth.

Federal and state governments are placing a greater emphasis on the rehabilitation concept, defined as a process of restoring the handicapped individual to the fullest physical, mental, social, vocational and economic usefulness of which he is capable.[1] The increased use of this approach in meeting the needs of disabled people reflects the public's growing recognition of a social obligation to help disabled people move toward their independence and self-sufficiency and at the same time the increasing realization of the economic benefits that come as a result of the rehabilitation process. Also, there appears to be an emerging consciousness of the purely humanitarian aspects of rehabilitation. In 1964 Mary Switzer, former Administrator of the Social and Rehabilitation Service, Department of Health, Education and Welfare, stated the following:

> Vocational rehabilitation, like many other aspects of human affairs, has evolved through three stages of public attitude—compassion without action, followed by willingness to act for economic reasons, followed by willingness to act for social reasons. It seems to me that we are at a transitional stage between the last two, with almost universal acceptance of the economic soundness of returning disabled people to employment and a slowly growing philosophy that an advanced civilization like ours should so order its system that all disabled people will be restored as fully as possible regardless of economic benefits to anyone.[2]

The U. S. Congress, in 1965, literally doubled the financial support of the Federal Government and at the same time extended rehabilitation services to the "socially" handicapped. In 1968, Congress passed unanimously the Vocational Rehabilitation Amendments which again increased financial support to the states and provided for state construction and operation of work adjustment centers to serve physically and mentally handicapped people and those persons termed "disadvantaged." Vocational rehabilitation regulations define the disadvantaged "as individuals who are handicapped because of their age, low educational attainment, ethnic or cultural factors, prison or delinquent records, or other conditions which constitute a barrier to employment."[3] John Gardner, former Secretary of Health, Education and Welfare, in establishing the Social and Rehabilitation Service in 1967, stated that he wanted to expand the concept of rehabilitation to extend the principles and techniques of rehabilitation to all people in trouble. "We can salvage many more lives. We can help restore a sense of belonging to those outside the mainstream of society— the people in the urban ghettos and rural slums, the needy and disadvantaged."[4] Another trend in this remarkable growth of rehabilitation is seen in the establishment of numerous joint or cooperative programs with special education units; state mental hospitals and centers for the mentally retarded through the departments of mental health; adult and juvenile correctional rehabilitation units; and cooperative agreements with social service departments, alcoholic rehabilitation units, sheltered workshops, local guidance clinics, the social security disability fund, local general hospitals, university service units and others.

Russell A. Nixon, Associate Director of the Center for Study of the Unemployed, New York University, in a major address to the National Rehabilitation Association's annual conference in New Orleans in 1968, stated the following:

> It is increasingly clear that vocational rehabilitation of the disabled cannot advance in isolation from the social and economic strains, problems, and convulsions which challenge our country today . . . these changes (1968 amendments in vocational rehabilitation) arising in these troubled times add to the traditional mission of rehabilitation in several difficult and very challenging ways. . . . A new mandate is given to reach and service adequately the toughest cases . . . to provide services to families of the handicapped, and to raise to a new level the vocational and work adjustment services of rehabilitation. . . . The experiences, processes and resources of vocational rehabilitation are now to be extended beyond the traditional physically and mentally disabled to serve the needs of those suffering socio-economic handicaps . . . fully implemented, this new legislature mandate will make vocational rehabilitation a central factor in the toughest and most intractable part of our national manpower, urban and anti-poverty problems—the vocational rescue of the hard core unemployed. . . . In size—from a program of $116 million five years ago to a program already authorized by Congress to start spending around $1.25 billion annually in 1971. . . . In content—from a well-conducted but relatively small program performing magnificent services for a special group of especially needy persons, to a major program in the center of the socio-economic storm, significantly involved in the labor market, in the anti-poverty, ghetto, minority participation, and urban decentralization problems that stir our society. This expanded and changed role of vocational rehabilitation is . . . the inevitable consequence of public policy and program experiences which have validated the rehabilitation philosophy and process and the best way to meet many of our most difficult human problems.[5]

It can be seen, then, that the concept of vocational rehabilitation offers hope to many in politics and government for a solution to some major social problems. Problems come, however, from the fact that there are few charts or guidelines available to those who are responsible for the expansion of the program. Through a more comprehensive understanding of the past, the rehabilitation concept will be less likely to be misinterpreted and new decisions will result in an improved program of services for handicapped people.

The vocational rehabilitation program in America began on June 2, 1920, with the passage of a minor act in the Sixty-sixth Congress, Public Law 236. The act opened with these words, "that in order to provide the promotion of vocational rehabilitation of persons disabled in industry or in any legitimate occupation," and the act provided a first attempt in defining the terms: "the term 'person disabled' shall be construed to mean any person who, by reason of a physical defect or infirmity, whether congenital or acquired by accident, injury, or disease, is, or may be expected to be, totally or partially incapacitated for remunerative occupation; the term 'rehabilitation' shall be construed to mean the rendering of a person disabled fit to engage in a remunerative occupation."[6] A twofold program of vocational guidance and vocational education for physically handicapped people, as contained in this act, was evidence of the Federal Government's early concern for the welfare of individuals. It was also the result of a greater awareness in this country of the need to conserve human resources for economic benefit to society as a whole. For an understanding of this new legislation, it must be viewed in the light of the historical forces and social movements of the late nineteenth and early twentieth centuries, during the period that has been described as the second phase of the Industrial Revolution.[7]

INDUSTRIALIZATION AND THE REHABILITATION MOVEMENT

Within a thirty-year period (1890–1920), the demands made on society by industrialization, immigration and urbanization created new individual and social needs which could be met only by a responsive federal government, a government based on the philosophy that every individual has the right of life, liberty and the pursuit of happiness as guaranteed in the American Constitution. "The history of vocational rehabilitation is the history of a long struggle to establish dignity and opportunity as a right of disabled persons, just as history in general is the story of the long struggle to establish dignity and opportunity as a right of every human being."[8]

The origins of the vocational rehabilitation movement can be found in an examination of some of the historical forces at the turn of the century. Historical perspective can be gained by an analysis of some of the social movements which were developing prior to (and parallel with) the program of vocational rehabilitation.

With an increasing industrialization of America, all social problems became more complex. The immigration movement contributed to the labor needs of a rapidly growing industrial nation, but a *laissez-faire* system of government in the nineteenth century created serious vocational and educational problems for immigrants. "Immigration had transformed the entire economic world within which they (the immigrants) had formerly lived. From surface forms to inmost functionings, the change was complete. A new setting, new activities, and new meanings forced the newcomers into radically new roles as producers and consumers of goods. In the process, they became, in their own eyes, less worthy as men."[9]

Labor unions were organized as a protest to this feeling of alienation as well as a revolt to the long hours, low pay and poor working conditions which prevailed at the close of the nineteenth century. Samuel Gompers (an immigrant himself) provided leadership for the new American Federation of Labor which became a major force in raising the standards of American Labor.[10] Prior to the activities of Gompers and other labor leaders in the early years of the twentieth century, many of the social ills caused by the Industrial Revolution were accepted as necessary evils by the government: "The accident toll taken by heedless negligence, and the damage done to workers' health by poor ventilation and lighting, dust and fumes, were all charged off as the cost of progress.[11] When the government intervened at all in the nineteenth century, it was to extend loans, grant subsidies and provide public resources for industry. Gompers emphasized the need for the government to regulate working conditions through safety and insurance programs; and he saw labor's major responsibility as gaining higher wages. He, unlike more radical leaders, felt that labor should accept the capitalist system and win for itself a legitimate position within that economic world. Another group of workers who felt the anguish of this period of industrialization were the farmers who began to migrate to the cities. America had gradually become an urban nation. Even in 1890, there were as many industrial wage earners as farm laborers, tenants and farm owners combined. New adjustments were required of these farmers as they took jobs in the factories and mills, just as with the immigrants from overseas.[12]

Industrialization increased the division of labor which produced additional problems for the workingman:

> First, it resulted in the breakdown of craft skills into a series of mechanized operations. Each special-purpose machine created a new job . . . the development of interchangeable parts led to an increase in the number of narrowly specialized jobs in assembly operations . . . the size of the work force required by the rapidly growing factories. . . . The growth of cities also increased the division of labor since a great many more service activities are required in urban than in rural areas.[13]

This increasing and more complex division of labor and the break that came from a change in the traditional bases of status and power were a part of the basic conditions that would be necessary for the later development of an interest in vocational guidance matters:

> The job was regarded as a sacred calling, and success at work was evidence that one had been chosen for salvation. . . . With an increasingly differentiated occupational structure serving as the basis for status distinctions instead of land holding or aristocratic birth, which had been more important earlier, the foundation was established for the elaborate occupational status structure characteristic of modern industrial societies.[14]

In a thirty-year span (1890–1920) population in the United

States increased over 100 percent, with more of the increase occurring in the cities. "The growth of the people of the United States is one of the remarkable phenomena in history. . . . Immigration increased from 50,262,000 in 1880 to 76,129,000 in 1900, to 107,180,000 in 1920."[15] As technical invention and technology proceeded along with this growth, higher qualified workers in all fields were in demand, as well as a greater variety. Also young women were able to become employed as wage earners.

URBANIZATION AND THE REHABILITATION MOVEMENT

"The city, with its immense need for new facilities in transportation, sanitation, policing, light, gas and public structures offered a magnificent internal market for American business. And business looked for the sure thing, for privileges, above all for profitable franchises and for opportunities to evade as much as possible of the burden of taxation. The urban boss, a dealer in public privileges who could also command public support, became a more important and more powerful figure."[16] One urban boss, George Washington Plunkett, who became a millionaire as a Tammany leader, enjoyed telling how he made his fortune through politics:

> Everybody is talking these days about Tammany men growin' rich on graft, but nobody thinks of drawing the distinction between honest graft and dishonest graft. . . . Yes, many of our men have grown rich in politics. I have myself. I've made a big fortune out of the game, and I'm gettin' richer every day, but I've not gone in for dishonest graft. . . . I might sum up the whole thing by sayin': I seen my opportunities and I took 'em. Just let me explain by examples. My party's in power in the city, and it's goin' to undertake a lot of public improvements. Well, I'm tipped off, say, that they're goin' to lay out a new park at a certain place. . . . I go to that place and buy up all the land I can in the neighborhood . . . and, there is a rush to get my land, which nobody cared particular for before. Ain't it perfectly honest to charge a good price and make a profit on my investment and foresight? Of course it is. Well, that's honest graft.[17]

Pressures for reform in politics and government mounted—not only to eliminate "honest" as well as "dishonest graft" from the city governments but also to promote assistance from the Federal Government for the welfare of individuals who were victims of the system. These pressures were expressed in the Populist-Progressive political movement, which began in the 1890's and continued to the beginning of World War I. This effort in political reform is considered "the first modern political movement of practical importance in the United States to insist that the federal government has some responsibility for the commonwealth; indeed, it (populism) was the first such movement to attack seriously the problems created by industrialization."[18] This political movement gave support to the fight for women's suffrage, led by Susan B. Anthony and other women pioneers in the late nineteenth and early twentieth century. "In January of 1886, a bill to enfranchise women was presented to the Senate for the first time and suffered its first defeat. Through the years the same measure was submitted to Congress regularly, until the number of Congressmen favoring women's suffrage grew to a majority. In June, 1919, with President Wilson as an ally, the Nineteenth Amendment was passed, and ratification of the amendment by thirty-six states occurred in August, 1920."[19] The employment of larger numbers of women in industry and business during this era already had provided women an increasing economic independence which helped in the preparation for this new political freedom. There were many women who had become prominent in literature and the arts who contributed to this new climate of acceptance. Also, the women involved in social reform who were concerned about the plight of women workers in industry were helping in the crusade for women's suffrage. The final passage of the amendment, however, was due to the aggressive work of key leaders such as Miss Anthony,[20] whose major concern was in the field of women's rights.

The progressive movement in politics was maintained by a new journalism being practiced in the United States during this period. Technical advances in the communication field (for example, rapid printing machines and the telegraph) and the emergence of newspapers and magazines provided the expression for reform; and the financial resources that were made available to the muckrakers helped to draw nationwide attention to the need of reform.[21] "Progressivism fed on indignation, and the turn of the century witnessed a revolution in journalism and literature which made it easy for conscientious people to stir up indignation."[22] *The Jungle* by Upton Sinclair and the writings of Jack London are examples of the literature of the period which contributed to the public's recognition of a need for reform.

MEDICINE AND THE REHABILITATION MOVEMENT

The striking progress made in technical inventions and science in this era contributed to the development of modern medicine which is ascribed to the period 1870 to 1920. Medical science began to offer a means of preventing disease and disability and also offered hope for the cure and rehabilitation of disabled people. Excess wealth accumulated over the years prompted many millionaires to contribute large amounts of money to the support of medical research and education.

> This era was the great turning point in the history of American medicine. After three centuries of dependence on European science, American medical research attained a status equal to that of the better European centers. After an equally long period of mediocre or inferior training, medical education attained a level similar to that reached in the old world. And, last, but not least, the average practice of the younger, native physicians became at least as reliable as that of their counterparts in Western Europe.[23]

This new medicine in America and its technical advances facilitated the establishment of large and improved hospitals, research institutes, medical schools, medical societies and professional publications. It can be seen that the development of a vocational rehabilitation program would be dependent on a medical science which could provide an optimistic way of helping disabled people.

The establishment of the Public Health and Marine Hospital Service in 1902 provided a federal base for extending public health services to meet the health demands of an increasingly complex society. Progress in science and medical practice gave public health leaders the knowledge and skills needed in the development of programs in sanitation, immunization and other preventive procedures; and in 1912, the United States Public Health Service was set up in the Federal Government.[24] The emphasis was placed on preventing disease and health problems for the masses rather than stressing a social medicine program that would be concerned with the individual. The public health leaders may have felt that the promise of sanitation and immunization would eliminate disease entirely and there would be no need for direct care to individuals.[25]

DEVELOPMENT OF WORKMAN'S COMPENSATION

At the close of the nineteenth century, industry followed the common law which stated that the master or employer was responsible for the injury or death of employees when the employer was negligent. With the expansion of production, the number of accidents increased and the law suits made against employers to prove "negligence" also increased. Many states, between 1900 and 1910, by judicial decision, adopted a rule that employees need not accept responsibility for disabilities resulting from work, and in 1910, the first complete workmen's compensation law in the United States was passed in New York. By 1921, forty-five of the states and territories had passed legislation for workmen's compensation. They were not all the same as they varied in scope, benefits and administration.[26] State legislators attempted to enact laws that would cover the following points:

1. provide compensation to victims of work accidents and their dependents,
2. free the courts from delay, cost and work load,
3. relieve public and private charities of the financial drain,
4. eliminate economic waste in the payment of fees to lawyers and witnesses,
5. to supplant the practice of concealing the fault by a spirit of a frank study of the causes to provide a program of prevention.[27]

The initial laws on workmen's compensation did not include services for vocational rehabilitation, but the people who supported legislation for workmen's compensation also supported the concept of vocational rehabilitation. It was clear to them that help was needed for injured workers to return to employment, but specific legislation was to come later. Dr. R.M. Little, active in the workmen's compensation movement and the first director of vocational rehabilitation in New York, felt that the leaders in workmen's compensation programs and in organized labor were more influential than others in the early discussions of vocational rehabilitation and that neither education nor social work took the lead in the development of legislation.[28]

Efforts by industry to prevent accidents and preserve the health of employees were based on the profit motive—how to avoid loss in production resulting from the workers' temporary or permanent absence. Large industries were the first to introduce industrial medicine programs for employees. Public health measures and laws such as those in workmen's compensation placed on the employer the responsibility for the elimination of hazards and for the medical care and compensation of injured workers. In 1909, Sears Roebuck and Company set up one of the first programs for periodic physical examinations of all employees, and, in that same year cooperation between voluntary health agencies and employers began when the Milwaukee Visiting Nurse Association placed the first nurse in an industrial plant. "By 1915, although most states had not as yet passed workmen's compensation legislation, occupational health programs maintained on a voluntary basis by industry had so far developed that industrial doctors met to form the American Association of Industrial Physicians and Surgeons."[29]

PSYCHOLOGY AND THE REHABILITATION MOVEMENT

From the 1890's through 1915, there was a corresponding growth in the new field of psychology. American psychology was influenced by the European movement, but Americans also made their own unique contributions to this developing profession. For example, William James, America's first prominent psychologist, stressed the individual rather than the social goals of education. He helped to bring psychology into the classroom by stressing its application to everyday problems.[30] G. Stanley Hall, the first president of Clark University and a professor in psychology, established the *American Journal of Psychology*, and in 1892 he helped found the American Psychological Association. Hall emphasized in his studies of children and adolescents the uniqueness of the individual. His studies brought about great public interest and led to the establishment of the child study movement.[31] Also, in 1909, Hall invited Sigmund Freud to Clark University for a series of lectures which provided American psychologists an opportunity to examine Freud's use of psychoanalysis as therapy for individuals with mental problems. Many of the American pioneers in psychology were present, including William James, and Freud's lectures were published in American psychological journals.[32] At about the same time, considerable interest was shown in America in the objective measurement studies by the French psychologist, Alfred Binet. These studies of individual children's intelligence led to the development of the first intelligence scale—the Binet-Simon IQ Test. In 1916, Louis Terman adopted the intelligence quotient (IQ) in his work at Stanford University as he revised the Binet Scales; consequently, the well-known Stanford-Binet Test for intelligence[33] was developed.

This national interest in psychology and its application to work with individuals contributed extensively to the developing concern for the lot of the individual in America. The principles of psychology and objective measurement techniques were to be utilized by industry in the new field of industrial psychology. In 1911, Professor Hugo Munsterberg of Harvard was employed by the Boston Elevated Railway to develop psychological tests for the selection of streetcar operators.[34] As Brewer states in his history of guidance, these developments and the growing complications of technology helped to set the stage for the need of vocational guidance, although they did not lead directly to the development of a vocational guidance movement. Frederick W. Taylor, the father of "scientific management," the forerunner of industrial psychology, represented the early concern for individual workers on the part of industry. In commenting on Taylor's early work, Brewer states:

History of the Rehabilitation Movement in America

The movement for scientific management concerned as it was with time and motion study and other intricate analyses, did serve to emphasize the fact that care must be exercised in adjusting the man to the job. Nevertheless, this very care in fitting the man to the job put the emphasis not on the man and his talents, desires, choices, but on the job as the center, to which the man was to be made to adjust in the interest of efficient production.[35]

Other parallel events were taking place in the general field of psychology during this thirty-year period, and the developing movement in mental health was significant. In the late nineteenth century, Dorothea Dix, in her concern for a more humane treatment of people with mental illness, led the drive to build state hospitals for the mentally ill in this country. "From thirteen institutions for the mentally ill in 1843, the number had risen to one hundred and twenty-three in 1890 of which seventy-five were state owned . . . in the founding of thirty-two of the seventy-five state hospitals, Dorothea Dix had had an intimate part."[36] Clifford Beers, a former mental patient, wrote a book in 1908 describing his experiences in two state mental hospitals in Connecticut. This book, *A Mind That Found Itself,* facilitated the growth of the mental health movement, and Beers, with the help of psychologists, psychiatrists and private citizens, established a national organization that became the National Association of Mental Health. William James, on reading the manuscript for *A Mind That Found Itself,* wrote the following in a letter to Beers:

> The book ought to go far toward helping along that terribly needed reform, the amelioration of the lot of the insane of our country, for the Auxiliary Society which you propose is feasible (as numerous examples in other fields show) and ought to work important effects on the whole situation. . . . You have handled a difficult theme with great skill, and produced a narrative of absorbing interest to scientist as well as layman.[37]

RELIGION AND REHABILITATION

There were other movements, in addition to those in mental health, which provided a stimulant for an awakening of the American social conscience. Religion, at the height of industrialization in the late nineteenth century, with its chief concern for the spiritual needs of people, was dedicated to individualism and the doctrine of *laissez faire,* in the main. Henry Ward Beecher, a prominent Protestant minister, preached the theory of Social Darwinism—survival of the fittest in the economic world.[38] Later, a few Protestant clergymen, responding to the social crises, began to preach the need for social reform and the concept of good works which led to the movement known as the Social Gospel. One of the leaders of that period, F. Ernest Johnson, held this idea about the need for reform:

> The point is that the Christian ideal of life is definitely blocked, thwarted, and travestied by the all-pervading influence of economic self-interest and of the competitive struggle. The social gospel program aims at clearing the way for a new advance by the spirit of man.[39]

Since the new immigrants were predominantly Roman Catholic, the American Catholic Church of this period became the church of the city, the worker and the immigrant. The papal encyclical *Rerum Novarum* of 1891 pointed out social ideals and responsibilities that supported the social views of many Americans. Earlier, James Gibbons, in Rome to be installed as a cardinal, defended the cause of American labor before the Holy See.[40]

Roman Catholics and Jews, because of their smaller numbers in the total population, were not as influential in the social reform movement as were the Protestants in their total effort; however, in some ways, they were more effective on specific issues because they were less restricted than the Protestants with their close alliance with the economic system. Reverend Johnson stated in his social gospel book:

> I have often envied my Catholic friends their ability to cite unquestioned, authoritative doctrines of vast social import in support of their preachments. The Jewish tradition likewise lends itself to a more active support of social idealism than has characterized Protestantism.[41]

Despite the problems, many of the new social programs emerged from the Protestant faith. The Salvation Army came to America from England in 1879 with a goal of reaching the city's poor people. Using evangelistic methods, they preached repentance to "rumdom, slumdom, and bumdom."[42] They also added a social program to bring welfare relief with the gospel. The growing concern in the Protestant church for the poor can be seen in the first program of Goodwill Industries, established in 1902 by Dr. Edgar James Helms, a Methodist minister in Boston. The idea of hiring unemployed persons to do the renovation and repair work on clothing and materials donated by the public and paying the workers from funds derived from the sale of these repaired products was developed. It was in 1918 that the Board of Missions of the Methodist Church took over Goodwill Industries, continuing the nondenominational approach and also emphasizing a sheltered workshop program for the physically handicapped.[43]

In tracing the historical development of the influence of the Jewish community on social ethics, Sidney Goldstein describes the major Jewish religious philosophy on social welfare issues: "It is only when mysticism becomes a pseudo-communion between the individual and God, an experience to be sought for itself and a form of emotional indulgence, that it fails to move men to social action. The legitimate, the necessary, the inevitable expression of the religious spirit in Judaism is the social passion . . . a more powerful expression of communion than is either creed or ceremony or the Commandments."[44] B'nai B'rith, a welfare and educational organization established by American Jews in 1843, developed rapidly during the late nineteenth and early twentieth centuries. Its present program in vocational guidance and its sponsorship of various nondenominational vocational training centers for the handicapped grew from this experience of B'nai B'rith during the early years of this century.[45]

In addition to these church-based or church-connected charitable programs, there were other eleemosynary organizations active during this period. For example, there was encouragement from the government; Rockefeller set up the Rockefeller Foundation; the Carnegie Corporation was established in 1911; and Woodrow Wilson, in 1913, pointed out the human cost of the industrial achievements of the country and suggested that industry should help to alleviate some of the misery created in its development. Many of the volunteer health, education and welfare organizations were established to provide a variety of services for people in trouble: The American Red Cross (1881), with its Red Cross Institute for Crippled and Disabled Men in New York City and its early sponsorship of Braille transcriptions for the blind (later to be administered by the Library of Congress); The National Tuberculosis Association in 1904; the National Easter Seal Society for Crippled Children and Adults which began in Ohio in affiliation with local Rotary Clubs; and the National Association of Mental Health founded by Clifford Beers in 1909.[46]

SOCIAL REFORM AND REHABILITATION

Jane Addams, the most famous of the early pioneers in social work, created the first organized secular program of social welfare in America in 1889; Hull House in Chicago, which was established to help educate immigrants and to protect them from exploitation. It was at Hull House that Miss Addams developed the casework approach in helping individuals adjust to their environments—family, school, neighborhood and country. "It was her method of approaching political and social questions that distinguished Jane Addams from other reformers. Like other progressives, she wanted to substitute explanation and analysis for moral exhortation. Therein lay her originality and the originality of her generation."[47] Some of the reforms with which she helped were the first 8-hour day laws for women, the first state child-labor laws and the first juvenile court. She was a strong supporter of reform in education as well. "Jane Addams' ideas paralleled and supported the educational theories of John Dewey. It is difficult to say whether Dewey influenced Jane Addams or Jane Addams influenced Dewey. They influenced each other and generously acknowledged their mutual obligations."[48] Dewey served on the first board at Hull House and one of his teachers was a resident of the settlement house. It was later that Miss Addams became the first president of the National Conference of Charities and Corrections (which was to become the National Conference of Social Welfare). Lillian Wald, founder of the Henry Street Settlement in New York, was the first person to propose that a children's bureau be set up in the Federal Government, and the first two heads of that agency came from Miss Addams' program at Hull House. The authors of *The National Experience* wrote:

It was these middle class reformers rather than the trade unions that launched the movement for social legislation in America. They led the agitation that put through the first child-labor laws and they helped to focus the nation's attention on the evils of the slums.[49]

A great system of free public education was developing in America during this period—1890 to 1920., "The cause of free public education was advanced as a practical necessity to fill the needs of a growing industrial America while serving as a fulfillment of a dream never before translated into action on a national scale."[50] That dream was to give every child a free education. By 1900, thirty-three states had passed statewide compulsory attendance laws and others were to follow, so that by 1920 all states had these laws.[51] Efforts made toward federal aid to education in these early years of the twentieth century were unsuccessful; however, certain legal precedents were set in such legislation as the Morrill Act of 1862, which offered states land grants to endow colleges of agriculture and mechanical arts.[52]

In the period from 1890 through 1920, one man stands out in the public school movement—John Dewey, the famous American psychologist and philosopher who had been a pupil of G. Stanley Hall. Interested in a child-centered school (that is, progressive education), Dewey established a laboratory school in Chicago which was the first school based on a psychological theory and it became one of the most influential schools in the Western World. Dewey's experiment continued for eight years (1896–1904) and much of its theory was published; also, thousands of educators from all over the world visited the school. The emphasis was on the individual child and the conditions necessary for its growth.

Five basic conditions were sought:

1. Freedom for the child to investigate and experiment.
2. Choice of school experiences to fit the child's changing interests, attitudes and stages of growth.
3. The program built around the solving of problems—considered important beyond all the rest.
4. The use of scientific material and the scientific way of working.
5. Provision for cooperative activity, because the school is a minature community.[53]

THE VOCATIONAL EDUCATION MOVEMENT

Many of the educational leaders (as well as industrial leaders) saw the unique opportunities presented by an industrial arts or a vocational education program in the public schools. Dewey's support is seen in this statement as he expressed the need for an integrated rather than an isolated approach in vocational education or manual arts training: "They (the manual arts) afford the most permanent and persistent occupations of the great majority of human kind. They present man with his most perplexing problems; they stimulate him to the most strenuous putting forth of effort."[54] There were, however, only isolated vocational education programs in the public schools in the early years of the twentieth century. Vocational training, for the most part, was confined to industrial schools for poor and delinquent children and in correctional institutions.

> It took the need for skilled labor, made manifest by World War I, to win from Congress federal support of vocational education. The Smith-Hughes Act became law in February, 1917, inaugurating a succession of enactments that reimbursed states for the teaching of vocational agriculture, home economics and industrial arts.[55]

Through federal support, vocational education became a part of most curricula in the public schools. The principles of vocational education, derived from this experience in the public schools, were fundamental to the development of vocational rehabilitation.

Special classes or special schools for handicapped children developed in the public schools in the latter part of the nineteenth century, although most of the programs were located in large cities and they were few in number. Earlier in the nineteenth century, private schools for deaf mutes and blind children were established: Thomas Gallaudet, a pioneer in work with the deaf, opened the first school for the deaf in 1817 in Connecticut and the Perkins Institution and Massachusetts School for the Blind were started in 1823.[56] These private schools and their special programs for handicapped children led to the development of numerous state schools or institutions for handicapped children in the late nineteenth and early twentieth centuries. These public institutions for indigent children who were blind, deaf or mentally retarded, placed an early emphasis on vocational training, but later this emphasis changed as the institutions, in the 1900's, became, for some years, "asylums" where stress was placed on custodial care.[57] Classes for handicapped children in the public schools began during the latter part of the nineteenth century: Special classes for the mentally retarded were instituted in Springfield, Massachusetts, in 1896; the first class for blind children was started in Chicago in 1900; and the Detroit Day School for the Deaf was organized in 1900 with two classes for the deaf.[58] Special education, as a distinctive profession within public education, was slow to develop. Beck provides one answer for this: "Agitation for special provision for the education of the handicapped was noticeably minimal, at least in the United States. Voluntary groups of laymen, of parents, did not organize; perhaps parents of handicapped children were too ashamed to make their plight public."[59]

Vocational education and vocational guidance were indicated in the original Vocational Rehabilitation Act in 1920 as the two services which would be provided physically handicapped people. Of greatest impact on the developing vocational rehabilitation program would be vocational guidance, a relatively new discipline. Only twelve years before, Frank Parsons, a social worker, organized and established the Vocational Bureau in Boston (1908), the first organized vocational guidance program in America. "It was his concern that the strengths and weaknesses of individuals be understood and brought into harmony with vocational opportunities."[60] In his book, *Choosing a Vocation,* Parsons stated three broad factors in outlining a theory of vocational guidance: "1. a clear understanding of yourself. . . . 2. a knowledge of the requirements and conditions for success . . . in different lines of work, and 3. true reasoning of the relation of these two groups of facts."[61] Parsons' intelligent spirit of reform and his far-seeing vision are reflected in this passage from his book:

> Not till society wakes up to its responsibility and its privileges . . . shall we be able to harvest more than a fraction of our human resources, or develop and utilize the genius and ability that are latent in each new generation. When that time does come, education will become the leading industry, and a vocation bureau in effect will be a

part of the public-school system in every community—a bureau provided with every facility that science can devise for the testing of the senses and capabilities, and the whole physical, intellectual, and emotional makeup of the child, and with experts trained as carefully for the work as men are trained today for medicine and law.[62]

The movement in vocational guidance grew out of the efforts of pioneers in the public schools as well. Eli W. Weaver, in 1904, set up a program in Brooklyn, New York, to help high school boys in job placement, work for the summer and part-time work after school. Jesse B. Davis, from 1898 to 1907, while principal of the Central High School in Detroit, provided counseling for students relative to their vocational and educational problems.[63] David S. Hill, an early leader in educational research in New Orleans, thought that the educational system should be based on scientific research. "Hill used more complete methods to study individuals than any of his contemporaries. He utilized the techniques of medical science to examine the physical fitness of boys and girls who were referred to his research bureau, he used the newest psychological tests including the Binet individual intelligence test, and he sent a trained social investigator into homes to learn about the environments of children. Society, according to Hill (1907), was constantly evolving, and it was necessary for an individual to adapt himself to the changing conditions within the society in order to survive."[64] Hill felt that the application of scientific principles would help education and industry move toward a greater cooperation that would result in progress for the whole society.[65]

As these concepts in vocational guidance spread, educators, social workers, business and government leaders and psychologists —those who were interested in applying its principles—joined together in founding the National Vocational Guidance Association in 1913, the forerunner of the American Personnel and Guidance Association.[66] An observation by the authors of *Guidance: A Developmental Approach* indicates the direction that guidance would take in the public schools as it became a major concern of American education:

> The optimal development of the individual became a concern of the affluent society, still bridled by many severe problems, but saddled

more precariously with the vast majority of normally or adequately functioning individuals who could improve their level of living. Indeed, this was an area for prime consideration by school staff. It would be different from the secondary school guidance offered by Jesse B. Davis, in Detroit Central High School, at the turn of the century.[67]

The First World War (1914–1918) provided an opportunity for increased emphasis on the need "to choose the right man for the right job" which Parsons stressed in his vocational guidance theory. Selective tests were devised to determine aptitude as well as intelligence. The first group of intelligence tests, the Army Alpha and the Army Beta, were used for literate and illiterate recruits, respectively. Tests were constructed also to measure skills in the various trades: "These tests were of three kinds: questions on materials, tools and processes (what to do), questions based on pictures, and performance assignments. Scores gave a four-fold classification in some eighty occupations: novices, apprentices, journeymen and experts."[68] Following World War I, these techniques and methods would be extended to all areas of vocational guidance, including the new program in vocational rehabilitation.

THE VOCATIONAL REHABILITATION ACT

Legislation passed by the Congress during World War I led directly to the enactment of Public Law 236 which established the state-federal program in vocational rehabilitation. The National Defense Act of 1916 indicated the importance attached by Congress to the area of vocational training: "In addition to military training, soldiers while in active service shall hereafter be given the opportunity to study and receive instruction upon educational lines of such character as to increase their military efficiency and enable them to return to civil life better equipped for industrial, commercial, and general business occupations. Civilian teachers may be employed to aid the Army officers in giving such instruction, and part of this instruction may consist of vocational education either in agriculture or the mechanic arts."[69] On February 23, 1917, the second session of the Sixty-fourth Congress passed the Smith-Hughes Act which set a precedent for federal funding of educational programs of all types and also established a pattern for vocational education in the United States. The act created the Federal Board for Vocational Education which later administered the vocational rehabilitation program for World War I veterans and the state-federal program in vocational rehabilitation.[70] The Soldier Rehabilitation Act of 1918 was passed by the Sixty-fifth Congress on June 27, 1918. The Federal Board for Vocational Education was authorized to operate a program of vocational rehabilitation for veterans: "an act to provide for the vocational rehabilitation and return to employment of disabled persons discharged from the military or naval forces of the United States and for other purposes."[71] Eligibility for services was outlined and a disabled veteran was defined as one who "is unable to carry on a gainful occupation, to resume his former occupation or to enter upon some other occupation, or having resumed and entered upon such occupation is unable to continue the same successfully, shall be furnished by the said board, where vocational rehabilitation is feasible, such course of vocational rehabilitation as the board shall prescribe and provide."[72] This act which became known as the Smith-Sears Veteran's Rehabilitation Act was signed by President Wilson on June 27, 1918. The passage of this act, and the previous enactment of the Smith-Hughes Act in 1917, helped gain support for vocational rehabilitation for civilians. Many of the same legislative and lay leaders who supported this earlier legislation for veterans were also committed to a program of vocational rehabilitation for civilians.[73] In order to avoid a delay in the passage of the veteran's bill in 1918, these leaders decided to wait for another time, and this time came only three months later (September, 1918) when Senator Hoke Smith of Georgia and Representative William Bankhead of Alabama first introduced their bill to set up a program for the vocational rehabilitation of civilians. Before this bill would become law (1920) many hearings would be held and the following men were among the key spokesmen: Dr. R. M. Little, of the United States Employment Compensation Commission, whose interest was in extending the state workmen's compensation programs; W. F. Faulkes, a supervisor of vocational education in Wisconsin, who represented the growing interest in vocational rehabilitation by state education departments (Faulkes would later become the first state director of vocational rehabilitation in Wisconsin, and as president of the National Rehabilitation Association (1924-1927), he would become a national leader for federal legislation in this field); Dr. Charles A. Prossner, Director of the Federal Board of Vocational Education, who was interested in following the same administrative pattern as had been established with the Smith-Hughes Act and the Smith-Sears Act—administration by the Federal Board of Vocational Education in partnership with the state vocational education department[74]; Lieutenant Colonel Harry E. Mock of Surgeon General's office and a distinguished orthopedic surgeon who argued for a more extensive bill which would have provided a program in prevention, medical care, compensation and insurance, vocational training and reemployment; and, Douglas C. McMurtie, Director of the Red Cross Institute for Crippled and Disabled Men in New York, whose organization was active in research and demonstration projects in the rehabilitation field and also in promoting state legislation for vocational rehabilitation. (A few states had some form of vocational rehabilitation programs prior to the enactment of the federal act in 1920.[75])

Following the passage of the Vocational Rehabilitation Act of 1920, thirty-four states within an eighteen-month period had passed acceptance or enabling legislation and had taken steps to organize a program of services to accommodate the federal funds which were made available on a fifty-fifty matching ratio through the Federal Board of Vocational Education.[76]

Prior to the federal legislation in June, 1920, several states had enacted vocational rehabilitation laws to accept provisions of the anticipated federal act.

> The first legislative action occurred in Massachusetts in 1918 with the passage of an act to provide for training and instruction of persons whose capacities to earn a living had been destroyed or impaired through industrial accident. Other states soon followed and by June, 1920, twelve had enacted vocational rehabilitation laws.[77]

Usually the states' legislation consisted of a few brief statements amending a public law dealing with vocational education. This procedure represented only an acceptance act; no attempt was made to define the scope of the work or to advise the state boards of vocational education on procedures to follow; and all regulations and policies were left entirely with the federal legislation. Funds were appropriated to match the federal monies made available in the act on a fifty-fifty federal-state matching ratio.

The Federal Board for Vocational Education issued a statement of policies for use by states in the administration of the vocational rehabilitation act in September, 1920. This publication made it clear that the Federal Government was reluctant to establish a new federal program.

> Under this act the Federal Government does not propose to undertake the organization and immediate direction of vocational rehabilitation in the states, but does agree to make substantial financial contributions to its support.[78]

Congress, by passing only temporary legislation, probably held the opinion that the funds would stimulate the development of programs carried on entirely by state governments at some future time. This first policy statement reflects the philosophy of responsible officials in the federal vocational education agency who viewed vocational rehabilitation as being synonymous with vocational education, except that this new area would be concerned only with handicapped people. The authors of the bulletin state:

> The industrial rehabilitation law provides practically the same administrative procedures as is required in the administration of the vocational education act. In so far as possible, the same methods of administration and relationships with state boards will be maintained.[79]

Requirements for the states' participation, which were based on the federal act, were provided in the bulletin:

1. the expenditure of funds in the state must be equal to the amount expended in federal funds (a fifty-fifty matching formula established with all states);
2. the development of a state plan for approval by the federal agency (guides were provided but emphasis was placed on each state developing an individual plan which would meet its unique needs);
3. submission of an annual report to the federal board;
4. administration of the state program placed under the state vocational education board and a cooperative agreement established with the state's workmen's compensation commission or bureau;

History of the Rehabilitation Movement in America   29

5. a prohibition of expenditure of funds for buildings or equipment (setting the early policy of a "purchase of service plan").[80]

Information was also provided on the forms to use in statistical and financial reporting. A question and answer section was included in this early bulletin to provide an interpretation of the law by the various state departments of vocational education:

> The board interprets the term "vocational rehabilitation" as used in this act not to include the work of physical rehabilitation, although such work may be necessary preliminary to or accompaniment of vocational rehabilitation.[81]

The question of purchasing artificial appliances was presented since the experience of workmen's compensation programs showed the majority of serious industrial accidents resulted in amputations. This question was answered in a somewhat ambiguous way which may have helped to set a pattern for the future establishment of a comprehensive physical restoration and treatment program: "In such a case it would be clear that this would be outside the purview of vocational rehabilitation, since like medical care and occupational therapy, it is physical restoration. . . ."[82]

But, in response to the question of providing "specialized" vocational prostheses, the authors of the bulletin replied, "If in these instances they are real supplies of an instructional nature necessary for the individual in training, it is possible. . . ."[83] The question regarding the provision of job placement only was answered in the negative, and this, for many years, resulted in the reluctance of rehabilitation workers to assist a handicapped person who needed only counseling and job placement services:

> A rehabilitation agency which contemplates placement only is not in harmony with the spirit of the Federal Act. The emphasis is laid by the act upon courses of studies, supervision, etc. and it is made clear that the chief thing in mind was the vocational re-training of the disabled.[84]

In answer to the question of a minimum age, the Federal Board provided an answer that was accepted as a policy in all states: "The Federal Act does not specify a minimum age. It is evident, however, that the minimum age in any state would be the minimum age of legal employability in that state."[85] Rigid adherence to this interpretation (and not to the law) over the years hampered efforts to provide counseling and other services of a prevocational nature to people under age sixteen. The answer given to the following question was answered affirmatively, "What about homemaking as an occupation? Persons engaged in homemaking, whether working for a wage or not, will be considered as engaged in a legitimate occupation."[86] This interpretation, however, was based on the vocational education act which had included home economics as a major educational program and the implications for the future development of vocational rehabilitation services for housewives and other unpaid family workers were not foreseen. It is clear that an action and service-oriented program was envisioned from the beginning. In answer to a question about the use of funds for preliminary surveys (research) prior to establishing a program, the federal official stated:

> The general principles on which the work should be constructed are fairly well recognized and are easily ascertainable. Further progress depends upon the contacts with individual cases, and actual work in vocational rehabilitation. A preliminary survey should include contacts looking toward an early beginning of training since the Federal Act has clearly in mind a definite undertaking of the work of vocational rehabilitation. Such a survey would be only incidental to the actual starting of the work.[87]

The last statement may have been needed in order to encourage a pioneering-type activity which was necessary in the development of a new program; however, it may have been somewhat shortsighted in the exclusion of an early emphasis on research and study which could have accompanied the developing service program to provide the data needed for improvement of services and sound planning for the extension of services in future development and growth.

The Federal Board for Vocational Education issued its second bulletin on vocational rehabilitation during March, 1921, months before most of the states had established programs. Additional interpretive data for the states to follow in setting up new programs were provided in this second bulletin. The first clear statement on the techniques and methods to be used by rehabilitation agents (later called rehabilitation counselors) was included. This was a case method approach adopted from the social work field. The employment of federal supervisors to work specifically in vocational rehabilitation and the experiences of a few states in attempting to rehabilitate people helped to establish this method.

Even before the state agencies began to function, the methods for providing services moved from those of instruction, supervision and courses of studies to the case method technique. Vocational guidance and vocational testing are not mentioned in this second bulletin; however, early vocational guidance principles were implied by stating that the purpose of the person contacting handicapped people was

> to inspire the disabled man with a feeling of receptivity and . . . of confidence. This may be accomplished by tact in giving encouragement, and proffering assistance, and by acquainting the injured man with the achievements and accomplishments of others who have suffered from similar or other disabilities. There should be induced, so far as possible, a mental state of hopefulness which will tend to counteract the almost inevitably discouraging effects of accidents or illnesses.[88]

A discussion of specific case procedures to be followed in the management of services was provided: (a) Determination of eligibility is made by the agent in three distinct areas—age, physical disability and feasibility. (b) Determination of the job objective, "the whole interview should be so conducted that the disabled person rather than the agent is led to make a decision as to the selection of a job objective," and yet stress was placed on what the agent does for the handicapped person: "In order to determine what particular occupation or employment is best in the case of any disabled person, it is necessary that an intensive study be made of the case (no mention is made of an objective appraisal by tests).[89] (c) Formulation of a tentative plan of rehabilitation, "when a specific employment objective has been determined upon, the agent of the State Board will be face to face with the issue of making at least a tentative plan of vocational rehabilitation for the disabled person."[90] (d) Follow-up during training and the determination of employability: "This follow-up on the job must continue until, beyond a question of a doubt, the disabled person is independent, confident, and happy, and all reports show that he is producing at his maximum efficiency."[91]

THE EARLY ROLE OF THE COUNSELOR AND REHABILITATION

In these early bulletins, no information was provided on the qualifications of rehabilitation agents nor was any concern shown for their training other than the distribution of various policy statements. Perhaps the federal supervisors followed the tradition established in the Federal Board's work with states on the Smith-Hughes legislation, which, for the most part, left selection and training of vocational education personnel to the state boards and departments of education. The directors of these state programs were also in charge of planning and implementing a program in vocational rehabilitation and, in many states, the director of vocational education, for many years remained director of vocational rehabilitation even though he delegated most of his authority to a supervisor of vocational rehabilitation.

In 1927, Homer L. Stanton, Supervisor of Vocational Rehabilitation in North Carolina (one of the early pioneers who served as the fifth national president of National Rehabilitation Association (1922–1930), in his history of the agency's work refers to his experience in this area during the first six years of the program:

> In the early experience of rehabilitation, three divisions were made of the work: counsel and advisement, training, and placement. However, experience soon taught that counsel and advisement is not a service that only needs to precede other steps in rehabilitation, but must accompany all other processes to the conclusion of the rehabilitation program. Since the whole aim is fitting the handicapped individual to the most suitable vocation, we may well call this service Vocational Guidance.[92]

Stanton continues later in this section of his study:

> ... the report of the sub-committee on vocational guidance of the Commission on Reorganization of Secondary Education admirably describes the process as applied to Rehabilitation. 'Vocational guidance should be a continuous process designed to help the individual to choose, to plan his preparation for, to enter upon, and to make progress in an occupation.'[93]

This statement indicates the direction rehabilitation work was taking—moving from an educational emphasis to a social work approach, then to the field of vocational guidance, while retaining parts of all three areas in attempting to meet the needs of a neglected group in America, the physically handicapped, the states were urged to find the means to get the necessary medical assistance they needed.[94] Dr. Henry H. Kessler, a prominent physician in New Jersey and consultant to the New Jersey Workmen's Compensation program, which administered the vocational rehabilitation program in that state, helped to pioneer in the development of national legislation for these services to be included in the federal act. His views were representative of many orthopedic surgeons and other physicians who felt a mistake had been made in excluding medical services. New Jersey established a physical medicine program in its vocational rehabilitation act of 1919. Kessler commented on the federal act of 1920 in his book, *Rehabilitation of the Physically Handicapped:*

> The attendant newspaper publicity stressed the vocational benefits to be obtained, but completely ignored the fact that in the case of the disabled World War I veterans, physical reconstruction had already been cared for in the veterans' hospitals. This oversight on the part of the publicists, and the unwillingness of the educational group to broaden their vision and see rehabilitation in its true perspective, was to lead to a long drawn-out controversy as to whether or not vocational rehabilitation should be preceded by physical rehabilitation in the case of the civilian handicapped. . . .[95]

However, many of the early leaders in the states gave support to physical medicine for adults with vocational handicapping conditions and showed an early concern for preventive medical programs for crippled children which brought many benefits to the agency and to its clients. One significant result was the development of close ties with physicians which established a firm base for future development of physical restoration services in the states. Another important development originated with the rehabilitation affiliated clinics: a strong alliance with volunteer, nonprofit groups interested in helping crippled children and adults. From the beginning, sponsors for the clinics were found in the Kiwanis, Rotary and Lion's Clubs. Involvement by volunteers in civic clubs set the state for alliances with the newly developing private organizations for the physically handicapped.

Obermann's review of this period reflects the kinds of activities in which the state rehabilitation leaders participated:

> The years from 1921 to 1926 were filled with the spirit of development and growth for the state-federal vocational rehabilitation program. The national conferences in St. Louis, Washington, and Cleveland reflected this in their programs and proceedings. The philosophical base for the new movement was being formulated, the administrative machinery was being established, definitions were being agreed upon, the limitations of operations under the federal act were being explored, and the techniques of rehabilitation practice were discussed.[96]

The first sectional meetings for the professional staff in vocational rehabilitation were held at the National Society for Vocational Education Annual Conference at Buffalo, New York, in 1923. At one of these sectional meetings, leaders from the state-federal vocational rehabilitation agencies established the National Civilian Rehabilitation Conference; and, in 1925, this organization began operating as a separate organization as it held its first annual meeting in Cleveland, Ohio. In Memphis, Tennessee, at its annual conference in 1927, the name of the organization was changed to the National Rehabilitation Association.[97]

The objectives of this new organization were listed as follows:

> (a) to provide through its meetings a forum in which all phases of vocational rehabilitation of disabled civilians and problems incidental thereto may be discussed, (b) to conduct a campaign of education to bring the general public to an adequate understanding of the importance of the civilian rehabilitation movement, (c) to further so far as possible and desirable agreement upon the principles and practices in the field of civilian rehabilitation and to promote comity between the various agencies, (d) to set up a medium through which expression may be given to the views of the membership upon pending legislation and public policies affecting the civilian rehabilitation movement.[98]

The other national forum for state supervisors and directors of vocational rehabilitation was provided by the Federal Board for Vocational Education as it sponsored national conferences on vocational rehabilitation.

At its second National Conference in Washington, D.C., in 1924, the first statements on qualifications for rehabilitation agents (counselors) were recorded:

"There is no place in vocational rehabilitation for a routine worker or one who is contented with his present knowledge and methods of rehabilitation."[99] The report continued with the outlining of the duties of a rehabilitation professional worker:
1. interviewing applicants,
2. setting up feasible plans of rehabilitation,
3. supervision of training,
4. job placement,
5. soliciting funds for areas not covered,
6. securing cooperation of individuals and agencies.[100]

The reports then described the kinds of personal qualities needed to carry out these duties as:

Tact, careful observation, patience and sympathy tempered by good judgment . . . a complete knowledge of the rehabilitation laws, policies and best practices, thoughtfulness, alertness, resourcefulness, ingenuity, and common sense, . . . one must have a liberal education in order that he may meet all classes favorably and deal with them on their own level. One must be socially agreeable, that is, be able to get on well with people. This requires courtesy, tact, poise, cheerfulness, and a good sense of humor. He should be a graduate of a standard college and should have some experience in rehabilitation, social services or other work that has given him experience. . . .[101]

Later one member spoke to this "necessary qualifications" list:

Someone may say that we can't afford the type of men described, I want to say that you can't afford any other type of men. The success of the work depends upon the kind of men who are administering it, the largest item of expense in the rehabilitation work, is, and, rightly so, that of administration (salary). The poorest economy that can be practiced in rehabilitation work is the employment of cheap and incompetent officers. The effectiveness of the work in any state will depend upon the ability of the staff that is in charge of the program.[102]

From 1926 to 1930, the vocational rehabilitation movement remained stable with little growth reflected either in the number of people rehabilitated or in the addition of staff members. Obermann provides, in his history of vocational rehabilitation in America, various reasons for this more static period of growth:

1. limited federal appropriations for federal staff and administrative activities,
2. vocational rehabilitation regarded by Federal Board for Vocational Education and the state boards as an extension of its programs in

vocational training rather than as a unique program requiring new methods and techniques,
3. administrations of Harding, Coolidge and Hoover were conservative, and
4. federal agency supervisors were anxious to make the program appear very successful rather than to point out the problems resulting from a lack of funds.[103]

The development of a special vocational guidance discipline for the physically handicapped can be seen in two documents published in 1928. One, the first national study made of rehabilitated people (1927), indicates that six years after the state-federal program began the emphasis continued to be placed upon serving people with orthopedic disabilities.

> It will be seen that a majority of the rehabilitated cases had disabilities affecting the lower limbs . . . 2,616 or 40.8% of the total number of cases had leg disabilities . . . 1,194 cases or 31.2% of the total number had disabled arms or hands . . . 688 persons were disabled by partial or total loss of vision . . . 108 by tuberculosis. It will be noted that the number of persons injured by heart disease and other disabling conditions was relatively small.[104]

The second publication, a report of the proceedings of the fifth national conference held in Milwaukee in 1929, indicates that vocational counseling and guidance had emerged as the dominant professional force. Dr. A. H. Egerton of the University of Wisconsin spoke to the conference in the "counsel and advisement" section. He commented on the changes he had observed in rehabilitation:

> Perhaps the most significant change which has taken place in counseling includes your specialized form of counseling. I refer to the change in attitude, namely, from counseling for individuals to counseling with them.

Egerton also suggested ways that certain tests might be helpful in vocational guidance. In a discussion that followed this presentation, it was necesesary for some to defend the use of tests in counseling since the majority of those rehabilitation agents present were opposed to using any of these new devices in helping people. A Dr. Fairies, a psychologist representing the Institute for

Crippled and Disabled Men in New York City, stated in this discussion:

> Having received my psychological training or training in psychology long before there was such a thing as a psychological test, I am not capable myself, having not kept up with psychology in the later years of its development, to give a test, but I do believe that every rehabilitationist should take advantage of the very best thought on the subject, because a great deal of attention is being paid to these tests.[105]

During these years, the state leaders who were acting as rehabilitation agents themselves (as well as supervisors) were establishing highly centralized state programs. The reasons for this highly centralized and authoritarian-type management provided by confident leaders are clearly seen:

1. A tight control of all activities prevented serious errors that could have harmed substantially the reputation of an unknown minor governmental agency attempting to grow and develop.
2. This type of management was encouraged by state government and was the approach used by industrial psychology and other personnel work in this period of time.
3. New Staff, inexperienced in the field with no special college training, would benefit by acquiring skills needed to operate a limited program of services for a relatively large number of people.

Some of the disadvantages in administration are obvious, but perhaps the greatest disadvantage was the fact that a rigid pattern of administration was established early which would, at a future time, become obsolete.

By 1930, there was a clear and strong design developing for the foundations of rehabilitation counseling, as a distinct professional area in the field of vocational guidance and counseling. Years later (1951), R. C. Thompson, an early leader and for many years director of the Maryland agency, wrote an article on the history of the National Rehabilitation Association and commented on the early concepts developing:

> ... at Milwaukee in 1929, the efforts of some leaders such as Terry Foster to commit the Association to the scientific approach to rehabilitation through vocational guidance and aptitude testing had disclosed an alarming cleavage still existing in our ranks as to the basic concept of our profession.[106]

Despite the growing body of knowledge that contributed to professionalization of the work of the rehabilitation agent during this period, little growth, in terms of the number of people served, took place in the early 1930's. These early depression years created conditions that restricted growth and, on some occasions, threatened the very existence of this small state-federal program which was not well known by the general public, nor by many of the politicians. This more static and inactive period did provide an opportunity for consolidation of gains made in the development of a new concept. The framework for future growth was built as rehabilitation leaders were called on to participate in some of the Federal Government's attempts to improve the plight of America's middle class as well as its poor who were suffering from a major economic depression.

Vocational rehabilitation, in 1933, became involved with the administration's total governmental effort to combat the Depression, President Franklin D. Roosevelt's New Deal. A monthly national allotment of $70,000 was made available through the Federal Emergency Relief Administration to the state vocational rehabilitation programs for the purpose of extending rehabilitation services to the unemployed handicapped people who were on relief.

> These funds could be expended for appliances, tuition, supplies and equipment for trainees; their travel to attend training centers; and their maintenance while in training. Administration of these funds for vocational rehabilitation was divided between the state's Emergency Relief Fund and the state supervisors of vocational rehabilitation.[107]

People on relief who received vocational rehabilitation services also were provided living expenses while they were in training. This inclusion of maintenance for a limited group led to legislation and regulations which came later when the total rehabilitation program was made more comprehensive.[108]

When the functions of the Federal Board for Vocational Education were transferred by an executive order by President Roosevelt to the Department of the Interior in 1933, the Secretary of the Interior assigned the vocational rehabilitation division to the Office of Education.[109]

Terry Foster was the author of the first rehabilitation bulletin published by the Office of Education in the Department of the Interior. This bulletin, written in 1934, presented "a manual of instructions, policies and practices for the guidance of case workers in the field of vocational rehabilitation." Sample forms for record keeping and reporting were based on those developed by Foster and the director of the vocational rehabilitation program in Pennsylvania. For example, Foster wrote guidelines for counselors to use in making decisions about "re-opening" cases, stating that a case could be re-opened but "careful investigation should be made however before re-opening such cases."[110]

BROADENING THE SCOPE OF REHABILITATION

Until 1935, emphasis was placed on the indigent "crippled" person, even though some services were available to people in all economic groups, for example, counseling and guidance and tuition for training; and limited services were also available to people with disabilities who were not crippled or orthopedically handicapped. It is clear that this program in 1935 was a limited one and a priority of service was necessary, therefore, the needs of the indigent person with an obvious disability that could be corrected or minimized received the highest priority.

The Social Security Act of 1935 provided the first permanent base for the federal vocational rehabilitation program.[111] "The Social Security Act thus accomplished three objectives of rehabilitation officials, namely a permanent authorization, increased grants, and increased support for federal administration."[112] This bill which was drafted by the House Ways and Means Committee in 1935 contained an authorization for a 75 percent increase in the grants to states ($1,938,000); and the federal administrative budget was increased from $80,000 per year to $102,000. "The report of the Ways and Means Committee declared that the provision for increased federal aid for vocational rehabilitation was made in recognition of the importance of such work in a permanent program for economic security."[113] Representatives of the National Rehabilitation Association appeared at the hearings to argue for this inclusion of vocational rehabilitation in the social security legislation, emphasizing to committee members that the bill already included services for crippled children.

In 1936, a new publication from the federal office provided additional information in the development of a vocational rehabilitation philosophy. John Kratz, chief of the federal division, wrote *Vocational Rehabilitation of the Physically Handicapped* and in one section stated:

> Of fundamental importance is the principle that from the inception of a rehabilitation case to its conclusion only one agent should deal with the disabled person. Functional handling of cases was tried in the soldier (sic) rehabilitation work, and it proved a failure.[114]

Kratz expressed his ideas on the importance of counseling:

> One of the most important services given by a rehabilitation agent is that of counsel and advisement. It is a continuous service designed to assist the disabled person in choosing, preparing for, entering upon, and making progress in an occupation . . . Such devices as psychological, individual, group, trade and intelligence tests have been used only to a limited extent, but it is not likely that they can ever be used in all cases as a general procedure in rehabilitation. A practical common sense trial and error process has been the procedure followed in most cases. . . .[115]

Kratz also provided a statement that reflected the growing recognition of the need to look at a client as a person of worth and dignity and, yet, as someone who still needed some manipulation and direction:

> It is far better procedure to have the person assume a measure of initiative and responsibility for the development of his own rehabilitation . . . the rehabilitation supervisor must be skillful in assisting the applicant to appraise his own abilities, capacities and deficiencies.

And, yet he goes on to say:

> If the agent is skillful, he leads the disabled person to follow his guidance and to enter into the rehabilitation plan which the agent suggests, as freely and as enthusiastically as if he himself had suggested and originated it.[116]

In this same bulletin, Kratz commented on the problems of administration and outlined the types of administration observed in the states without making a recommendation for the use of any particular kind. There were two basic types of organization: a central office which handled all services in the smaller states and a central office with district offices established throughout a larger state. In addition, Kratz mentioned two basic approaches used in administration—a centralized program with all or most decision-making taking place in the central office and a decentralized program which provided for some autonomy in the district offices.[117]

Many chose the centralized approach for the delivery of services statewide, and, as Kratz outlined in his paper, most matters were cleared and handled in the central office with little autonomy found in district offices.

The Federal Security Agency was established in July, 1939, and all education, welfare and health organizations were transferred to this new department. The Office of Education moved from the Interior Department to the new agency; and vocational rehabilitation was set up as a separate division within the Office of Education. "Thus, administrative reorganization, rather than legislative change . . . ended the subordination of vocational rehabilitation to vocational education . . . It remained within the Office of Education, however, an agency concerned with different problems."[118]

The first annual report of the Federal Security Administration was published in 1941 and, while very brief, it pointed out the new strength of this division: Congress that year (1940) increased the appropriation for the states from $1,938,000 to $3,500,000. Provision was made for the extension of services to physically handicapped people who were not eligible before—services for the severely handicapped group who were either homebound or employed in a sheltered workshop. A new policy adopted during 1940 authorized the state agencies to provide services to handicapped people who needed them to maintain a job; earlier, services were available only to people who were unemployed at the time of application. Moreover, for the first time, a limited program for paying living expenses for handicapped people while participating in a rehabilitation plan was made available to the state agencies.[119] These new policies combined with the legislation passed by Congress in 1940 had a liberalizing effect on vocational rehabilitation programs in the states.

World War II affected the vocational rehabilitation agency in many ways as it influenced all activities in the nation and the world. The consequences of this war, for rehabilitation, however, were different from the effects that the war had on other peacetime programs supported by the government; federal legislation passed by Congress at the height of World War II resulted in the greatest period of expansion in the twenty-year history of vocational rehabilitation.

The 1941–1942 and 1942–1943 annual reports published by the Federal Security Agency provide information which indicates the expansion of services: "The number of people rehabilitated during the fiscal year 1942 showed a 48 percent increase over the preceding year, and an 81 percent increase over 1939–1940...."[120] "On December 22, 1942, the Federal Security Agency, acting on instructions from the President, called a meeting of the administrators of all related federal agencies for a program for the rehabilitation of the war disabled. Recognizing that this problem would intertwine with that of supplying disabled civilian workers to war industries, steps were taken to plan a combined program for the rehabilitation of disabled civilians for employment in war industries and essential civilian industries both now and after the war."[121] In this same report, the agency announced that a new and completely separate administration known as the Office of Vocational Rehabilitation was established for the program on July 6, 1943.[122]

These events in the early years of the war, led to the development of a new federal act for vocational rehabilitation in 1943. Known as Public Law 113,[123] this law was to have the greatest impact on the growth of the program since the original act was passed by Congress in 1920.

Obermann, in his history, states that:

> It was a time when rehabilitation workers and their disabled clients were being given the opportunity to demonstrate to a broad and receptive audience that disability need not be an employment and productive handicap.... The tragedy of the war, and the new approaches to personnel practices required by it (the need to seek out all workers who could be productive, e.g., "Rosie the Riveter") was advancing the cause of vocational rehabilitation far faster than would have been possible under conditions of peace and labor surpluses.[124]

During the war, the agency's services were in demand by industry and business because of the serious manpower shortage. Governmental agencies began to increase referrals to vocational rehabilitation by substantial numbers. The Selective Service Agency referred people who were rejected for the armed services because of disability and the Employment Security Commission and the War Manpower Office referred people who were needed as productive workers despite their disabilities.

The major changes in the Barden-LaFollette Act of 1943 were:

1. all administration and guidance and placement costs, including salaries for professional and clerical staff, were paid by the federal government. This led to a rapid expansion of staff in the state program. (Services to clients remained on a fifty-fifty matching ratio.)
2. the use of federal funds for physical restoration services including hospitalization, surgery, and therapeutic treatment.
3. maintenance for living expenses and occupational tools and equipment was authorized.
4. the mentally handicapped were included so that mentally retarded and mentally ill people for the first time were eligible for vocational rehabilitation services.[125]

The objectives of this new legislation were clear: "During the year (1943-1944) the two primary objectives defined by the Federal Security Agency on establishing the Office of Vocational Rehabilitation have been foremost: first, to channel disabled manpower into war production and essential business as rapidly as possible and, second, to provide a comprehensive service to enable the disabled to prepare for and secure employment in peacetime pursuits."[126] For the first time, the state vocational rehabilitation programs were given the opportunity to develop a comprehensive service program for disabled civilians.

It was during this period in the middle and late forties that a more sophisticated view of rehabilitation counseling emerged. For the first time in its publications, the Office of Vocational Rehabilitation in Washington provided a clear statement on the professional role of the counselor in the rehabilitation process and reported that an emphasis was placed on the training of staff beyond regional and national conferences. In the 1944-1945 Annual Report of the Federal Security Agency, one section of the rehabilitation report shows the federal agency's growing concern for trained professional staff:

> Counseling or advisement is an essential service extended throughout the rehabilitation process to all disabled clients. Furthermore, counseling is the one service extended to disabled people directly by the state rehabilitation agencies. As such, counseling becomes the very core of the rehabilitation process around which all other services revolve. . . . Because of the value of this service to disabled persons, effort has been directed toward improving the quality of this service through orientation institutes, preparation of staff development materials for use by the States, and in-service training by State agencies; major emphasis was devoted to improving the quality of counseling.[127]

In the states, opportunities were provided for orientation and in-service training through short-term institutes and workshops developed through extension divisions of the colleges and universities. These training programs were provided for experienced staff members as well as for the new rehabilitation counselors.

In August 1945, Congress passed a joint resolution which established the President's Committee on Employment of the Handicapped and designated the first week of October as National Employ the Physically Handicapped Week.[128] N.E.P.H. Week provided an opportunity for a continuing program in public information to promote the employment of handicapped people by business and industry. Most of the states followed this action by establishing governors' committees on employment of the handicapped. The promotional materials emphasized the ability that handicapped people have rather than the disability, and these materials were distributed to employers and personnel managers throughout the nation.

THE DEVELOPMENT AND IMPACT OF PUBLIC LAW 565

In the federal program of vocational rehabilitation in the early fifties, events were taking place which would lead to the enactment of the most significant legislation since the amendments of 1943. Miss Mary E. Switzer, a long-time government administrator in related programs, was named Director of the Office of Vocational Rehabilitation in the Federal Security Agency in 1951. In 1953, President Eisenhower appointed Mrs. Oveta Culp Hobby as Secretary of the newly organized Department of Health, Education and Welfare and Nelson Rockefeller as Undersecretary.[129] Eisenhower's philosophy of "dynamic conservatism"[130] fitted in well with the vocational rehabilitation concept of helping handicapped or dependent people help themselves to a productive life, thus bringing about economic benefits to the nation. Mary Switzer presented to Mrs. Hobby and Mr. Rockefeller a greatly enlarged program in vocational rehabilitation which had the potential of performing a humanitarian service for the welfare of handicapped citizens and, at the same time, providing an opportunity for the government to "do something about what was considered by the administration as an increasing dependence of citizens on the welfare state."[131] Mrs. Hobby was impressed with possibilities presented by Miss Switzer; and Nelson Rockefeller was able to recommend this program to Mrs. Hobby as he had worked with Miss Switzer on committees previously and was a strong supporter of the vocational rehabilitation goals and objectives.[132] When the Health, Education and Welfare proposals were presented to the President and the Cabinet in 1953, they were approved and plans were made to ask Congress for the greatest expansion of rehabilitation services in its history.[133]

Public Law 565, cited as the "Vocational Rehabilitation Amendments of 1954," became law on August 3, 1954.[134] The purpose of this new act was stated in the Department of Health, Education and Welfare Annual Report of 1955:

> The law's avowed aim is to assist "the states in rehabilitating physically (and mentally) handicapped individuals so that they may prepare for and engage in remunerative employment . . . thereby increasing not only their social and economic well-being but also the productive capacity of the nation. . . .[135]

Public Law 565 authorized $30 million for federal grants-in-aid for 1955; the use of federal funds for the training of doctors, nurses, rehabilitation counselors, physical therapists, occupational therapists, social workers and other specialists to meet the personnel needs of the expanded rehabilitation program; extension and improvement grants and special project grants for research and demonstration.[136]

In addition to the greatly increased federal funds authorized for services to handicapped people, this 1954 act established the foundation for the development of various rehabilitation facilities. The emphasis placed on in-service training of staff as well as the new graduate degrees available in rehabilitation counseling also helped the agency in its future growth and development. "In 1954, no plan for expanding rehabilitation services was realistic unless it took into account the serious shortages of professional personnel required to render these services . . . Public Law 565 recognized this need and authorized a training program to provide funds for short-term specialized courses and long-term degree training."[137]

A stronger financial structure allowed for federal funding for case services and administration to be determined by a formula which gave consideration to the state's per capita income and population. This new formula eliminated the previous funding in full by the Federal Government for salaries and administrative costs; however, the new formula for allotment of federal funds to states helped the poorer states, particularly those in the Southeast. No major changes were made in the policies regarding eligibility nor were any new definitions provided for terms such as "disability" and "handicapping condition" which might have extended services to new groups. The state agency was allowed, for the first time, to use its funds in expanding or remodeling buildings to make them suitable for the rehabilitation of severely disabled persons, for example, rehabilitation centers and sheltered workshops.[138]

One organizational requirement in the new act was significant. The 1954 act permitted, for the first time, for state agencies to move from vocational education boards to other administrative units or to set up an independent agency of vocational rehabilitation. If they were to continue under the state boards for vocational education, however, the state directors of vocational rehabilitation were to have direct access to these boards.[139]

An analysis of the 1956–1957 fiscal year for one state-federal program provided information which was characteristic of this period. Seventy-one and seven tenths percent of the 2,930 people rehabilitated that year received surgery and/or treatment; 13 percent received training; 62 percent received hospitalization; 26.6 percent, artificial appliances; 12.9 percent received maintenance; and 3.5 percent received tools and equipment.[140] The positive effects of this greater emphasis on medical services during these years are obvious. Thousands of citizens were able to receive free medical care and attention from doctors, hospitals and facilities meeting exceptionally high professional standards. Thus, these thousands of individuals were able to begin or return to employment, thus maintaining their independence. Arrangements were made for these services by a more experienced staff who were being trained in counseling and psychological techniques. The negative effects are also clear. Rehabilitation counselors became, in this period, coordinators who provided less and less vocational counseling and guidance services. These counseling skills were not entirely forsaken by the staff, but the emphasis placed on providing medical services to large numbers of people meant that handicapped people who were in need of counseling services and job placement were many times referred to other agencies and professional individuals, and, as a result, severely physically handicapped persons and mentally handicapped people were quite often excluded from services. It is possible that the tempo of the times combined with the lack of sufficient funds and trained staff justified the shift to a service of coordination for those handicapped people who could have their disabilities removed or minimized and return to productive work. Medical expenses became increasingly high and it was difficult to provide one severely handicapped person with a rehabilitation program when the same amount of funds would allow ten to twenty other less handicapped people (who were also dependent) to become productive citizens. Whatever the opinion on the justification of this course of action, one significant result was the establishment of a coordinator's role for rehabilitation counselors generally. Perhaps the greatest problem for the emerging profession of rehabilitation counseling and for the more severely handicapped clients was the possibility of individual counselors losing a "counselor's attitude" as stated by McGowan in his book, *An Introduction to the Vocational Rehabilitation Process:*

> The danger of holding to the Coordinator model is that the rehabilitation counselor *could* lose his perception of the client as a unique individual. That is, there seems to be a danger that the Coordinator would become too *product oriented* and begin to mechanically provide services without considering the personality dynamics involved in a client's problems. He then would be providing the services a client was entitled to by law without consideration of the client's individuality or needs....[141]

Before the rehabilitation counselor can recognize the needs of his clients and adequately "coordinate" the indicated services, he needs to have all the skills associated with a professional counselor.[142]

REHABILITATION IN THE 1960'S

An unprecedented period of growth in the vocational rehabilitation movement in the 1960's was due to increased state support, joint program agreements for the mentally ill and several other jointly administered units; for example, public school special education programs, private and public rehabilitation facilities, et cetera. Three key events which occurred in three of these years—1965, 1967 and 1968—influenced the course and the great potential of this extraordinary era of expansion.

First, the Vocational Rehabilitation Amendments of 1965 were passed unanimously by Congress.[143] Obermann states that these new expansive amendments "could almost have been written by an enthusiastic professional in the state-federal vocational rehabilitation program."[144] The new amendments provided for a substantial increase in federal spending and also provided a broader base for extending services to additional handicapped people with "socially handicapping conditions" as determined by a psychologist or psychiatrist; for example, juvenile delinquents and adult public offenders were eligible without regard to a specific physical or mental diagnosis. An extended plan for evaluation was authorized in the new act, which, in effect, permitted the agency to waive the third item of eligibility: a reasonable expectation that vocational rehabilitation services may render the individual fit to engage in a gainful occupation. This 1965 act also provided special grants for construction and operation of sheltered workshops and other rehabilitation facilities to the state agencies or to private agencies which held joint program agreements with the official agency for vocational rehabilitation.[145]

The second of these events occurred in 1967 when the Department of Health, Education and Welfare was reorganized and the Social and Rehabilitation Service was established to provide a rehabilitation emphasis to many of the welfare and health programs in the department.[146] John W. Gardner, who was Secretary of Health, Education and Welfare, asked Mary Switzer, Commissoner of Vocational Rehabilitation, to head up this new administrative unit. "To better coordinate the programs, Health, Education and Welfare Secretary, John Gardner has gathered five major welfare agencies under one office, named the Social and Rehabilitation Service (SRS). To Washington's surprise, Gardner went over the heads of HEW's brightest young men and selected as the first boss of SRS a 67-year-old spinster . . . Mary Elizabeth Switzer has spent forty-six years in government, the last seventeen as the highly successful head of the Vocational Rehabilitation Administration, which aids the handicapped."[147] In addition to the new Rehabilitation Services Administration (RSA), the Children's Bureau, Administration on Aging, Medical Services Administration (Medicaid) and the Public Welfare Assistance Payments Administration, were consolidated in the new Social and Rehabilitation Service.[148] The reorganization, which favored a rehabilitation concept, provided greater visibility and a national recognition for the total state-federal program, and, occurring just two years after the 1965 federal legislation, it strengthened the federal base for future growth at the state level.

The third major event of this period occurred when Congress passed the 1968 Vocational Rehabilitation Amendments. Among the important changes and additions contained in this act were

1. substantial increases in appropriations with the basic programs moving from a 75-25 matching ratio to a new formula for all states (80% federal-20% state, effective 1969);
2. approval for Vocational Rehabilitation to expend funds in new construction of rehabilitation facilities;
3. the definition of rehabilitation services was completely rewritten to

include follow-up services in maintaining an individual in employment, services to families of the handicapped individual when services can contribute substantially to the rehabilitation of a group of individuals; and

4. the state was permitted to amend its state plan to enable it to share funding and administration responsibility with another state agency to carry out a joint project (a policy already established in many states, informally).

In addition, the agency was recognized as having responsibility for assisting with the administration's efforts to combat poverty for this specific purpose, Section 15 was added to the amendments. This authorized 90 percent of the costs for the establishment of vocational evaluation and work adjustment centers for "disadvantaged" individuals, who were defined "to include the physically and mentally handicapped and other individuals disadvantaged by reason of age, youth, low educational attainments, ethnic, or other factors such as prison and delinquency records."[149]

Dramatic progress (as seen in the 1960's) is not evident today as this author surveys the rehabilitation movement in 1971. However, as the events listed above in the chronology show, Obermann's optimism of 1965 does not appear to be unwarranted:

> It is reasonable to expect that support for this movement will be progressively increased to the point where it will be practical to insure that every disabled and handicapped person will receive the assistance he needs to make an optimum adjustment to his handicap. While it is comforting to the professions in the movement to know that they are working in an atmosphere of almost unlimited acceptance and approval, at the same time this enormous privilege carries with it a very sobering responsibility. There is now required a level of leadership, imagination, skill, and devotion to match the opportunities that have been provided.[150]

There are many obstacles, however, for vocational rehabilitation to overcome in order to respond to the challenge of a new mission in the coming decades. Perhaps the greatest challenge the agency faces today and in the future is the problem associated with change. Carl Rogers, in an article on possibilities for the year 2000, stated:

> I am going to sketch possibilities, alternative routes which we may travel. One important reason for refusing to make predictions is that

History of the Rehabilitation Movement in America

for the first time in history man is not only taking his future seriously, but he also has adequate technology and power to shape and form that future. He is endeavoring to choose his future rather than simply living out some inevitable trend. . . . Before I try to sketch some of these possibilities, I should like to point to the greatest problem which man faces in the years to come. It is not the hydrogen bomb, fearful as that may be. It is not the population explosion, though the consequences of that are awful to contemplate. It is instead a problem which is rarely mentioned or discussed. It is the question of how much change the human being can accept, absorb, and assimilate, and the rate at which he can take it. Can he keep up with the ever-increasing rate of technological change, or is there some point at which the human organization goes to pieces? Can he leave the static ways and static guidelines which have dominated all of his history and adopt the process ways, the continual changingness which will be his if he is to survive?[151]

We may ask the same questions of organizations as well as their individual members. Vocational rehabilitation's major challenge is the adaptation to change that is required to provide new and additional services for new clients who can benefit from them. The growth of the vocational rehabilitation program from 1921 until 1963 was an orderly process (except for those beginning years) with the first major expansion occurring twenty-two years after it started in 1943, prompted by war needs, and, then, in 1954, eleven years later, in answer to the government's search for an answer to the mounting welfare and dependency problems. There was time for consolidation of gains made and sufficient experience to make a case for new needs. In the more recent period (1964–1968) the situation was much different. As one prominent contemporary leader in rehabilitation said, "There is a sense of urgency not only in our own field (rehabilitation) but throughout the American society.[152]

John Gardner, in a Harvard lecture, offered one solution to this need for agencies to adopt to ever-increasing change:

Each reformer comes to his task with a little bundle of desired changes. The implication is that if appropriate reforms are carried through and the defects corrected, the society will be wholly satisfactory and the work of the reformer done. That is a primitive way of viewing social change. The true task is to design a society (and institutions) capable of continuous change, renewal and responsiveness. . . . We must dispose of the notion that social change is a process that alters a tranquil *status quo*. Today there is no tranquility to alter.[153]

It is obvious that the rehabilitation agency in the future will need to accommodate change if growth of services to the handicapped is to continue. A whole new structure will be required to help rehabilitation counselors maintain a quality of services needed by handicapped people. Patience and tolerance of change and a clear understanding of the desperate need for change in vocational rehabilitation will be required of all staff members.

SUMMARY

An attempt has been made in this chapter to provide significant facts about the growth and development of the rehabilitation movement. The concept of rehabilitation is much broader than the story of the legal state-federal partnership might reflect. A concept of the total rehabilitation movement in this country has developed from the basic values of our system of government—the ideals, customs and traditions of the American people—which found expression in the public support of vocational rehabilitation services for handicapped people. This chapter is written with the hope that a review of the past can lead to understanding and wisdom on the part of all who attempt to help others through the broader concept of rehabilitation.

> Time present and time past
> are both perhaps present in time future,
> and time future contained in time past.
> T. S. Eliot,
> *Four Quartets, Burnt Norton.*

REFERENCES AND NOTES

1. McGowan, John F, and Porter, Thomas L.: *An Introduction to the Vocational Rehabilitation Process.* Washington, D. C., (Rehabilitation Services Administration, U. S. Department of Health, Education and Welfare, 1967, p. 4.
2. *Rehab Rec,* Vol. I, 1964, p. 14.
3. National Rehabilitation Association: *Newsletter,* 23 (No. 4): 2, August 1968.
4. Gardner, John W.: To extend the concept of rehabilitation *J Rehab,* 34 (No. 1):12, January-February 1968.

5. Nixon, Russell A.: Rehabilitation-human reinforcement in a troubled world. *J Rehab, 35 (No. 2)*:14, March-April 1969.
6. *United States Statutes at Large,* Vol. 41, Sixty-sixth Congress, 1920, p. 735.
7. Blum, John M. (Ed.): *The National Experience, A History of the United States,* 2nd ed. New York, Harcourt, Brace & World, Inc., 1968, p. 437.
8. Obermann, C. Esco: *A History of Vocational Rehabilitation in America* Minneapolis, T. S. Denison & Co. Inc., 1965, p. 47.
9. Handlin, Oscar: *The Uprooted.* New York, Grossett & Dunlap, 1951, p. 94.
10. Morrison, Samuel Eliot: *The Oxford History of the American People.* New York, Oxford University Press, 1965, pp. 770-772.
11. Blum, *op. cit.,* p. 456.
12. *Ibid.,* pp. 437, 458, 464.
13. Faunce, William A.: *Problems of an Industrial Society.* New York, McGraw-Hill Book Co., 1968, pp. 21-22.
14. *Ibid.*
15. Landis, Paul H., and Hatt, Paul K.: *Population Problems.* New York, American Book Co., 1954, pp. 27-28.
16. Hofstadter, Richard: *The Age of Reform.* New York, Alfred A. Knopf, 1956, pp. 173-174.
17. Riordon, William L.: *Plunkitt of Tammany Hall.* New York, McClure, Phillips & Co. 1905, p. 405.
18. Hofstadter, *op. cit.,* p. 61.
19. Burnett, Constance Buel: *Five for Freedom.* New York, Abingdon Press, 1953, pp. 311-312.
20. *Ibid.,* p. 317.
21. Hofstadter, *op. cit.,* p. 186.
22. Mayer, George H., and Forster, Walter O.: *The United States and the Twentieth Century.* Boston, Houghton-Mifflin Co., 1958, p. 51.
23. Shryock, Richard H.: *Medicine in America, Historical Essays.* Baltimore, The Johns Hopkins Press, 1966, p. 32.
24. Hanlon, John J.: *Principles of Public Health Administration.* Saint Louis, The C. V. Mosby Co., 1955, pp. 49-50.
25. Galston, Iago (Ed.): *Social Medicine.* Cambridge, Harvard University Press, 1949, p. 36.
26. Obermann, *op. cit.,* pp. 120-121.
27. *Analysis of Workmen's Compensation Laws.* Washington, D. C., United States Chamber of Commerce Publication, January 1958, p. 3.
28. Obermann, *op. cit.,* p. 123.
29. Maisel, Albert Q. (Ed.): *The Health of People Who Work.* New York, The National Health Council, 1960, p. 4.
30. Watson, Robert I.: *The Great Psychologists, From Aristotle to Freud,* 2nd ed. New York, J. B. Lippincott Co. 1968, p. 354.

31. *Ibid.*, pp. 375-377.
32. *Ibid.*, p. 355.
33. *Ibid.*, pp. 335-336.
34. Maisel, *loc. cit.*
35. Brewer, John M.: *History of Vocational Guidance.* New York, Harper & Brothers, 1942, pp. 4-5.
36. Marshall, Helen E.: *Dorothea Dix, Forgotten Samaritan.* Chapel Hill, University of North Carolina Press, 1937, p. 245.
37. Beers, Clifford: *A Mind That Found Itself,* 3rd ed. New York, Longmanns, Green & Co., 1913, p. 244.
38. Blum, *op. cit.*, p. 473.
39. Johnson, F. Ernest: *The Church and Society.* New York, The Abingdon Press, 1935, p. 64.
40. Blum, *op. cit.*, p. 474.
41. Johnson, *op. cit.*, p. 33.
42. Blum, *loc. cit.*
43. Obermann, *op. cit.*, p. 104.
44. Goldstein, Sidney E.: *The Synagogue and Social Welfare, A Unique Experiment 1907-1953.* New York, Bloch Publishing Co., 1955, p. 321.
45. Baron, Salo Wittmayer: *A Social and Religious History of the Jews.* New York, Columbia University Press, 1937, III, 165.
46. Obermann, *op. cit.*, pp. 91-102.
47. Lasch, Christopher: (Ed.): *The Social Thought of Jane Addams.* New York, Bobbs-Merrill Co., Inc., 1965, p. 124.
48. *Ibid.*, pp. 176-177.
49. Blum, *op. cit.* p. 472.
50. Glanz, Edward C.: *Foundations and Principles of Guidance.* Boston, Allyn & Bacon, Inc., 1964, p. 26.
51. Beck, Robert Holmes: *A Social History of Education.* Englewood Cliffs, Prentice-Hall, Inc., 1955, pp. 89-90.
52. Blum, *op. cit.*, p. 347.
53. Rugg, Harold, and Withers, William: *Social Foundations of Education.* New York, Prentice-Hall, Inc., 1955, pp. 502-503.
54. Archambault, Reginald D. (Ed.): *John Dewey on Education. Selected Writings.* New York, The Modern Library, Random House, Inc., 1964, p. 420.
55. Beck, *op. cit.*, p. 91.
56. Baker, Harry J.: *Introduction to Exceptional Children.* New York, Macmillan Co., 1959, pp. 201, 326, 369.
57. Obermann, *op. cit.*, p. 85.
58. Baker, *loc. cit.*
59. Beck, *op. cit.*, p. 124.
60. Farwell, Gail F., and Peters, Herman J.: *Guidance Readings for Counselors.* Chicago, Rand, McNally & Company, 1960, p. 2.
61. Brewer, *op. cit.*, p. 61.

History of the Rehabilitation Movement in America 55

62. Parsons, Frank: *Choosing a Vocation.* Cambridge, Houghton-Mifflin Co., 1909, p. 165.
63. Brewer, *op. cit.,* p. 51.
64. Smith, C. E., and Mink, O. G. (Ed.) : *Foundations of Guidance and Counseling.* New York, J. B. Lippincott Co., 1969, p. 12.
65. Hill, David S.: *Introduction to Vocational Education.* New York, Macmillan Co., 1920, p. 402.
66. Moser, Leslie E., and Moser, Ruth Small: *Counseling and Guidance An Exploration.* Englewood Cliffs, Prentice-Hall, Inc., 1963, p. 4.
67. Peters, Herman J., and Farwell, Gail F.: *Guidance: A Developmental Approach,* 2nd ed. Chicago: Rand, McNally & Co., 1967, p. 28.
68. Brewer, *op. cit.,* p. 203.
69. *United States Statutes at Large,* Vol. 39, Sixty-fourth Congress, 1916, p. 186.
70. *Ibid.,* Vol. 39, Sixty-fourth Congress, 1917, p. 929.
71. *Ibid.,* Vol. 40, Sixty-fifth Congress, 1918, p. 617.
72. *Ibid.*
73. Pattison, Harry A.: *The Handicapped and Their Rehabilitation.* Springfield, Charles C Thomas, 1957, p. 844.
74. Obermann, *op. cit.,* pp. 216-226.
75. Patterson, C. H. (Ed.) : *Readings in Rehabilitation Counseling.* Champaign, Stipes Publishing Co., 1960, pp. 25-26.
76. *Ibid.*
77. Blauch, Lloyd E.: *Vocational Rehabilitation of the Physically Disabled,* The Advisory Committee on Education, Staff Study Number 9. Washington, D. C., U. S. Government Printing Office, 1938, p. 4.
78. *Ibid.,* p. 12.
79. Federal Board for Vocational Education: *Industrial Rehabilitation—A Statement of Policies to be Observed in the Administration of the Industrial Rehabilitation Act.* Bulletin No. 57, Industrial Rehabilitation Series No. 1. Washington, D. C., U. S. Government Printing Office, September 1920, p. 9.
80. *Ibid.,* p. 13.
81. *Ibid.,* p. 31.
82. *Ibid.*
83. *Ibid.*
84. *Ibid.,* p. 33.
85. *Ibid.,* p. 37.
86. *Ibid.*
87. *Ibid.,* p. 33.
88. Federal Board for Vocational Education: *Industrial Rehabilitation— General Administration and Case Procedures.* Bulletin No. 64, Industrial Rehabilitation Series No. 2. Washington, D. C., U. S. Government Printing Office, March 1921, p. 31.
89. *Ibid.,* p. 33.

90. *Ibid.*, p. 36.
91. *Ibid.*
92. Stanton, Homer L.: The Rehabilitation of Disabled Civilians in North Carolina Carolina. Unpublished Master's thesis, North Carolina State College of Agriculture and Engineering, Raleigh, North Carolina, 1927, p. 14.
93. Stanton, *op. cit.*, p. 8.
94. Obermann, *op. cit.*, p. 231.
95. Kessler, Henry H.: *Rehabilitation of the Physically Handicapped.* New York, Columbia University Press, 1947, p. 227.
96. Obermann, *op. cit.*, p. 246.
97. Obermann, *op. cit.*, pp. 354-358.
98. Obermann, *op. cit.*, pp. 357-358.
99. Federal Board for Vocational Educational: *Proceedings of the National Conference on Vocational Rehabilitation of Civilian Disabled Persons.* Bulletin No. 8. Washington, D. C., U. S. Government Printing Office, 1924, p. 123.
100. *Ibid.*
101. *Ibid.*
102. *Ibid.*, p. 127.
103. Obermann, *op. cit.*, pp. 247-248.
104. Federal Board for Vocational Educational: *A Statistical Analysis of 6,391 Disabled Persons.* Bulletin No. 132, June, 1928. Washington, D. C., U. S. Government Printing Office, 1928, p. 12.
105. Federal Board for Vocational Education: *Proceedings of the Fifth National Conference on Vocational Rehabilitation of Disabled Persons.* Bulletin No. 136, Vocational Rehabilitation Series, No. 18. Washington, D. C., U. S. Government Printing Office, September 1928, pp. 104-120.
106. Thompson, R. C.: Hotel continental. *J Rehab, 17(No. 5)*:15, September-October 1951.
107. Blauch, Lloyd E.: *Vocational Rehabilitation of the Physically Disabled.* Staff Study No. 9, The Advisory Committee on Education. Washington, D. C., U. S. Government Printing Office, 1938, p. 8.
108. Blauch, *loc. cit.*
109. McDonald, Mary E.: *Federal Grants for Vocational Rehabilitation.* Chicago, University of Chicago Press, 1944, p. 97.
110. United States Department of Interior, Office of Education: *Manual for Caseworkers.* Bulletin No. 175, Rehabilitation Series No. 23. Washington, D.C., U.S. Government Printing Office, 1934, p. 47.
111. Pattison, Harry A. (Ed.): *The Handicapped and Their Rehabilitation.* Springfield, Charles C Thomas, 1957, p. 845.
112. McDoanld, *op. cit.*, p. 80.
113. *Ibid.*, p. 79.

History of the Rehabilitation Movement in America 57

114. United States Department of Interior, Office of Education: *Vocational Rehabilitation of the Physically Handicapped.* Bulletin No. 190, Vocational Rehabilitation Series No. 25. Washington, D.C., U.S. Government Printing Office, 1936, p. 44.
115. *Ibid.,* p. 49.
116. *Ibid.,* p. 50.
117. *Ibid.,* pp. 68-69.
118. McDonald, *op. cit.,* p. 100.
119. The Federal Security Agency: *First Annual Report.* Washington, D. C., U. S. Government Printing Office, 1941, pp. 26-27.
120. Federal Security Agency, Annual Reports for fiscal years, 1941-1942 and 1942-1943. Washington, D. C., U. S. Government Printing Office, 1944, pp. 27-28.
121. *Ibid.*
122. *Ibid.*
123. *U. S. Statutes at Large,* Vol. 57, Public Law 11e, Seventy-eighth Congress, 1943, pp. 374-376.
124. Obermann, *op. cit.,* p. 289.
125. Pattison, *op. cit.,* p. 849.
126. The Federal Security Agency, Annual Report for the Fiscal Year, 1944-1945. Washington, D. C., U. S. Government Printing Office, 1945, p. 151.
127. Federal Security Agency, Annual Report, 1944-1945. Washington, D. C., U. S. Government Printing Office, 1945, p. 154.
128. *United States Statutes at Large,* Vol. 59, Public Law 176, Seventy-ninth Congress, 1945, p. 530.
129. Morison, Samuel Eliot: *The Oxford History of the American People.* New York, Oxford University Press, 1965, p. 1082.
130. *Ibid.,* p. 1084.
131. Obermann, *op. cit.,* pp. 311-312.
132. *Ibid.*
133. *Ibid.*
134. *United States Statutes at Large,* Vol. 68, Public Law 565, Eighty-third Congress, 1954, p. 652.
135. United States Department of Health, Education and Welfare, Annual Report 1954-1955: *Office of Vocational Rehabilitation.* Washington, D. C., U. S. Government Printing Office, 1955, p. 182.
136. *Ibid.*
137. McGowan, *op. cit.,* p. 31.
138. Obermann, *op. cit.,* p. 316.
139. *Ibid.,* p. 317.
140. State Department of Public Instruction, Division of Vocational Rehabilitation: *Reach, 1 (No. 1)*:1, July-August 1953.
141. McGowan, John F., and Porter, Thomas L.: *An Introduction to the*

Vocational Rehabilitation Process. Washington, D. C., U. S. Government Printing Office, 1967, p. 147.
142. McGowan, *op. cit.,* p. 147.
143. *United States Statutes at Large,* Vol. 79, Public Law 89-333, Eighty-ninth Congress, 1965, pp. 1282-1294.
144. Obermann, *op. cit.,* p. 323.
145. National Rehabilitation Association: *Newsletter 23 (No. 4):*2, August 1968.
146. Gardner, John W.: To extend the concept of rehabilitation. *J Rehab 34 (No. 1):*12. January-February 1968.
147. The administration. *Time Magazine, 90 (No. 9):*14, September 1, 1967.
148. Gardner, *loc. cit.*
149. National Rehabilitation Association: *Newsletter, 23 (No. 4):* August 1968.
150. Obermann, *op. cit.,* p. 324.
151. Rogers, Carl R.: Interpersonal relationships: U.S.A. 2000. *J Appl Behav Sci, 4 (No. 3):*265-266, 1968.
152. Hamilton, Kenneth W.: Perspectives and prospects in rehabilitation. *J Rehab, 34 (No. 1):*19, January-February 1968.
153. Gardner, John W.: Toward a self-renewing society, Godkin Lectures, Harvard University, "Time Essay." *Time, 93 (No. 5):*40, April 11, 1969.

2

Philosophical Considerations in Rehabilitation and Work

William R. Phelps

Historical Perspectives
Why People Work (Man's Concept of Work)
Work and Rehabilitation
Summary and Conclusion
References

HISTORICAL PERSPECTIVES

DURING THE PAST SEVERAL DECADES, numerous research projects and books have devoted their attention and efforts to work and theories of career development, work as a social problem, work alienation, work and social organization, work and leisure-time activities, the sociology of work, work and social change, and the psychology of work. Yet, only recently has society dealt with work and its relationship to the problems of the disabled and handicapped.

Little is known about the very early beginnings of work. In fact, writers of the Old Testament reveal to us that as consequences of expulsion from Eden, man must earn his bread through the sweat of his brow. Throughout history, work has had its darker as well as its brighter sides. Very little of the older historical literature praises work as such. However through centuries of the acculturation process, work has taken on a more positive meaning in the lives of all men. Work also has had meaning in role identification and self-identification—that is, how one perceives himself and is perceived by others. Work also has been one of the major reasons for man's conflicts as well as his vast talents for effective cooperation.

As early as 1911, Taylor became interested in the technology of work and became the recognized pioneer in the United States in time-and-motion studies. As a result of the Hawthorne studies (1939), the "human relations" movement in work came into existence. These studies by Roethlisberger et al.[11] were felt by some to be a panacea in the "interpersonal relationship" area which would increase productivity with less conflict and tension on the part of workers.

Marx (1887) felt that the manner in which members of society made their living was the primary determinant of everything else —its systems of religious beliefs, social systems and social structure, political philosophies and critical aspects of art and literature. Therefore, the human worker becomes the key figure in history.

In American democracy we live in a work-oriented society. It is expected that when man reaches a certain maturity he will engage in work. More and more women are encouraged to work and full employment is a national goal. Through social change over many centuries, work began to be perceived by the masses as "good" (the advent of the Protestant Ethic) as opposed to evil, a curse or punishment (Hebrews, Greeks). Work also began to be perceived as a natural right, duty and responsibility, having religious value (John Calvin), creative intrinsic good, with dignity. Along with this, in American democracy it is felt that every individual should have the freedom to choose his life work. There is a history of legislation designed to eliminate any social barriers to the exercise of this freedom.

WHY PEOPLE WORK (MAN'S CONCEPT OF WORK)

Many studies have been undertaken of work as a human necessity and problem. Roe's[10] personality theory of career development; Holland's[5] career typology theory of vocational behavior; the Ginzberg, Ginsburg, Axelrad and Herma theory;[4] the psychoanalytic conceptions of a career choice;[4] Super's[13] developmental self-concept theory of vocational behavior, psychological needs and career choice;[7] and social systems and career decisions (the situational approach)[2] have all made significant contributions to career development, the meaning of work, work and human behavior, the adjustment to work, and work in a democracy. The underlying common theme in all these theories is the essential nature of work in our culture.

To the Greeks and Romans of the classical period, work was perceived as more or less a curse and something to be avoided. For the ancient Hebrews, work offered man a way to atone for sin and a means to regain lost spiritual dignity. For the early Christians, no significant intrinsic value was recognized in hard labor. In early Catholicism, work was not exalted as something of value in itself but rather as an instrument of purification, expiation and charity. However, with the advent of Calvinism, work was seen as the will of God; diligence, industry and prosperity came to be considered as signs of God's grace. A dislike for work to the Calvinist might suggest that elections to God's grace was doubtful. To pursue one's occupation with all of one's conscience was a religious duty. Max Weber in his classic study, *The Protestant Ethic and the Spirit of Capitalism,* holds that the Protestant Ethic was instrumental in the development of capitalism.

Some writers[15] show a decline in the religious meaning of work in the modern era. Unlike the era of the Protestant Ethic, when consumption and indulgence prevailed, the present period has been characterized as sensate and pleasure seeking. Other writers have focused on the importance of leisure[6] and the decline of the work ethic in the United States. Yet, the cultural meanings attached to work in a relatively affluent society appear to have their effect on the disabled and handicapped population. This appears to be true, even though[3] it is pointed out that "production for the sake of goods produced is no longer very urgent." As a result of the role of the disabled in a society of affluence and some changes in the meaning of work, vocational rehabilitation agencies will need to be alert to future trends and changes. However, in 1970, even though we have the capacity to produce more than the necessary material goods for all our culture, the society still expects that the disabled should fill productive roles in order to justify their share of their surplus products. The existence of this seemingly inconsistent stance toward the disabled in our society forces the rehabilitation practitioner to take into account the cultural meaning attached to work in order to insure the most meaningful program of services to his clientele.

WORK AND REHABILITATION

During 1970 over 200,000 individuals were rehabilitated by state rehabilitation agencies in the United States. The federal agency describes its success in terms of persons "rehabilitated into employment," which explains the percise meaning of rehabilitation success. Most research has focused on employment outcomes in rehabilitation, although there have been isolated efforts to develop success-failure criteria other than the vocational. Since we live in a strongly work-oriented society which stresses the ability to perform in remunerative employment as an indicator of full citizenship, work as a way of life has become for most of us an internalized concept for becoming autonomous and independent. They may account for the close ties of the rehabilitation movement in the United States and issues bearing upon work and employment.

Evolving from the close relationship between work and rehabilitation have come needs for vocational and psychological assessment of work potential, the psychosocial theory of work,[12] techniques of work assessment,[8,9] the work sample, situational assessment[9] and the rehabilitation workshop movement.[8] After all of these efforts techniques of work assessment are still relatively weak. They have pointed out the need for a broad spectrum of sheltered, semi-sheltered, and slightly sheltered work situations, which would meet the needs of persons who cannot quite cope with unprotected employment or would provide a transition between substantial gainful employment and unemployment.

It may be that society has made us set our goals and expectations too high and often disabled persons bear the consequences of failure to meet its standards. Possibly our criteria need to consider degrees of vocational adjustment and success. Practitioners of the future will need to attempt to find the solution to what appears to be somewhat of a dilemma at the present time.

SUMMARY AND CONCLUSION

Environmental deprivation along with industrial and technological change has had considerable impact upon many disabled individuals. Accident or illness sometimes destroys vocational or occupational skills as well as the potential for its development or redevelopment. This may be particularly true depending upon the length of interruption or duration. After suffering varying periods of vocational deprivation growing out of forced illness, limited opportunities and lack of access to certain realistic but socially denied employment objectives, many disabled persons appear to be vocationally unmotivated.

If vocational development is dependent upon how one uses his capacities in life situations,[13] then disuse may result in occupational stagnation and retardation. In some instances, vocational inactivity may be as crippling as the direct effects of the disability itself and indicates to the rehabilitation counselor the urgency of early case finding and early reentry into meaningful work. Thus, the identification of transferability of past skills becomes crucial.

Although some clients, especially those disabled in early life, are confronted by lifelong vocational development problems related to their disabilities, a substantial proportion are handicapped by an interruption in their vocational development process. For many of the disabled, work has to some extent been a meaningless concept, and with the advent of the "age of cybernation" work may well lose some of its centrality for an even larger proportion of the population. One could ask, what will there be to take its place? Historically, not working has been looked upon as a sign of personal incompetence or deficiency. Work has fulfilled unsatisfied needs for self-esteem and self-actualization, and the possibility for fulfilling these needs outside of some type of institutional setting are limited. Not only are these unsatisfied needs personally disruptive but socially as well.

An affluent society cannot draw upon the past for applicable guidelines to solve the problems of rapid sociological change relative to the world of work, but it must face the necessity of dealing with changing concepts.

Rehabilitation practitioners may need to consider new ways of satisfying fundamental needs of their clients through means other than the historical concept of work. Since work appears to satisfy some basic needs and since social and technological change in the future may reduce the number of workers needed to perform society's tasks in an affluent society, should not attempts be made to satisfy these needs for the disabled through other means?

All the social, technological and ideological shifts in our society are undoubtedly changing the meanings imputed to work. Work may also be losing some of its intrinsic virtues, mass production and increasing mechanization prevail. However, probably none of this implies any immediate risk that work will become a negligible part of human existence. What the remote future holds in prospect would be very risky, at best, to attempt to predict. Innovation presently is taking place at a breakneck pace and will likely continue in the future. Work continues to be a major life sphere and will continue to be so indefinitely. The rehabilitation counselor needs to be aware of present and future trends as these relate to work and rehabilitation, since work is still very far from being eliminated as a major human enterprise.

REFERENCES

1. Brill, A. A.: *Basic Principles of Psychoanalysis.* Garden City, Doubleday, 1949.
2. Borow, H.: *Man in a World at Work.* Boston, Houghton-Mifflin Co., 1964.
3. Galbraith, John Kenneth: *The Affluent Society.* Boston, Houghton-Mifflin Co., 1958.
4. Ginzberg, E., Ginsburg, S. W., Axelrad, L., and Herma, J. L.: *Occupational Choice: An Approach to a General Theory.* New York, Columbia University Press, 1951.
5. Holland, J. L.: *The Psychology of Vocational Choice.* Waltham (Mass.), Blaisdell, 1966.
6. Kaplan, Max: *Leisure in America.* New York, John Wiley & Sons, 1960.
7. Murray, Henry A.: *Explorations in Personality.* New York, Oxford University Press, 1938.
8. Neff, Walter S.: *Work and Human Behavior.* New York, Atherton Press, 1958
9. Neff, Walter S.: Work and rehabilitation. *J Rehab 36 (No. 5):* 16-22, Sept.-Oct. 1970.
10. Roe, Anne: *The Psychology of Occupations.* New York, John Wiley & Sons, 1956.

11. Roethlisberger, F. J., and Dickson, W. J.: *Management and the Worker.* Cambridge (Mass.), Harvard University Press. 1939.
12. Suinn, Richard M., and Paulhe, Richard M.: A Psycho-Social Theory of Work, April 1970, Research Paper, The Clearing House, Rehabilitation Counselor Training Program, Oklahoma State University, Stillwater, Oklahoma, 10 pages.
13. Super, Donald E.: *The Psychology of Careers.* New York, Harper & Row, 1957.
14. Taylor, F. W.: *The Principles of Scientific Management.* New York, Harper & Row 1911.
15. Tilgher, Adriano: *Work: What It Has Meant to Men Through the Ages.* New York, Harcourt, Brace & Co., 1930.

3

Changing Rehabilitation Manpower Utilization

Edward Newman

The Rehabilitation Generalist
A Rehabilitation Manpower System
A Three-Level Staffing Pattern
Staff Development
Career Opportunities in Rehabilitation
Tomorrow's Manpower—A Look Ahead

THE PROCESS OF REHABILITATION incorporates change and movement—a handicapped person's ability to perform meaningful work changes. His physical and mental capacity changes. His attitude changes. His life style changes. He changes.

The rehabilitation worker's role within the rehabilitation process is to assist the client to undertake the changes he must to achieve maximum independent functioning or self-sufficiency. Over the years, the role of the public rehabilitation worker appears to have been largely immune from change.

The public rehabilitation program has grown rapidly. The client group has been expanded from an exclusive concern with the physically handicapped to a broad responsibility for serving all of the physically and mentally disabled, with special emphasis on the disabled disadvantaged. The services available under the public rehabilitation program have similarly been extended from a specific vocational training authority to the provision of a full range of restoration, adjustment and supportive services. Yet, in spite of this growth, the system for delivering the services has not

---

Note: This article appeared in the *J Rehab, 36 (No.5)*:45-48, 1970.

dramatically changed in many states and the office-based agency rehabilitation counselor is still generally representative of the rehabilitation service provider.

Fundamental changes in the way we organize to deliver services are demanded. This is a challenge we must meet. Intrinsic in any change in our service delivery system will be a change in the way we structure and utilize rehabilitation manpower.

In rehabilitation, we are trying to find ways to bring services closer to the places where community residents work and live. The National Citizens Advisory Committee on Vocational Rehabilitation suggested that if we are going to reach our goal, traditional appointments will have to be supplanted by new service roles which would include, among others, mobile teams, indigenous case finders, and information and referral personnel available on a round-the-clock basis.

The way we structure and utilize our manpower should satisfy two primary objectives. First, our manpower system should enhance our ability to attract increased numbers of direct service personnel. Second, the system should attract the kind of personnel best able to understand and communicate with the kinds of clients receiving our services.

THE REHABILITATION GENERALIST

Rehabilitation is an interdisciplinary process which focuses on the individual. We call it a client-centered approach: one in which the client is a party to the process and not merely a specimen which is "done to." In order to ensure that the rehabilitation process is fully effective, the talents and skills of all types of rehabilitation workers must be utilized: physicians, counselors, nurses, occupational therapists, physical therapists, psychologists, speech therapists, vocational evaluators and many others. These professionals have learned to work together as a rehabilitation team. However, it is the rehabilitation workers who are generalists—the workers in the public and private agencies who try to integrate the whole rehabilitation process—who form the basis of the rehabilitation effort.

The rehabilitation counselor is the model rehabilitation generalist and he is called on to perform an extraordinarily varied range of functions. The counselor must be familiar with the medical aspects of disability. He must be able to integrate and evaluate psychological information. He must understand what work means and be able to develop custom job opportunities and avenues for self-employment. He must be able to interview and test clients and interpret his findings to them. He must be able to counsel clients to help them with personal problems. He must be a community organizer and public relations specialist, able to educate the community about rehabilitation and its services. He must be familiar with the contributions of related disciplines such as speech therapy, occupational and physical therapy, and the many allied health professions, and he must be able to serve as the focal point of all their services. He must understand the functions of sheltered workshops as well as other types of rehabilitation facilities and their appropriateness for his client.

On the other hand, this need for a broad spectrum of skills is reflected in our expectation that counselors serving in the public and private rehabilitation agencies have completed graduate training. On the other hand, this wide scope of required knowledge and practice also argues towards defining new patterns of personnel organization in the delivery of services. We are now forced to question whether it is reasonable or economical to expect one kind of staff person to perform so many different kinds of duties and possess so many different kinds of skills.

Rehabilitation counseling is a young profession which like so many other professions has been seeking to develop a tradition to set it apart from other professions. Because of our concern with a high standard of service, we have been trying to restrict full professional status to those practitioners with master's degrees and have encouraged agencies to employ only those practitioners with graduate education.

The evidence surrounding the rehabilitation manpower crisis forces a reappraisal of our position. It is clear, for example, that in spite of our efforts, most rehabilitation counselor positions in public rehabilitation agencies are filled by persons who do not possess graduate degrees. Our expanding role in new social welfare legislation related to the vocational rehabilitation program places new kinds of demands on our staff and points out a need for a qualitative enrichment. Other social welfare programs have demonstrated that less well academically trained indigenous personnel can be effective in providing social services. How slowly we have accepted this approach in rehabilitation!

How should we cope with our manpower dilemma? Some suggest we should reduce the time it takes to earn a master's degree and thereby increase our supply of graduate counselors. Others suggest that if we double or triple our support of university counselor education programs, we can assure an adequate supply of counselors. Neither of these proposals is consistent with current trends. Most rehabilitation educators feel that two graduate years of education are in fact not enough to master the enormously complex and varied kinds of knowledge necessary to perform a counseling function. It seems unlikely that either federal financial resources or school faculty resources can make possible a dramatic expansion of counselor training programs in the immediate future.

The most likely answer for the immediate future would seem to lie in the development of a systematic plan for the differential utilization of generalist personnel—a plan in which several levels of personnel can be used to complement each other's contributions and a plan in which a new kind of rehabilitation team can be organized.

There is also nothing particularly new about the concept of subprofessionals in rehabilitation. We have been familiar with the idea for many years, and yet when the National Rehabilitation Association surveyed state vocational rehabilitation agencies this year, it turned out that fewer than half of our rehabilitation agencies were experimenting in any way with the utilization of preprofessional personnel. Relatively little analysis has been made of the functions and tasks to be performed in rehabilitation and to relate them to the required qualifications. But we do know that a considerable portion of what professional people do could be accomplished by individuals whose education and skill are less than is expected of the professional. In fact, we even seem willing to accept the possibility that some of the tasks which professionals attempt to perform might be done better by those with less or different kinds of educational and experience background.

A serious effort should be made to analyze the counselor's job; to break it down into tasks; to restructure rehabiltation jobs; and to develop rehabilitation career ladders. Some interesting work has certainly been done in this area. Muthard and Salomone, for example, reported in the special October 1969 issue of the *Rehabilitation Counseling Bulletin* some significant findings on the use of support personnel. It seems that rehabilitation counselors are willing to delegate only the most routine and repetitive tasks to support personnel but feel comfortable when other professional workers, such as social workers, perform many of the tasks generally identified with rehabilitation counseling. Yet, the same survey indicated that only one third of a counselor's time is spent in counseling and guidance activities; 25 percent in recording and clerical tasks; and 7 percent in placement efforts. A majority of counselors believe a master's degree should be held by those doing affective counseling, group procedures and test interpretation, while on-the-job training is viewed as sufficient preparation for such duties as medical referral and vocational counseling. This contrast is reflective of the deep-rooted attitudes prevalent among practitioners today.

Within the field of rehabilitation, several different kinds of auxiliary personnel have been identified. Some assist the professional by performing office tasks. These are indigenous to a particular racial or cultural subgroup and act as liaison between the community and the agency.

Our manpower problem is perhaps related to the fact that there is such a wide gap in rehabilitation between these subprofessionals and the professional graduate counselor. There is no fully recognized intermediate position.

A REHABILITATION MANPOWER SYSTEM

In rehabilitation, we need a manpower system that provides a structure into which employees with different academic and social backgrounds may be fitted. Our system should provide for a progression into positions of greater responsibility for employees who have demonstrated unusual ability, regardless of their formal degrees or credentials. Our system should reward attainment of education but should nonetheless place a special value on achievement of techniques relevant to the field of rehabilitation. It should provide for a training continuum from the lowest entrance level in the hierarchy to the highest levels of employment and should include formalized training programs spaced at intervals along the progression. It should provide a means to utilize available manpower effectively. Our system should fill the gap between the professional and subprofessional levels.

A THREE-LEVEL STAFFING PATTERN

The new kind of rehabilitation team, a vertical generalist team, should possess three levels of employment ranging from the basic aide and subprofessional levels through a middle specialist level up to a professional leadership level. This means taking a hard look not only at our willingness to hire aides, indigenous personnel, or outreach personnel but also at the total structure of rehabilitation practitioners.

The "New Careers" concept implies staff development and mobility at all levels. Russell Nixon of New York University said at the 1968 NRA Conference:

> "New Careers" is a phrase of art—legislatively validated—which describes a program of major change in the recruitment, training and education, occupational advancement, status and utilization of nonprofessional personnel—it has profound implications for the entire system of service delivery, for the definition and reconstruction of occupations, for the conventional requirements of degrees and licenses as credentials necessary for work, and for change and enhancement of the role of the professional.

What is frequently missing in rehabilitation and related fields is an intermediate position for the progression of the support personnel and aides and for the entry level, the junior college graduate and the inexperienced holder of a four-year degree.

Hylbert and Kelz have suggested a rehabilitation manpower plan based on a three-level approach using counselor, case manager and aide.

The rehabilitation counselor reviews all records and conducts screening interviews with all clients to determine whether and to what extent counseling is needed. For clients needing counseling services, the counselor, with the assistance of other professionals, is responsible for evaluating physical, psychological, social, educational and vocational characteristics of the client. He identifies the personal and environmental changes which can be instituted to facilitate rehabilitation and enhance personal-social adjustment. He plans the rehabilitation strategies for the client and formalizes all recommendations for the rehabilitation plan. The counselor acts in a consultative relationship with other staff and exercises a degree of quality control over the implementation of the rehabilitation plan. The rehabilitation counselor provides direct counseling to the client, of course, at any time during the rehabilitation process when either the client or the lower-level agency staff feel it necessary.

The rehabilitation case manager is the intermediate position. It is the case manager who is responsible for such things as case finding; program explaining, distributing literature and forms; intake interviewing; securing case histories; arranging for routine psychological and medical examinations; obtaining pertinent information from hospitals, schools, and other agencies and institutions in the community; scheduling counseling sessions with the rehabilitation counselor; case recording, other than related directly to counseling; coordinating and authorizing services, and contacting vendors; authorizing payment for services; supervising clients in training, checking on client progress; providing continuing supportive client contact at the guidance level; making necessary statistical reports; and providing follow-up services.

The rehabilitation aide is a flexible lower-level position. The aide may perform any of the functions assigned to the case manager and such other duties as his abilities, education, experience and interest may enable him to undertake. The aide may specialize in certain areas such as outreach, follow-up or family services, or he may be utilized in providing a broad range of services in order to enrich his experience.

The key aspect of this system is that through experience and provision of an agency staff development program, the aide can eventually achieve the case manager status. The case manager similarly may have the opportunity to become a rehabilitation counselor.

At each level, one of the main responsibilities of the rehabilitation worker is to be an advocate for those disabled. It is clear that the rehabilitation program has the potential to perform on behalf of all handicapped individuals this advocacy function. In the rehabilitation process as carried out under the state-federal program, we determine whether the individual is eligible, arrange with the individual for the development of a plan for his rehabilitation, manage the arrangements for the necessary service, counsel and guide him and try to provide him with satisfying opportunities through successful placement on the job. What better description could be given of the role of a client advocate? The rehabilitation worker has the potential to enable all handicapped clients to play productive roles in their social environment and assist them to locate all the services needed to achieve a goal of productivity.

The rehabilitation aide can be especially valuable in helping the vocational rehabilitation agency to assume the advocacy roles.

STAFF DEVELOPMENT

Implicit in the staffing plan is a more intensive and broader commitment to staff development and an acceptance of the fact that manpower development is a continuous process. We need to look closely at what it is we do; study our service system; analyze our jobs into tasks; restructure our jobs where necessary and then build career ladders and provide the opportunities for our staff to climb these ladders.

We need to make both a personnel and financial commitment to this task. In the rehabilitation field, people—and their improvement—are everything. We should reflect this in our personnel budgets. As we enter a new kind of cooperative relationship with other programs, interagency training should be emphasized. Staff should be encouraged to attend short courses, seminars and professional meetings. New staff should have a special training program. Personnel at all levels should be encouraged to continue their education and educational leave opportunities should be expanded.

CAREER OPPORTUNITIES IN REHABILITATION

We have a continuing responsibility to attract new people into the rehabilitation field. There is a large reservoir of potentially capable professional people in urban slums and ghettos and rural backwoods settings who should be encouraged to enter the rehabilitation field. Special effort should be made to ensure that there are employment opportunities for workers representing all the minority groups whom we serve. High school and college students should be offered the opportunity to work in rehabilitation settings through summer internship programs. Just as investment in scholarships is a usual part of the recruitment programs of industry, it should also be considered for careers in rehabilitation.

For older new employees, there is the opportunity for immediate entry at the aide level with a clear potential for upward movement within the agency.

Although job progression is basic to this kind of manpower utilization plan, it is important to point out that something has to be done for those superior employees, at all levels, who are thoroughly satisfied with their duties and are not interested in pursuing the additional training necessary for upward movement. A special salary range should be established to reward superior counselors who wish to remain in direct client services rather than becoming supervisors and those superior case managers who do not wish to become rehabilitation counselors.

Quality of performance needs to be rewarded as much as seniority and academic qualifications. Successful and active rehabilitation workers should be rewarded for their enthusiasm, involvement, concern and sensitivity.

TOMORROW'S MANPOWER—A LOOK AHEAD

A three-level rehabilitation team provides one opportunity for enriching agency potentials at the same time that high professional standards are maintained. There will always be a basic demand for highly trained professionals in the rehabilitation field.

Even though little experimentation has taken place in restructuring the counselor's job, almost no attention has been given to other new responsibilities which may develop for the public rehabilitation program in the future.

Consider the implications for the allocation of manpower tasks if the public program were to commit itself to a comprehensive advocacy approach to *all* handicapped persons residing in a community or geographic service area. Efficient and workable referral services would have to be established and manned. Rehabilitation workers would find themselves, for example, not only finding housing and transportation for clients, but also stimulating and nurturing housing and transportation resources for all handicapped people. Some rehabilitation workers will act as consultants to other health, education and welfare workers—helping these care-giving and human development workers to understand their roles in helping their handicapped students, clients or patients.

Maximizing the potential for each handicapped person implies a broader conception of professional tasks than personal counseling and seeking out appropriate resources on behalf of clients. It implies a responsibility to analyze the extent, organization and quality of community institutional arrangements and resources for meeting the basic needs of our handicapped citizens.

To my knowledge, we do not yet train people nor have we begun to conceptualize the knowledge base or job requirements for new challenges which face us in this new area of community development for handicapped people.

We must recognize the shortcomings of our present reliance on the professional and face up to what John Gardner calls "professionalism" or "credentialism." In his book, *No Easy Victories,* Mr. Gardner says, "Professions are subject to the same deadening forces that affect all other human institutions: an attachment to time-honored ways, reverence for established procedures, a preoccupation with one's own vested interests, and an excessively narrow definition of what is relevant and important." In rehabilitation, we cannot afford to fall into this trap.

Beyond this, rehabilitation workers should be taking the lead in facilitating better communication and working relationships among all human service career fields. This could begin with consultation and collaborating with other professional manpower systems.

4

Developing Trends in Rehabilitation

Corbett Reedy

An Emergency Commitment to Rehabilitation
Fifty Years of Growth
Rehabilitation Comes of Age
Developing Trends and Rehabilitation Practice

AN EMERGENCY COMMITMENT TO REHABILITATION

REHABILITATION, as an endeavor of man, is a relatively new development. While health services, education programs and institutional care have operated for centuries, rehabilitation as an identifiable human service scarcely spans three generations. Five decades cover the bulk of its history.

Slowly "rehabilitation" as a philosophy has replaced a long era of "exploitation." Natural resources have been consumed in a most wasteful way with little thought of the future. The farmer moved to new clearings after having worn out his original acreage. Coal and timber resources have been extracted to reflect only the highest profit to the harvester.

Even people were treated with equal disregard. Injured or unfit workmen were left to fend for themselves. The chronically ill and disabled experienced either an early death or were kept by families or the state in a totally dependent and hopeless state.

Gradually this heartless waste of human and natural resources began to weigh on the conscience of man. As new lands became scarce it became more important to reclaim the old. The toll of human disablement came to be regarded both as inhuman and as economically wasteful.

Only in the last thirty years has rehabilitation of the disabled become a significant factor in national social policy. Many of the pioneers of the movement are still living.

Today rehabilitation is more than a profession, a process or a program. It has become a profound, pervasive, vital movement in our society. The level of success now attained in this movement is as much the promise of the future as it is the achievement of the present.

Beyond the rehabilitation movement itself, forces are at work which will reshape many of our social and economic patterns and in the process will influence the entire rehabilitation field. The search for better ways of meeting peoples' needs in social welfare, health, social security, education and employment goes on continuously—often in controversy, always intensively—and the rehabilitation program could not escape its involvement even if it wished.

A new climate has been created in which rehabilitation efforts operate today. Until recently, the provision of rehabilitation services was largely optional and seldom a sense of obligation to an individual or to groups to produce services "on demand." Today there is less and less option and instead an increasing volume of feeling among all citizens that rehabilitation, like education, medical care, welfare and many other services, shall be available when needed.

We have moved out of the period in which a comparative handful of dedicated leaders alone promote the cause of the disabled person and advocate rehabilitation as the methodology of choice in combating the problems and burden of disability; it is a broadly-based, spontaneous demand generated by the increased knowledge among the public generally that something constructive can be done about disability and the problems it creates.

This means that plans for the future of rehabilitation must be constructed not solely in terms of what rehabilitation leaders want but in terms of what the American people want. The dimensions of rehabilitation efforts during the coming years will be vastly expanded; the total cost is certain to rise sharply; professional and technical resources will be strained to keep pace; technical and professional competencies of workers will have to increase; and organizational, administrative and operating structures and methods—including the proper "meshing" with other programs—to meet the steadily growing demands for rehabilitation.

The New Economics of Disability

The financial impact of widespread dependency caused by neglected disability in this country "hits" every taxpayer. Obviously, not every disabled person can be restored to activity and work; some are victims of conditions which cannot be improved. Even with this recognition we still are faced with hundreds of thousands of disabled people who either can be restored to the status of workers and taxpayers or can be moved up the scale from total dependency to the independence—and consequent cost reduction—that follows the restoration of ability to care for one's self.

Rehabilitation and Skilled Manpower

The loss of technical skills and manpower resources because of disability is a serious deterrent to sound national economic and social planning. Under present circumstances we get along without these skills and resources, not having learned the value of conserving and utilizing them.

In one recent year, through the public rehabilitation program, over 300 engineers and more than 1,400 teachers completed their rehabilitation programs and went to work at a time when civic, business, professional and governmental leaders were frantically trying to produce more qualified workers in these shortage fields. The approximately 3,500 persons (included in these two groups) who were rehabilitated into professional jobs offer a clue to the tremendous possibilities which reside among the unrehabilitated millions of handicapped persons for adding to our pool of professional and technically trained manpower.

Income Maintenance and Rehabilitation

Most of our income maintenance programs have come into existence in the last forty years through workmen's compensation, social security, veterans pensions, union retirement plans and so forth. However inadequate, they may now be adjudged, for millions of persons it has meant the difference between starvation and survival. The social gain, within its era, has been tremendous.

We find increasing willingness to discharge the public responsibility to the disabled by writing a check, but little willingness to earnestly consider whether this should be society's principal response. Should a permanent money payment be the first aim or should it be the last resort when all restoration efforts have failed.

Continuing cash payments to the disabled—because they are disabled and unable to work—now impose a cost in excess of $20 billion on the working population of this country. When we realize that total public expenditures within the rehabilitation program in FY 1970 were less than $0.7 billion, we can appreciate the tremendous imbalance that exists in our use of resources for income maintenance and rehabilitation. When loss of earnings of potentially rehabilitable persons are added to other contributions from family and "care" programs, the comparison is even more staggering.

We cite here the results of well-documented, substantial experimental rehabilitation programs which show:

1. Early prevention rehabilitation attention to younger disabled persons of school age can effectively prevent unemployment and disability in adulthood.

2. Institutional rehabilitation programs for the mentally ill and mentally retarded provide a tested means for bridging expensive, futile institutional living and productive community adjustment.

3. A one-time expenditure on rehabilitation of disabled welfare recipients, averaging less than the cost of one year's assistance payments, can remove a large percentage of such persons permanently from welfare rolls.

4. Rehabilitation efforts in behalf of disabled beneficiaries of social security, financed in large part by a small allocation of trust funds, demonstrates that rehabilitation saves money for the "fund."

5. Experimental rehabilitation projects in correctional insti-

tutions show that for both youthful and adult offenders (the behaviorally disabled) employment and community adjustment is speeded and recidivism is dramatically reduced.

FIFTY YEARS OF GROWTH

Fifty years is a relatively short span of time but it encompasses the historical development of rehabilitation programs in this country. Although the history of rehabilitation is treated more definitely elsewhere in this scheme, it is necessary to identify significant developments of the part to understand current trends in this field of human service.

In a quick review of the background of our present rehabilitation program five distinct periods stand out in significance: 1900 – 1920, 1920 – 1943, 1943 – 1954, 1954 – 1965, and 1965 to the present. Except for the first period, important national legislation, representing significant advances in the national commitment to rehabilitation, sets the stage for each of these periods of growth and provided the program with unique opportunities and challenges to serve disabled persons.

The Period 1900–1920

This period is significant in that it marked the emergence of the concept of rehabilitation, expressed largely in small programs under private auspices. Small demonstrations were developed in various locations in the country giving credence to the idea that rehabilitation of the disabled was not only possible but was also socially desirable and economically feasible. A national effort based on the principle of public funding was just around the corner.

The Period 1920–1943

The initial national legislation, Public Law 236, was passed in 1920. Support was based on a year-to-year basis until 1935 when rehabilitation achieved permanent status under legislative amendments to the Social Security Act. Initially services were provided only to the *physically* disabled and limited to counseling and vocational guidance, job training possibilities and job placement.

Such a limited program appears woefully inadequately today, but a beginning had been made!

After gaining much valuable experience in organizing and providing rehabilitation services during these early years, leaders were able to advise with the Congress to broaden the scope of services and to expand its scope to cover all categories of disability.

The Period 1943–1954

A significant "breakthrough" came with the passage of Public Law 113 in 1943. Three distinct gains were made, altering significantly the future character of the public rehabilitation program, as follows:

1. It broadened the concept of rehabilitation services within the program to include physical restoration services.

2. For the first time the mentally handicapped were made eligible to receive services.

3. A substantial expansion of financial support for the program was provided by increasing the federal share of program costs.

The meaning of these changes was that it was no longer necessary to work around a disability that could be removed or reduced by physical restoration measures; counselors learned medical aspects of disability, gained knowledge about restoration services and learned to work with physicians in the provision of the new physical restoration services and state legislatures were more responsive to the request for funds to match federal monies thus permitting substantial increases in numbers of the disabled served and rehabilitated.

It can be said that during this period rehabilitation became firmly established in the national policy dealing with disability.

The Period 1954–1965

In this period rehabilitation truly "became of age."

Two new acts of great significance were passed. The first was Public Law 565 that brought forth from President Eisenhower at the signing ceremony these words:

This law is especially noteworthy in two aspects. In the first place it re-emphasizes to all the world the great value which we in America place upon the dignity and worth of each individual human being. Second, it is a humanitarian investment of great importance, yet it saves substantial sums of money for both Federal and state governments.

In addition to providing greatly increased funding for servicies, Public Law 565 contained authority for:

1. A nationwide system of training grants to colleges, universities and other appropriate training grantees to increase the supply of rehabilitation workers.

2. Make grants to rehabilitation agencies and to nonprofit organizations and institutions to help bear the cost of conducting research into the problems of disability and rehability or demonstration projects to test and model new approaches to rehabilitation.

3. Provided means whereby federal aid could be extended, through state agencies, to community rehabilitation projects.

4. Further liberalized federal matching and enlarged the allotment of federal funds to the states to encourage rapid expansion.

In a parallel action, further impetus was given to the rehabilition effort through the passage in the same year of the Medical Facilities Survey and Construction Act. This Act provided for grants-in-aid to assist states in construction of rehabilitation facilities, now held to be absolutely vital to successful rehabilitation programming.

Further Expansion Demanded

Gains in rehabilitation in the first forty years as shown in Figure 1, while comparatively impressive was held to be only a token effort in comparison to the growing need. Consequently in early 1960 the then Office of Vocational Rehabilitation developed and gave limited distribution to a document entitled, *Rehabilitation in the Decade of the 60's—A Report of the Task Force on Program Development.* This report developed the thesis that "rehabilitation of the disabled is in the public interest, is in fact a public imperative." Ambitious goals in the form of sixteen recommen-

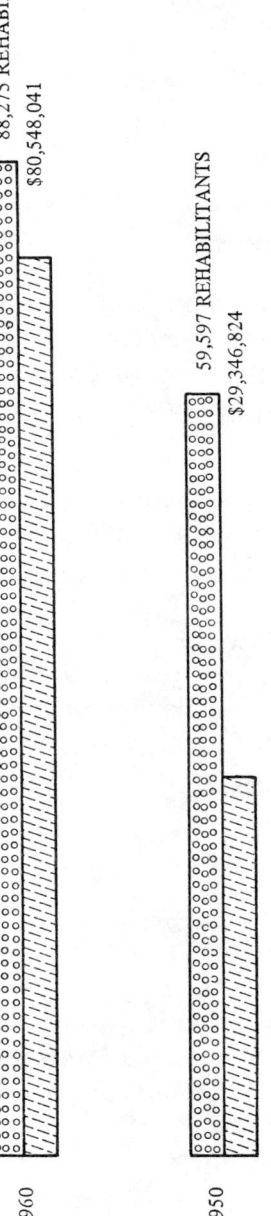

Figure 1. Increase in number of rehabilitations and financial support. Ten-year intervals: 1920-1960. State-federal vocational rehabilitation program.

dations (appended to this chapter) were proposed which to the top leaders in the field became the "new charter of rehabilitation program developments."

Immediately thereafter an ambitious new legislative program was launched with sponsorship by the Administration, the States Council of Rehabilitation Administrators, and the National Rehabilitation Association. This program had widespread endorsement and support from a host of national state and local organizations, agencies and institutions.

The Period 1965 to the Present

In 1965, Public Law 333 was passed, the most liberal and far-reaching piece of national legislation ever enacted. It focused interest on evaluative techniques and services, community sheltered workshops and rehabilitation facilities, "self-care" rehabilitation and new, greatly expanded goals. Behavioral disabilities and factors of cultural and economic privation as facets of disability and handicap were established.

This is the period of greatest expansion in rehabilitation—numbers of persons served and rehabilitated, financial support, and rehabilitation resources and facilities. The rehabilitation "system" was greatly expanded by the mechanism of "cooperative programming" bringing rehabilitation agencies into new productive relationships with a host of public and private agencies and organizations. Community rehabilitation projects and rehabilitation facilities spring up by the hundreds, solid evidence of widespread citizen support and involvement.

REHABILITATION COMES OF AGE

Current challenges to rehabilitation are of a magnitude and urgency never before experienced. More people know about rehabilitation and its results. The disabled want rehabilitation and they want it now. They bring new rehabilitation problems to the program and expect prompt service of a high quality to be provided. Physicians, labor leaders, social agencies, schools and a host of others now have become advocates for their disabled constituents in securing prompt attention from rehabilitation agencies.

Role of Leadership and Coordination

During the last decade there has been tremendous increase in knowledge about disabilities and rehabilitation and in the development of services and facilities that provide rehabilitation services. This has resulted in a myriad of activities under a variety of sponsorships, even in a single community that has not always given the best return for the investment. The major ingredient lacking has been that of leadership in the planning and development of such programs and facilities and a coordinating force which would prevent wasteful overlapping and duplication of effort. It is often difficult to marshall for the individual disabled person the right kind of service when he needs it. The state agency, having a background of fifty years' experience in the rehabilitation field can and should play the key role in providing leadership at the community level as well as the state level. State agency administrators must recognize this role and give it proper weight in the development of agency staffing patterns.

The rehabilitation counselor with proper training can be the focal point of community leadership. He should see as a major responsibility the cultivation of community interests in solving its rehabilitation problems and join his efforts with others in the community in planning and initiating new service activities and resources. The strength of his leadership and of the program he represents should be infused into the dynamics of the community so that sound goals will be established and practical plans will be developed for achieving these goals. He should be empowered to make judicious use of the agency's resources, both financial and staff, to enable community rehabilitation goals to be realized. As the local office staff is augmented with other professional personnel—the physician, the psychologist and the social worker—this task of community leadership can be shared.

Consideration of rehabilitation goals and resources cannot be limited to the local community level. State agency personnel at regional and state levels also have a vital leadership and coordinating function to perform quite similar to the community role of the counselor. Our strong rehabilitation agencies today find it possible to encourage and strengthen the rehabilitation efforts of sister public agencies and to aid the private and voluntary agencies to find much-needed direction for their efforts. This exercise of leadership requires provision of sufficient staff at the state and regional levels to enable supervisory and consultative personnel to share meaningfully and effectively in the leadership function without serious impairment of their service to regular agency operations.

The leadership role can be exercised in many ways. One of its major challenges and contributions is to develop a greater appreciation of quality standards of service among all of those who are presently engaged in providing rehabilitation services to the disabled. The rehabilitation leader, both in his own agency and through consultation with others, will seek to bring about the development and acceptance of constantly higher levels of quality in techniques, personnel and facilities. The state agency is in the best position to lead the formulation of standards of service and in bringing about their acceptance since it is a statewide agency and is recognized by all as devoting its capabilities exclusively in the field of rehabilitation.

Many agencies of government and many voluntary organizations are beginning to emphasize rehabilitation in their programs. A multiplicity of small, unrelated rehabilitation programs would be uneconomical and inefficient. The state agency, as the principal channel of rehabilitation effort must coordinate the statewide effort.

The second important avenue for the exercise of leadership is in the development of public understanding and the building of public support of rehabilitation programs. While its own agency's services will be emphasized, this public relations effort should be on a far broader basis. It should emphasize the needs of the disabled and their potentiality for rehabilitation, the values of rehabilitation to families and communities—both socially and economically—and give emphasis to the importance of a broad attack on disability through many agencies and efforts—both public and private—leading to the achievement of the accepted objectives of rehabilitation for the locality. The state agency should spearhead this program of public understanding but should see that the task involves all agencies and individuals related to the rehabilitation movement.

Above all, the state agency should be the leader in performance. Its own service program to the disabled should constitute the core of the statewide, organized attack on the problem of disability and should point the way for meaningful participation and collaboration by other agencies and organizations having services and resources to offer in this field. We know of no other agency, public or private, which offers a comparable breadth of goals and service, or which devotes its energies so effectively toward the task of rehabilitating the disabled. The disabled want and deserve an agency devoted exclusively to their welfare. This challenges the state rehabilitation agency to have the best-trained personnel, the highest standards in performance and service, the most efficiently operated facilities and the most effective placement services and to be a dynamic, forward-moving agency responsive to the needs of people.

A Broadened Base of Eligibility

A public, tax-supported program of services must have standards of eligibility based on legislation and regulations. Since 1920 the vocational rehabilitation program has had only three basic eligibility requirements: the presence of a vocationally limiting physical or mental disability, the probability of employment following provision of rehabilitating services and a restriction limiting eligibility to those having reached or approaching legal employment age. Two of these, the age standard and the presence of a disability, can be established objectively and with relative ease. Our great difficulty has been experienced in evaluating the effect of the disability on potential employability of the disabled applicant. Trained evaluation teams operating in most favorable settings have been able only to reduce the margin of error, not eliminate it. Today, we know that the only truly effective method of determining work potential is through an actual trial rehabilitation experience for the disabled person.

Bound by the stern necessity of limiting the acceptance of cases because of shortage of funds and resources, state agencies

Developing Trends in Rehabilitation

have tended to accept those better prospects whose rehabilitation could be accomplished with a minimum of time and expense. Those with doubtful rehabilitation promise or who present a need for services that are expensive and long drawn out have been either rejected as a group or have been accepted only in trickles. More and more, however, our most progressive state agencies are working with assurance and success with persons with extreme severity of disability. Our problem is to make this a uniform practice.

Through all of this has remained, however, the requirement that no case be accepted which did not offer reasonable promise of eventual employment and self-support. Those with lesser goals, however worthy and meaningful to the individual, to his family and to the community, have been excluded from the public program of vocational rehabilitation and have had to turn elsewhere for help—the latter often a futile effort. Today, there is mounting demand that the public program of rehabilitation broaden its base of eligibility to include those who may not initially show promise of employment but who, with the provision of a reasonable amount of service, can acquire or regain ability for self-care and personal independence. This is an entirely worthy rehabilitation objective. To the disabled individual this means the achievement of that degree of self-sufficiency that can assure a reasonable satisfaction in living day by day. To the family it means relief from the daily, continuous investment of funds for care or the release of a relative who is bound by the needs of the disabled family member. To the community it may mean relief from an expensive and continuous burden of financial support to the disabled—either in his home or in an institution.

Who can say in the case of the individual most concerned—the disabled person himself—that these early efforts to regain personal independence may not be the beginnings of a more far-reaching level of progress that leads to a status of productive living, creativity and economic self-sufficiency as well? Without assuming responsibility for those who need long-term care and concentrating services to those who can truly become capable of caring for their personal needs in their own homes, state and federal rehabilitation statutes should immediately be liberalized to permit the state-federal program to accept for services those who can achieve such status of self-care.

Today, in our agencies for the blind, self-care rehabilitation is commonplace. These agencies have long since accepted the fact that restoration of self-care abilities and the achievement of a minimal level of personal and social adjustment require in family and community living is a requirement for successful efforts toward vocational rehabilitation. In a similar manner, our general agencies which serve such severely disabled cases as the paraplegic, the hemiplegic or the severe mental retardate have found it necessary to restore self-care skills before the more traditional "vocational" services are applicable. This liberalization of eligibility requirements to permit acceptance of self-care cases, as far-reaching and significant as it is, does not require new services not presently provided by our agencies. It simply means that we realign our service resources to meet the evaluation and treatment needs of this new group of eligibles and set out to secure the funds, facilities and staff required for the greatly enlarged case load. It is estimated that the full exploitation of the values of a self-care rehabilitation program will increase by 50 percent the potential case load in the average state.

Improving Capacity for Providing Service

As one state agency administrator aptly remarked, "A counselor is severely limited in the rehabilitation results he can achieve out of his briefcase."

Traditionally, the vital services of client evaluation, counseling, supervision and placement have been provided by the agency's own staff. It must now look to strengthening each of them. The agency itself must develop the staff resources and the facilities which will permit it to incorporate into its own operating procedure the very best of current knowledge and practice in regard to rehabilitation evaluation. This can be achieved through the organization within the state agency structure to supplement the counselors' function evaluation centers at district office levels, special client evaluation units at state-agency–operated comprehensive rehabilitation centers and broad use of specialists and consulting personnel whenever indicated. In no area of the rehabilitation process is the special experience and competency of the rehabilitation agency better established than in the area of evaluation.

Our responsibilities to the client do not end with evaluation. We must see that he has the rehabilitation treatment, training or other special services that are required to fit him for effective living, including employment, if possible. To do this the agency must make broad use of all existing community facilities and service resources. However, the usual community facilities serving the general population are not always adequate to meet the special rehabilitation needs of a large segment of the agency clients. This means that the agency must promote the development and use of special rehabilitation resources to serve the community, a region or the entire state.

As we continue to bring into our case loads a greater number of clients having increasing severity or disability, our skills in job placement must be improved to meet this need for special placement services. There must be far greater stress on job placement, job evaluation and job development skills for both new and experienced counselors in our training programs. The agency must make increasing use of sheltered employment and agency-managed business enterprise programs to accommodate the severely disabled and the homebound. Each of our larger agencies (those employing twenty or more counselors) should add to its staff a full-time placement specialist who will organize and direct appropriate activities designed to improve client employment. The smaller agencies may need to combine this function with others in a multiple purpose position. As General Maas, chairman of the President's Committee on Employment of the Physically Handicapped, has so well stated on many occasions, "to prepare a handicapped individual for a job and then fail to help him secure a job is a mockery."

New Areas of Service

As the state agency undertakes the rehabilitation of cases for self-care, it will result in many instances of the release of a family member who may then become the family breadwinner. The agency should not overlook the opportunity to achieve the potential economic gains that may result from rehabilitation of the disabled member. If we take a family approach to the problem we can easily see the logic of completing the rehabilitation of the family by helping the father, the daughter or the housewife to secure employment. This extension of service to include assistance to an able-bodied person is still related to the fulfillment of the goals of the disabled client and the family for independence.

It should make the services of its counselors and consulting staff available to render service to disabled children and youth at a much younger age than is the prevailing practice today. As our special education, health and welfare agencies seek to improve services of education, treatment and social adjustment for physically or mentally handicapped children, rehabilitation should contribute as fully as possible the value of its experience, knowledge and resources to support and strengthen these vital programs It should not hesitate to supplement by giving direct services where needed in physical restoration, prosthetics, guidance services and consulting services to individual disabled children when such services will influence the eventual rehabilitation prospects of such persons.

The rehabilitation agency also must accept additional responsibility in an area which we may call "maintenance in employment" for its clients. Our agencies for the blind have been far more realistic in this regard than the general agencies, having learned that blind rehabilitants often need continuing service and supervision in order to retain the initial gains of previous rehabilitation efforts. Many of our rehabilitated clients achieve a status of independence that makes it unnecessary for the agency to give further attention to them. This is a very gratifying result and is the highest measure of rehabilitation success. However, many of our other clients with marginal earning potentialities, with limited vocational, social and intellectual assets cannot meet, unaided, the continuing problems which they face following rehabilitation and thus in time regress to a former state of dependency, unemployment and defeat. The replacement of worn-out appliances, the replenishment of stocks, tools and work equipment at critical points, the provision of periodic rehabilitation treatment services, or the continuation on a supportive basis of personal counseling and encouragement through counselor contacts with such clients may make the difference between a long period of productivity and a relatively short one. The community rightfully should look to its rehabilitation agency to meet the continuing rehabilitation needs of disabled persons. What other agency is better suited to this task?

Rehabilitation Facilities: An Indispensable Resource

Rehabilitation facilities represent an indispensable resource in modern rehabilitation. Facilities provide the means for evaluating, treating and training the severely disabled who otherwise could not be effectively rehabilitated.

There are many types of rehabilitation facilities. Included are comprehensive rehabilitation centers, speech and hearing centers, optical aids clinics, rehabilitation centers for the blind, evaluation and treatment centers for the epileptic, halfway houses for the mentally ill and mentally retarded, and workshops. Some of the facilities are large; some are small. All disability groups may be served in a single facility or only selected groups. Regardless of the size of the facility each plays an important role in rehabilitation.

Facilities should not be regarded as mere appendages to the rehabilitation efforts of the state rehabilitation program. In actuality they represent the most important new tool for rehabilitation developed in recent years. Without adequate facilities the community is severly limited in its ability to meet the needs of its disabled citizens.

Rehabilitation Centers

Early proponents saw the center as a special type of rehabilitation facility which would join the many evaluative and therapeutic efforts of medicine and important nonmedical therapeutic services, including adjustment training, social and recreational training, vocational counseling, job tryout and vocational training. This combination of services makes it possible to give simultaneous consideration and treatment to the entire range of problems presented by the disabled individual. The setting frequently provides stimulation for a higher and more sustained form of motivation within the patient—a key factor in rehabilitation. Its rationale is based on the conviction that severe problems call for intensive effort and specialized skills working in concert.

Prior to the establishment of comprehensive rehabilitation centers, counselors were forced to secure various services piece by piece. The pieces were fitted together with his own counseling efforts. This approach to rehabilitation is no longer adequate for many of the disabled that must be served.

Rehabilitation centers exist in a variety of forms and are found in various administrative settings. A generally accepted classification of centers does not exist; however, they tend to fall in one of two major categories: the medically oriented center and the vocationally oriented center. The medically oriented center is generally a part of a general hospital or a medical school or hospital center. The medically oriented center as the term implies has a strong emphasis on medical and medically related services. Its counterpart is the vocationally oriented center in which medical services are supplemented in a major way by extensive services for vocational counseling, vocational testing and vocational training.

The modern comprehensive rehabilitation center today represents rehabilitation in its highest form of development. Herein are combined under a single management the broad range of services that are needed even by the severely disabled. These services include the following:

- Evaluation and counseling services
- Restorative services including the rehabilitation therapies, prosthetics, etc.
- Educational services for general educational and cultural development
- Social and personal development services including recreation and group living activities
- Counseling and treatment for emotional problems

- Vocational counseling, testing and training
- Sheltered work opportunities

Rehabilitation Centers and the Rehabilitation Process

It was the late Colonel John Smith, former Director of the Institute for the Crippled and Disabled in New York City, who called rehabilitation "a new composite science." Colonel Smith, often called the father of modern comprehensive rehabilitation, saw very clearly the contribution which special rehabilitation facilities could make in the rehabilitation process. In the rehabilitation center setting he saw a natural joining of the many therapeutic efforts of medicine—physical medicine, physical therapy, occupational therapy, speech therapy, prosthetics, drug therapy, psychotherapy—with other important nonmedical therapeutic services including adjustment training, social and recreational training, vocational counseling, vocational exploration and tryout, vocational training, sheltered work and special placement services, with the result that the disabled individual and his entire range of problems were being treated simultaneously.

Prior to the establishment of comprehensive rehabilitation centers, those who planned the rehabilitation programs of disabled persons were forced to secure the various services required piece by piece. Evaluation services, therapy, prostheses and vocational training were usually available only in widely scattered locations. This required that rehabilitation be a segmented process rather than a unified, coordinated one. This was costly in funds, in time, in patient morale and in results.

Rehabilitation centers have made their special and unique contribution to the rehabilitation of the severely disabled. The center for the first time provides an effective setting in which the full range of rehabilitation services required for meeting the entire rehabilitation problem of an individual are available to those who direct the rehabilitation of the disabled person. This permits proper timing and coordination of services and has lead to a new and more effective approach to rehabilitation. Not only has it meant that each individual service operates more effectively, but acting in concert with other services and with full knowledge of their contributions and activities, each rehabilitation modality has been able to make an intensified contribution.

One of the most important developments in the rehabilitation center in improving the process of rehabilitation for the individual is its ability to stimulate a much higher, more sustained form of motivation within the patient. For the first time the patient can have the assurance that all his problems are recognized and that a broad common sense approach is being taken to meet them. Also, his own sense of responsibility becomes sharp and clear because of the emphasis on patient activity and on the gains which he can realize from his own purpose and dedication. He is faced daily with a prospect of foreseeable specific improvement provided he invests proper activity and attention on his own part. When the patient is surrounded by skillful persons who understand the rehabilitation process, who realize the importance of patient effort, who do only those things for the patient which he cannot do for himself, a climate is maintained that keeps alive a sustained effort toward rehabilitation.

In the broad program in the rehabilitation center he engages more purposefully in physical rehabilitation activities because at the same time he is given opportunity for vocational training and social activity that gives real purpose to increase in physical functioning. Likewise, the fact that he is getting an improvement in his physical functioning gives him greater belief and assurance that he will have the physical ability to complete his training program satisfactorily and that he will in the end get to a job and achieve independence. The fact that those who work with him—his physician, his therapist, his vocational teacher, his counselor and his recreation director—all believe in him and in his prospects for the future and use their own special way of communicating this faith to him brings forth the level of effort that is lacking in other settings.

Not the least in this special climate of motivation is the influence of the great number of other disabled people who are undertaking rehabilitation at the same time and whose purpose, efforts and accomplishments are a daily and convincing demonstration to the new patient that if he will but have the same faith and make the same effort he can improve his own situation in like manner. Rehabilitation specialists in center setting often point to the fact that patients have been reached and stimulated for the first time to sincere effort only because of the help which comes to them from fellow patients.

While we think of the comprehensive rehabilitation center as being designed primarily with the severely disabled in mind, this does not lessen the effectiveness of such centers for persons who have only moderately severe disability or a single type of disability. The versatility of the rehabilitation center in meeting a broad range of rehabilitation problems—from moderate to severe, from single disability to very complex disability, from the moderate type to the more severe and discouraging forms—has meant the broad utilization of centers in the service of a high percentage of rehabilitation clients.

There is also increasing evidence that there is wisdom in planning centers that are not only comprehensive in service but which accept a broad range of disability problems. Many of the different disability problems have common elements in the need which they present for services. The modern well-planned rehabilitation center program today can make provision for the special needs of various disability types but meet their common needs through a common provision. This permits the development of a broader range of services for all disability problems. Experienced rehabilitation observers today believe that the social growth and development of the disabled person is better accomplished if he is in a more normal society providing opportunity for a normal cross-section of social contact and experience. This situation more nearly approaches the demands and opportunities of living in the society of which he hopes to return.

Rehabilitation Centers Less Expensive

In addition to its demonstration of a special quality and effectiveness of rehabilitation services, the comprehensive center offers promise also of a less expensive approach to the rehabilitation of the disabled. Although the question is open to dispute at present, there are clear indications that a well-planned center program which will keep in mind its proper relation to basic rehabilitation services with feeder hospitals can offer quality rehabilitation services at a much lower per diem cost than can such services be offered in a hospital setting.

There are many reasons for this fact. In the first place, the total emphasis within the hospital and within the rehabilitation center differs. The hospital is geared to meet acute problems of illness and injury, where for the sake of the patient's health and comfort no effort can be spared in the way of medical supervision, nursing care and the various other specialized hospital services to see that the patient survives and gets well. In the hospital, nursing care is directed toward meeting the patient's special needs while he is seriously ill or seriously injured, in a state of shock, and when the demands for the services of others are heavy. In this setting the nurse bathes the patient, aids him in self-care, brings him food and provides a large number of "care" services which the patient today qualifies as "good nursing."

In the rehabilitation center, however, the emphasis on nursing services is to provide only the minimum of care which the patient must have for health and comfort. Instead, the nurse is part of the team which constantly encourages the patient to do all he can for himself, even though it takes a long period of time—to walk, to bathe himself, to feed himself, to clothe himself, to shave and to attend meals as early as possible outside his room. Rehabilitation nurses constantly challenge patients to transfer their dependence for self-care and activity from the nurse to themselves.

Likewise, in the hospital the therapist is, more often than not, operating on a one-to-one ratio with the patient, seeing him at the bedside or in a special treatment room. In the rehabilitation center, however, procedures and methods have been developed which permit grouping of patients so that patients teach each other many of the skills of physical reconditioning and where the therapist can spread her skills and supervision over a large number of people.

In the typical hospital, the ratio of staff to patients may be as high as three, or four, to one. The emphasis on maximum self-care and independence on the part of each patient and less emphasis upon care by staff in the rehabilitation center makes it possible to revise this ratio without seriously affecting rehabilitation progress or potentiality for the individual patient.

Another important form of saving in the rehabilitation center is found in the less expensive physical facilities that are required. The use of multiple bed wards, the use of common toilet facilities and the use of central food service establishments where self-service is emphasized makes possible a reduction in the cost of providing facilities on the individual patient cost basis. These accommodations are designed to encourage the patients in the center to have social contacts with others and to overcome the tendency of many to withdraw to themselves. There is no evidence that rehabilitation activities are any more effective in settings in which elaborate buildings and equipment are used than in those in which modest facilities are provided.

Rehabilitation Facilities and the State-Federal Program

The state-federal program of vocational rehabilitation, now in its fiftieth year, has changed very radically in its five decades of development. Today, the rehabilitation administrator who takes a realistic view of his job and of his agency's responsibility is keenly aware of the indispensable role of rehabilitation facilities in serving the agency's clients. We may say with considerable truth that the effectiveness of state agency services is directly and inseparably related to the level of development and use of rehabilitation facilities. Those who have promoted this development of needed facilities are finding it possible to serve persons with greater and greater severity of disability. Those who have not done so must operate on a limited basis which brings into serious challenge the ultimate value of their services to the community.

As we develop more knowledge of the meaning and significance of disability problems and how they can be treated, and more understanding of the rehabilitation process itself, we have come to place increasingly greater dependence upon the special capabilities of the rehabilitation center for accomplishing some of our more demanding rehabilitation tasks. There is a very definite limit, for example, to the extent and effectiveness of the rehabilitation evaluation process when it is limited to that which even a well-trained rehabilitation counselor working alone can accomplish. Far too often the counselor is still faced with the necessity of carrying out the diagnosis and making the decision as to whether or not the person can be served largely on the strength of his own judgment, experience and courage. This is too great a responsibility for the resources of a single individual. The rehabilitation center, however, has been able to develop and offer to the counselor, a laboratory-type of rehabilitation evaluation which not only has the advantage of the employment of a wide variety of professional skills but which also makes it possible to extend the period of evaluation over a sufficient length of time that the disabled person needs and potentialities can be seen far more clearly. In this setting the client is given an appraisal of physical functioning by physicians and therapists who have specialized knowledge of such examinations and who use instruments and techniques of evaluation not available to the counselor in his own setting. Vocational exploration involving a far greater and more effective range of formal testing, job tryouts, trial training and an exposure to a wide variety of testing situations is possible within the special evaluative facilities of the center. In the center it is possible to bring together information regarding the total observation of the client as seen by many persons in many experience situations. A face-to-face discussion of these facts by the members of the evaluation team permits a weighing of those facts that inevitably lead to a clear understanding and more valid diagnosis.

The various forms of rehabilitation therapy that can be assembled and offered in the rehabilitation center has made it possible for agency clients to achieve a far greater degree of restoration. This professional service opens new possibilities for employment and adjustment to life. With the severely disabled it has been found that the small margin of improvement which can be accomplished in the rehabilitation center is often the difference between success or failure in getting that client into a selected job situation.

Although further studies are needed to substantiate this belief, many rehabilitation workers feel that the graduates of the rehabilitation centers who are prepared for jobs, enter living with a higher purpose, have more thoroughly developed physical and functional skills, have a better understanding of their disability, gained through a more intensive program of reeducation, retain their rehabilitation gains longer and make a contribution over a longer period of time as working producing members of society.

Providing vocational training required by the severely disabled clients has posed serious problems to the rehabilitation agency. Persons with moderate disabilities may often attend community training facilities used by the nondisabled with complete satisfaction. However, when there is a strong problem of motivation to undergo retraining, when the training itself must be geared to the special needs of the disabled person—either in timing, intensity, methodology or even in goals—it is found that special training classes and services are required. In the rehabilitation center setting it has been found possible not only to offer high quality vocational training in a great variety of skilled technical fields but that many less demanding forms of training more suitable to the needs of persons with limited intellectual, physical or educational levels can be designed. The needs of these latter can be met without expense to the former.

Rehabilitation agencies through the years have seen a substantial number of their rehabilitation clients fail in employment and in meeting the demands of living because of a lack of personal and social adaptability required to meet the demands of living on the job or in the community. In the traditional approach to training and treatment of rehabilitation clients little can be done specifically to meet this need for social and personality growth and adjustment. The rehabilitation process often served to make the client even more withdrawn and maladjusted. When he was placed in a training school he was often sent to live in the new surroundings of an impersonal boarding home where no one took the trouble to see that he did not shut himself away in his room. In the rehabilitation center, however, recognition can be given to the need for growth of the individual in sound personality development and in the matter of social skills and participation. Skilled directors of social activities and recreation make their unique contribution to the rehabilitation process so that many of our clients demonstrate an amazing development of social skills, social participation and social responsibility.

The rehabilitation center has other major values to the state agency as well. Although the average citizen has some vague idea as to what rehabilitation is, it has no real meaning to him until he can actually see it in operation, see its results and see the reaction of the disabled person who is undergoing rehabilitation. The rehabilitation center has made it possible to give real meaning to the process of rehabilitation, its possibilities and its results to both professional and lay individuals who can be brought into contact with the center program. The rehabilitation center has been called "the showcase of rehabilitation." The center is a concrete symbol of the state agency's services, a means of identification that becomes strong and clear in the minds of the community and of the state.

Development and Operation of Rehabilitation Facilities

It is a sign of the growing sophistication within the rehabilitation movement that more and more attention is being given to the development of special facilities for rehabilitation. At this stage, however, we have done little more than provide a good demonstration of the value which rehabilitation facilities have to a total rehabilitation program. If every rehabilitation bed were filled today, only a fraction of those persons needing such services could be accommodated. Therefore, as we discuss the development of rehabilitation facilities in connection with a full adequate rehabilitation program, we must envision a tremendous development of this particular resource.

Today we have only a few rehabilitation centers in the country that can qualify as broad comprehensive centers. The remainder of our institutions are those which offer either a single service or the more common services applying to a limited number of disability problems.

To what extent should we promote the development of rehabilitation facilities in the coming years? Vocational schools that serve the nondisabled should accept the disabled student without prejudice when the disabled person is able to use such facilities without difficulty. Those rehabilitation clients who can be handled satisfactorily in the modern community hospital should not be sent away from their home communities to special facilities. The very greatest stimulation should be given toward developing adequate training and treatment and diagnostic services for the whole population within each community.

Each modern community hospital must provide the full values of physical medicine and rehabilitation for its patients. Each institution caring for the chronically ill should have a strong rehabilitation unit which can accomplish maximum restoration of its patients. However, we must recognize that there are hundreds of thousands of potential rehabilitation clients who cannot be accommodated satisfactorily in the public and private vocational school, nor who can be diagnosed and treated adequately in the well-equipped and well-staffed community clinic or hospital. If we are not to leave these persons in their homes or in other permanent care institutions, then we must set out boldly to develop sufficient resources in the form of well-planned rehabilitation facilities that will augment the resources found in the average community and make rehabilitation a reality for even the complicated difficult case.

It becomes increasingly clear that there is tremendous advantage in locating the rehabilitation facility which gives concern principally to medical and restorative rehabilitation within the large general hospital or medical center. This is the natural and logical place for such a center in that it enjoys the full support of related services of the hospital, ensures adequate medical provision (which is one of the big problems of the small separate center), and it will share in the overall financial planning that goes into the operation of a hospital or medical center. Likewise, such a center being a part of the hospital, under a common administration, will enjoy a steady flow of clients who move from hospital beds to rehabilitation beds.

In the matter of comprehensive vocationally oriented rehabilitation centers the increasing weight of thinking today is that these should be away from hospital settings, that they should be of sufficient size to justify a broad program of services and that they should accept many disability types. It is also believed that these centers should increasingly become the responsibility of the public rehabilitation program. This will not mean that these facilities are exclusively for agency clients. They should serve the broader community. But, both to ensure financial support and to maintain a broad-balanced program of services, these centers should be identified with the public rehabilitation program.

In between the large comprehensive free-standing rehabilitation center and the hospital-based mentally-oriented rehabilitation center, there is need for a wide variety of smaller facilities usually for outpatients living in a more restricted community area. These may be in the form of therapeutic workshops, facilities for the diagnosis and treatment of special disabilities, such as speech and hearing, or any other specialized type of facility for which the community has great need and for which it has demonstrated its willingness to support. The same facility should be used by the major government agencies for their clients living in that locality, to the extent that they meet the needs of these clients and to the extent that those who operate the facilities will provide the services in kind and for a rate that state agencies can accept.

When rehabilitation leaders are considering the establishment of new rehabilitation facilities in a community, there are several important questions that must be answered: Is there a need for new services which this facility will offer, or is the community amply supplied with such services? What will be the relationship of the new facility to existing rehabilitation facilities or to other treatment resources such as hospitals, clinics, training schools, etcetera? What problems of disability and in what number is this new facility expected to serve? Who is the logical sponsor for the development and operation of the center? How can the development and operation of the center be financed? Will it be possible to secure the necessary professional staff to permit the center to operate in a satisfactory manner?

Thus it can be seen that the establishment of a center or a rehabilitation facility involves, in the first place, an intensive exercise in community planning, analyzing the community's needs, its resources and the special needs of disabled people that may be met in this manner. Taken into account also must be the resources and relationships of community agencies—both public and private—and the professional membership in the community that has an interest in the rehabilitation field. Generally, rehabilitation center planning should involve a broad cross-section of professional, public and lay representation so that when the decision is taken it will be a community decision and in effect involve a commitment for community use and support.

Being in most instances the sole agency devoting its resources and services exclusively in the field of rehabilitation, the state vocational rehabilitation agency, through its district and local representatives, assisted by its advisory committees and special consultants from the state office, offers a ready and effective resource for organizing and leading community planning efforts for rehabilitation facilities. No agency has a greater stake in the outcomes of rehabilitation center development than does the state agency, nor is any other group more knowledgeable about rehabilitation needs and possibilities. It is natural for voluntary workers who give only a portion of their time to this area of service to turn to the full-time trained rehabilitation worker to carry the major share of the burden of study, analysis, leadership, planning and eventual decision-making. Where the leadership role in center planning and development resides in a community group or in representatives of other agencies, the representative of the state agency should make his interest and services felt as positively as possible. Through working with his known case load he is in an excellent position to interpret and even dramatize the needs of the disabled person. He can bring realism into the understanding of other persons regarding the rehabilitation process, the organization of rehabilitation services, how these services can be financed, and the general resources to which they can turn for technical and professional assistance in bringing the new project into final shape. It would be a great mistake for the state agency not to exercise maximum influence in each community in this direction. The administration of the state agency must recognize its broad responsibility extending through all levels of personnel for such participation; it should see that its professional staff from the counselor to the highest level professional in the central office is thoroughly acquainted with rehabilitation center services and problems and organizational patterns, so that each recognizes the promotional and technical services in the development of a center as being one of his important professional responsibilities and that he is not only encouraged but directed to make available such time as is needed to give proper service to community effort in the development of facilities.

The financing of the establishment of rehabilitation centers has followed a great variety of patterns. Centers which are a part of a general hospital or medical center have been financed through the same source of funds as build the hospitals—Federal funds, state and local funds, and funds contributed by the community. Other centers have received substantial help through state-federal vocational rehabilitation funds. Many communities, through direct solicitation campaigns and through appropriations by local governing bodies, have aided in financing new centers. Many private agencies have devoted a major portion of their annual budgets to the establishment of facilities. This range of sponsorship and financial participation has resulted in a very unplanned and haphazard approach to the development of centers and facilities. Often too little care is taken to determine the type of center needed, the size of the facility and how its operation is to be financed. Centers with very narrow services, with expensive services, and whose operation is identified with a particular group makes successful operation very difficult. It would appear that there is great need now, and for the future, for more substantial government aid through both state-federal and local participation, in the planning and development of rehabilitation centers. Along with the acceptance of this public responsibility would come additional guarantees for sound planning, sound design and sound proposals for operation. Higher standards of service and a broader provision of service could be assured through the adoption of standards by state and federal authorities which must be observed in the establishment of such facilities. Only when government agencies recognize their responsibility for providing the facility to meet major human needs that are widespread in every community, as has been the case in the fields of health and education, can we expect rehabilitation programs and rehabilitation facilities to support such programs to develop in the sound substantial manner that the problem of disability would require.

The old experience in securing financial support for the construction of an institution or facility is well illustrated in the history of rehabilitation center development in that it has been proven far easier to finance the construction of centers than to finance their operation. It is possible through sustained intensive effort to develop a generous response by the community and the government agencies to bring into existence a new facility that is shown to be vital to the welfare of the community. Often, however, too little thought is given to the annual continuing expense involved in the operation of such facilities. The requirements for operation are often only vaguely understood by those who are promoting the center, or else in a naive faith they play down to the public the size of the responsibility that is being created through the establishment of a center. Even the small number of centers which we have in the various states today are already experiencing serious problems in financing a minimum level of operations. In fact, many centers that are badly needed have been forced to close their doors after two or three years of deficit operation. Others are operating at only a partial capacity level and having a severe financial struggle that takes the efforts of its sponsors to keep its doors open. Far too often to make ends meet the center curtails its services and thus discounts its real opportunity for broad service. This would indicate that major thought and planning must be given to the matter of financing the operation of rehabilitation facilities.

The principal considerations in the operation of rehabilitation facilities in regard to the meeting of the continuing problem of financing are the following: The size of the center seems to be a major consideration; a center of small capacity cannot offer quality services except at high unit cost; the small center which attempts to handle inpatients puts an additional strain on its financial resources. Far too often there is too little attention given to cost control. Very often those who operate centers are overly influenced by staffing and cost experiences of hospitals and make the mistake of imposing hospital standards and procedures in the rehabilitation center operations. Also, in many instances, centers have gone their own merry way insensitive to the needs and desires of those who would purchase services from them and who would thus contribute to the support of the center's operation. There seems to have been an unexplained attitude and philosophy that users of rehabilitation centers should take them as they find them, not raise too much question either about the cost of services or the kinds of services, even the matter of communication, information and cultivation of understanding has been in a very unplanned haphazard situation. Consequently, the center drops more and more out of the thoughts and plans of those who are working with the disabled, and its sources of support dry up. This is a tragic situation since in that same community there are hundreds of people who need center services and since this failure is likely to offer a setback lasting over many years in the development of a strong rehabilitation resource for the community.

Significantly, it has been the state agency developed and operated center that has had the greatest stability in maintenance of a broad program and in financing center operations. This is not difficult to understand when one looks carefully at the situation. The state agency has a direct and continuing interest in rehabilitation center services for its clients. It has a steady and increasing flow of clients. This flow being constantly heavier in terms of those who will require rehabilitation center services as it develops this aspect of the program. The rehabilitation agency is able to include in its appropriations request provision for financing rehabilitation center services just as it does for all the other types of rehabilitation services which it provides its clients. In its annual budget it is able to set aside an amount sufficient to finance a given number of clients in rehabilitation center programs.

It is suspected that voluntary and other community sponsors

have gotten into the picture in a majority of cases because of the unwillingness or reluctance of the state agency to become the sponsor of the rehabilitation facility program. It is strongly suspected that the voluntary agencies within the community and the other government agencies having some rehabilitation responsibility would welcome the opportunity to rally behind the state agency to develop a type of center and to give it stability that would give promise of permanence and at the same time which would make readily available to the special agencies and organizations the rehabilitation services that they would need to meet the particular needs of their clientele.

Mobility and Self-Care

A new priority in rehabilitation is emerging—that of reestablishing and maintaining mobility and self-care for the severely handicapped. This has special appreciation to the aged disabled.

Self-care rehabilitation was aggressively promoted in the early 1960's by the National Rehabilitation Association. It was not incorporated into the public rehabilitation program, as its sponsors advocated; probably "its time had not arrived." The idea, however, is undergoing a major revival.

Through new programs such as Medicare and Medicaid, the chronically ill and disabled are receiving a great deal of attention. Huge sums are being spent in long-term care that often leads to little else than permanent dependency. In fact we are facing the prospect of developing a new form of institutional care for such persons that has many of the same grim features as the old insane asylums of another century.

The chronically ill and disabled suffer a dual loss under such arrangements; they decline in functional ability and live under a growing feeling of isolation, abandonment and hopelessness. Costs are usually high, consuming the individual's or family's resources at a too rapid rate.

A large number of such persons can have mobility restored and can return to their own homes with assurance of being able to resume the familiar role in the community. The feasibility of such an approach has been fully demonstrated in thousands of cases. Rehabilitation hospitals emphasizing restoration of self-care abilities and return to family living such as those operated in Maryland by the state health agency have achieved impressive success.

Rehabilitation will have become fully mature as service area only when it moves to embrace all those needing rehabilitation services and can adjust to limited goals. Self-care rehabilitation embodies fully the social and economic values which have characterized rehabilitation through the years.

Rehabilitation as a Right

In view of the great concentration on "rights"—civil rights, rights to income, rights to health and medical care and so forth—it is amazing that so little stress has been placed upon "right to rehabilitation" for the disabled. From any point of view—social, economic, humanitarian, political—such a position is supportable.

The public often expresses its outrage at the growth burden of dependency, often including persons with current or potential ability for work and self-support.

As Dr. Ray L. Smith, former editor of the *Christian Advocate*, once said, "It is mockery to give a man a sermon when he needs bread." Similarly it is a mockery to criticize the handicapped for not working but to deny such persons the means through which they can prepare for and enter employment.

A serious question of public ethics is raised when services provided at public expense are provided a fortunate few of the disabled but some of the disabled who want services are turned away.

Quality education at public expense is now the rights and heritage of every American child. No school age child is turned away when schools open.

This is far from being the case in the opportunity for rehabilitation that exists for the disabled today. It is estimated that no more than one of three persons newly disabled can be served through the existing limited system. Thus we accumulate more backlog of unserved persons day by day.

We are on the brink of a new commitment of added billions of dollars for an "income floor" for the poor. Hundreds of poor are dependent because of disability—a condition for which rehabilitation is indicated but is not available. Surely the soundness of paralleling increased income maintenance support with added dollars to reestablish self-support through rehabilitation measures is not open to debate.

It is encouraging that there is a rising chorus of voices advocating that rehabilitation become a right and a reality for all disabled Americans as quickly as possible.

Rehabilitation and the Behaviorally Disabled

One of our most challenging new areas of rehabilitation is with the behaviorally disabled. Incorporated into national rehabilitation statutes in the 1965 Amendments, a modest beginning has been made in creating appropriate services for this group, usually under cooperative arrangements involving rehabilitation agencies and state or local correctional agencies.

Social maladjustment characterized by antisocial behavior does not fit the traditional concept of "disability." Generally all physical systems function normally. The "impairment" is persistent social dysfunction, whereby the individual demonstrates inability to develop wholesome relationships and to behave harmoniously with the usual rules of society. Although somewhat abstract in concept, it nevertheless produces symptoms that are as real and concrete as the more classical handicaps.

New modalities of rehabilitation must be designed and applied. New professional skills and insights are required. Research and experimentation in this field is sorely needed.

The problem is a massive one in which there is widespread interest today. All community institutions have a potential role in this developing area of rehabilitation. Thus far our principal efforts have been confined to institutional settings working with the confirmed case. Community-based programs that will combine the related goals of prevention and rehabilitation are critically needed.

Rehabilitation and the Addictive Disabilities

The disability resulting from alcoholism is quite familiar in medical and rehabilitation circles. Disability resulting from drug addiction is a relatively new phenomonen.

Rehabilitation efforts for the alcoholic have met with indifferent success, often frustration. Good programs do exist, however, with a sound methodology having evolved. Public rehabilitation programs have had only a limited involvement in such service efforts.

The dramatic growth in the use of hard drugs, particularly among the young, has produced its toll in deviant behavior, impairment and even death. As a people we stand thus far practically powerless to halt the use of drugs or to combat with success its permanent side effects.

Rehabilitation has an obligation to join with all those who are concerned with any aspect of the problem to develop the technique and resources required to rehabilitate the victims. Today parents and victims alike, through a sense of shame, prefer to remain as anonymous as possible. Activation of a treatment and rehabilitation program in the community, with high visibility which enlists the participation of parents and concerned citizens, will fill an important gap that now exists in the fight against drug abuse.

Rehabilitation and the Socially and Culturally Handicapped

In the human services field the most important development during the past decade has to be the fact that "poverty" has been rediscovered, exposed and dramatized to the shock of millions of Americans who somehow had managed to keep themselves insulated against this problem. Or if poverty was known to exist, it produced among the affluent such reactions as "the poor can only blame themselves," "in this country any person worth his salt can get a job" or "I've done my part—my taxes pay for those high welfare payments to the idle."

Americans at all levels—public, private, business; government and church officials, youth and just plain citizens—have become increasingly knowledgeable and sensitive to the plight of the poverty stricken. From a position of virtual neglect, "poor people" have become our priority targets for assistance.

The concrete help already given is impressive including such things as:

- Enactment of the Medicaid Program (Title XIX of the Social Security Act) giving the poor access to community medical services.
- Expanded work and training assistance to the poor, such as work incentive programs, under the auspices of the Department of Labor.
- Training and employment programs for the hard-core poor by major American corporations.
- Minimum social security payments have been more than doubled.
- Major federal subsidies to public education seek to improve education services to disadvantaged children.
- Creation of the Office of Economic Opportunity and hundreds of local antipoverty organizations to foster innovative community action on behalf of the poor.
- Consumer education and consumer protection programs.
- Increased emphasis on family planning services, making them available to all poor families who need them.
- Decentralization of service programs to new locations directly in poor communities.
- Expansion of nutrition programs such as school lunches, food stamps and surplus food programs.
- Organization of day-care services to permit mothers in poor families to receive job training and employment.

Despite this substantial effort, however, the number of hardcore poor and disadvantaged does not diminish. In fact at the present time when the country is undergoing such rapid change the number is increasing. Many of those who have been trained or otherwise treated have either remained in or reverted to dependency.

Why have these efforts been so ineffectual?

The problems of the culturally deprived handicapped are very complex. Generally there are combinations of low education, uncertain health and poor work history. There may be actual handicapping physical disability resulting from untreated disease or injury. There generally is a sense of social inadequacy that leaves the individual unable to cope with the mechanics of seeking help. Above all there are firmly established attitudes of failure, lack of worth, hostility and apathy growing out of years of poverty-level living and neglect.

The plight of the poor is dramatically presented in the following quotation from Michael Harrington's book, *The Other America:*

> In a sense, one might define the contemporary poor in the United States as those who, for reasons beyond their control, cannot help themselves. All the most decisive factors making for opportunity and advance are against them. They are born going downward, and most of them stay down. They are victims whose lives are endlessly blown round and round the other America.
>
> Here is one of the most familiar forms of the vicious circle of poverty. The poor get sick more than anyone else in the society. That is because they live in slums, jammed together under unhygienic conditions; they have inadequate diets, and cannot get decent medical care. When they become sick, they are sick longer than any other group in the society. Because they are sick more often and longer than anyone else, they lose wages and work, and find it difficult to hold a steady job. And because of this, they cannot pay for good housing, for a nutritious diet, for doctors. At any given point in the circle, particularly when there is a major illness, their prospect is to move to an even lower level and to begin the cycle, round and round, toward even more suffering.
>
> The individual cannot usually break out of this vicious circle. Neither can the group, for it lacks the social energy and political strength to turn its misery into a cause. Only the larger society, with its help and resources, can really make it possible for these people to help themselves. Yet those who could make the difference too often refuse to act because of their ignorant, smug moralism. They view the effects of poverty—above all, the warping of the will and spirit that is a consequence of being poor—as choices. Understanding the vicious circle is an important step in breaking down this prejudice.

To attempt to treat these individuals through the same processes, methods and settings as other disabled simply leads to failure. Certainly to gather them up in mass classes or groups without individual study, diagnosis and treatment has ended in failure.

They represent a true challenge to the use of the "rehabilitation" process—one which is designed around the peculiar needs of the deprived individual. Slow, patient effort is needed introducing as early as possible activities such as remedial education, health services and sheltered work. A key factor is use of some form of incentive wage so that very early the client begins to experience a sense of worth. In addition he may need considerable help in the beginning to solve such problems as clothing, transportation and family subsistence.

Many professionally trained middle-class rehabilitation workers find themselves powerless to achieve a positive response from these disadvantaged clients. The gulf separating them is too large —a fact often not appreciated by the worker. It has been demonstrated very conclusively that indigenous workers add substantially to the effectiveness of the rehabilitation team.

Furthermore the process cannot be hurried. The effects of a lifetime of privation cannot be erased in a six months' "quickie" rehabilitation plan.

New Models Needed

It is a serious mistake to believe that these new candidates for rehabilitation—the addict, the behaviorally disabled, the socially and culturally handicapped—can be rehabilitated using traditional methods and resources. They need their own models, developed and refined by experimentation and research.

It will require heavy emphasis on community-based programs in which the various resources of the community are brought to bear. Citizen help must be enlisted as must that of business, industry and the professions.

A special priority among these groups should be handicapped young persons. The outlook for many older dependent persons is bleak, regardless of the effort put forth, because time and neglect have done their work. With the young the outlook is different. "Hope springs eternal" is not just a poetic myth. New goals can be readily established and their spirit reawakened when faced with real opportunity for meaningful satisfying opportunity. Thus the school dropout, the poor achiever, the youthful offender and the youthful members of a poverty stricken home must become special targets for community action. The application of rehabilitation measures is surely the most promising course with this group.

DEVELOPING TRENDS AND REHABILITATION PRACTICE

While it is unlikely and even inadvisable to restrict publicly supported rehabilitation services to the economically disadvantaged, this group will for the next decade represent our top priority. The Federal Rehabilitation Agency only recently declared a policy naming disabled welfare recipients as its number one target group.

Disability and dependency go hand in hand. Vocational rehabilitation has been called the "original anti-poverty program."

Undoubtedly we are now embarked on an effort to provide rehabilitation services to massive numbers of new clients which compound the scope of present efforts. Actually, this emphasis on expansion is merely giving practical expression to the national mandate to bring rehabilitation services up to the level of sufficiency for all who need them. While this is a gigantic task, what other goal can a public service in a democracy adopt?

Need to Expand Rehabilitation Resources

This surely means better use of our present resources both public and private, using all methods of coordination and mutual reinforcements to move us more effectively toward our mutual goals. Undoubtedly, there is room for vast improvement in this respect.

But no one with any acquaintance in this field could argue that our problem will be solved purely through more efficient use of existing resources. There must follow a vast expansion of rehabilitation facilities of all types, a majority of them oriented to community needs, to accommodate the growing volume of candi-

Developing Trends in Rehabilitation

dates for service. The progressive state rehabilitation administrator of today has long since committed himself to a major investment in the creation of a network of facilities, workshops and other service resources to give counselors ready access to the services which they need for their clients. Such an administrator recently remarked, "The day that we would depend on an itinerant counselor traveling over an extensive district doing rehabilitation out of a briefcase is over."

In addition to the traditional types of facilities, there will be growing pressure for the creation of facilities and service resources designed specifically for the newer categories of disability —the alcoholic, the drug addict, the youthful offender and the confirmed welfare recipient.

Special Outreach Efforts

New legislation expanding coverage in welfare and social security will carry requirements for mandatory referral of the disabled and disadvantaged for rehabilitation and manpower services. Such referral systems could result in a massive flow of paper work with relatively little response on the part of the individuals concerned.

New outreach methods must be utilized to bring the potential clients from the ghettos or from rural poverty settings into the rehabilitation service system. Two new methods of promise are under development to solve this problem. Service offices are being located in poverty sections making it easy for clients to reach them. Outreach workers are being employed whose principal role is that of finding the persons who are in need of service and facilitating their contact with the service agency. The requirements for effective teamwork between such workers and trained professionals are obvious.

Unified Services Approach

Former HEW Secretary Gardner stated, ". . . we find that usually the trouble an individual or family is in is a combination of several related problems requiring a combination of approaches. These approaches, different though they may be, are all concentrated in that one person or one family. We must encourage a unified approach to the problems of all these groups. Each of its parts can draw on the strengths of the others and can be mutually reinforcing."

The trend is mounting to insure concerted planning and action in behalf of dependents, disabled persons through unification of effort on the part of health, welfare, rehabilitation and employment agencies. Workers in these agencies must learn to work with their counterparts in a team relationship. There must be flexibility and understanding on the part of workers which will put clients' need above agency vested interests.

As rehabilitation grows in prominence in our national effort to combat povetry and dependence, rehabilitation workers must bear heavy responsibility as the "spearhead" of the new movement. It must share generously its own knowledge, methods and resources with its new partners.

Significance for Rehabilitation Counseling

As we chart expanded goals and new plans, the problem of manpower looms as our most serious hurdle. Each new program or facility places its demand on our already inadequate manpower supply. Literally thousands of new workers will need to be recruited, and trained, and many of those already employed must be provided extensive reorientation, new knowledge and new skills.

Thus we can expect to see the emergence of manpower planning and programs aimed at recruitment, training and utilization of personnel to meet our expanding needs.

Rehabilitation counseling is central in this picture, having the potential of making one of the most significant contributions to the solution of this gigantic problem.

The pressures of an expanding national effort in rehabilitation, the higher expectations placed by the public on rehabilitation agencies for improved performance, and the added stress on rehabilitation for the severely disabled and unconventionally handicapped have created a number of issues affecting the future of rehabilitation counseling as a unique "helping" profession:

1. The product of the typical two-year graduate counselor training program does not perform up to expectations. This raises serious question as to the content, nature and method of training used.

2. There is a widespread feeling that counselor trainers express unfavorable judgments to students about the desirability of vocational rehabilitation agency employment and the lack of job satisfaction that is likely to be experienced in working in this setting.

3. There is a feeling by many that training is too sheltered—too academic—leaving students with little preparation to face the realities of working with real clients in real communities. One student expressed his reaction by saying that he was "petrified" when faced with his first real tasks.

4. There is lack of communication and understanding between agency officials and educators. Each uses a language that is not fully enlightening to the other. The student is caught in the middle. Other than formal conferences, there are few shared experiences between the agency representatives and the university instructors. Yet, they do have common goals.

5. Agencies have been unresponsive to needs of the university in creating quality training resources in work settings. The educator often can only see his student exposed to poor practice and poor instruction.

6. Agencies often have so little to offer in the way of continued training that students and instructors take a dim view of opportunities for continued growth and advancement in the agency setting.

7. Counselor trainees have little exposure to poverty and the poverty stricken. They both reject and are rejected when they face the necessity of working in the slums. Training does not seem to get at the barrier of middle-class value systems that characterize both student and staff in universities. This is especially serious in view of the fact that the greatest concentration of the disabled is in the group most culturally and economically disadvantaged.

8. Agencies and universities often have not found means

through which the resources of the universities are fully utilized in continuous staff development efforts. This has voided one strong possibility for achieving "togetherness."

9. A major issue lies in the conflict of views on long-term versus short-term training. Can any real training result from concentrated short courses? Are two-year degree programs really necessary?

10. How will the baccalaureate degree holder be received in counseling ranks? What about basic training in rehabilitation at the undergraduate level? What effect do offensive titles (as "subprofessionals") have on the motivation of promising young graduates entering the rehabilitation field? If, as many believe, we can *never* meet our staffing needs through unrealistically high academic standards for training for service professions, how do we bring about the formation of practical, constructive training and personnel policies in regard to utilization of baccalaureate degree holders?

11. Finally, there is the issue relating to counseling, itself, and its efficacy in solving problems of human needs. "Counseling" has been so idealized and romanticized, so covered with mystique and professional ritualism that it, like casework, is threatened with broad-scale rejection in service settings. We do not seem to face the fact that counseling is an element in a great variety of settings and relationships and is not the exclusive prerogative of any ordained group. Is one-to-one counseling a methodology which no longer meets the test of practicality? Will the counselor of the future be a facilitator and coordinator of services in the community becoming more of an intermediary between the disabled and the source of service needed than a primary therapist?

PART TWO

THE REHABILITATION PRACTITIONER

The Challenge of New Dimensions in Rehabilitation Counselor Education in the Seventies

The Professional Status of the Rehabilitation Counselor

5

The Challenge of New Dimensions in Rehabilitation Counselor Education in the Seventies

Beatrix Cobb

Review of the Controversial Roles and Functions of the Rehabilitation Counselor
Developments During the Sixties
History of the Movement of Rehabilitation Counseling toward Professionalism
New Dimensions of the Challenge for the Seventies
References

IN THIS golden year of the fiftieth anniversary of vocational rehabilitation,[30] there comes a clarion call for the consideration of new dimensions in the education of rehabilitation counselors. This appeal is based upon current social and political developments in our nation and research relative to the controversy over roles and functions of the rehabilitation counselor. The call concedes that the rehabilitation counselor has been a key figure in the delivery of the lauded rehabilitation services during the last fifteen of the fifty years that have witnessed the "acceptance of, growth in, and public mandates for" those services. The research describes this dedicated counselor as leading the vanguard of expansion (as a representation of his agency) into an ever-increasing array of new fields of need. Until, by the end of the sixties, he has carried the banner of rehabilitation, with purpose, dignity and effectiveness, into mental hospitals, welfare offices, public schools, drug abuse clinics, alcoholic units and socially disadvantaged areas and to the aged.

Certainly, the call for reevaluation must not be construed as a criticism of the counselor and his services through the decade. Rather, it congratulates him on a job well done in meeting the challenge of the sixties in the expansion of rehabilitation services to include persons and groups in need, never before served by rehabilitation. Thoughtful leaders in the field do, however, highlight a definite and urgent need for reevaluation of roles and training of the rehabilitation counselor in view of the counselor's experience in that decade and the proliferation of types of services now required of him.

In his keynote address to the 1968 National Rehabilitation Association Conference, Russell Nixon[16] stated this challenge succinctly:

> It now becomes necessary to go beyond attention to 'individual pathology and personal failure' or handicap into consideration of social and political factors [p. 17].

In 1969, Dan McAlees,[11] president of the National Rehabilitation Counseling Association, warned:

> As a result of the wide-spread and critical scrutiny to which professional education has been subjected during the last decade, some of the most strongly held beliefs about length and content of the course of study have been shaken, and on all sides curricular manipulation and program changes are evident. The time has come for an equally critical look at rehabilitation counselor education and preparation. . . .
>
> Rehabilitation counseling as a profession is rapidly approaching a critical period . . . it is mandatory that we reassess our present practices in professional education, staff development, and manpower utilization . . . [p. 22].

Sussman, Haug and Joynes[25] insist that if the rehabilitation counselor is to maintain his leadership role in the seventies, he must be prepared not only in counseling but also in "several new dimensions." Included in these new dimensions they would place in addition to counseling:

1. Knowledge of sociological theories of organizations and institutions, and the skills of creating linkages among them to benefit the client.

2. Ability to counsel agencies and institutions as well as in-

The Challenge of New Dimensions in Rehabilitation 125

dividuals. This area could involve skills of working in the ghettos, model cities, rural poverty areas, programs in family planning and so forth.

3. Information relative to the role of client advocate. This body of instruction would be concerned with the development of ability to "fend-off, fight, organize and manipulate dimensions of his (the client's) existence beyond their dyadic relationship."[25]

Further, they point out:

> Even if the counselor with traditional credentials would prove to be the superior practitioner in the counseling function, he still must face certain hard realities about the demands placed upon him. He must realize that service delivery in rehabilitation does *not* rest in expertise in the counseling process *alone* [p. 9].*

These challenges bring into focus the philosophy and content of our present training programs in graduate education for the rehabilitation counselor. As in the case of the counselor *per se*, this challenge is not a vicious criticism of the efforts and results of the educational programs serving the field since 1956. It is meant as a timely reminder that to rest in comfortable ruts of the best we had to offer in the sixties may not meet the educational and professional challenges of the progressive seventies. It is also an urgent plea that educators join counselors in taking a close look at the evolving functions of that profession as well as at the philosophy, content and directions of counselor preparation in the coming decade.

McAlees[11] also cautions the rehabilitation agencies that if they are to remain the "prime agencies" responsible for the rehabilitation of handicapped people "they must be involved in the identification of knowledge and skills which professional personnel must have that other counselors, or workers, do not require." To date, McAlees posits that the creation and current concepts of the role of the rehabilitation counselor have been necessarily formed by "applications of laws, regulations, administrative procedures, and fiscal policies, as opposed to some base in a systematic applied science."

Again this admonition is not reported critically. It is agreed

---

*Italicizing for emphasis by Cobb.

that rehabilitation administrators have performed an almost impossible feat over the past ten years in providing excellent and more and more services to more and more numbers and categories of clients with a shortage of personnel at any level, let alone professionally trained counselors. The situation does partially explain the mutual frustrations experienced by administrators and counselor educators over those years; because graduate programs have, perforce, been set up from a more professional (as opposed to pragmatic) perspective than the administrators could, by necessity, operate their agencies.

Moriarty,[12] at that time director of the Ohio Bureau of Vocational Rehabilitation, gave an insightful and tantalizing analysis of the baffling divergence of opinion between counselor educators and agency administrators as he visualized it:

> ... one still gets, by expression or implication, the feeling that some coordinators see state program administrators as essentially non-professional short-cut artists, giving only lip-service to the importance of research and training, and comfortably ensconced in soft warm cocoons ingeniously built of a monumental supply of paper from old R-9 closures, flow sheets, master lists, annual reports, and minutes of committee meetings. ... One also gets the feeling that some state program directors see university coordinators as long-term lessors of ivory towers, allergic to contact with economic, social and political reality, who see rehabilitation counseling not as a means to an end (the rehabilitation of a handicapped person) but always as a highly intellectual, usually sedentary, application of theory in a controlled clinical setting, the primary purpose of which is gratification of the professional ego of the counselor through discovery of and attack upon deep-seated and essentially unimportant problems within a client who could be gotten to work and adequate adjustment merely by meeting a very simple and obvious need [p. 8].

Later in his report, Moriarty stated that his own early concepts had changed through opportunity to interact with coordinators in the Joint Liaison Committee. He observed:

> ... one of my vague early concepts was the Universities should turn out counselors fully equipped to function in my program in all its detail. I now realize this cannot be the case—nor should it! Instead, I am now grateful to get from these programs counselors who have deliberately chosen to enter the field, and who have been given some measure of basic, fundamental foundational training on which, on

the job, we can build a sound superstructure of method and technique [p. 9].

And all three—the call for reevaluation of functions to counselors, the training challenge to counselor educators and the caution to agency administrators—are stated to underscore the urgency of the increasingly close cooperation and collaboration between pertinent educational institutions and agency leaders in the further elucidation of roles, functions and educational preparation of rehabilitation counselors for the seventies and beyond. As Moriarty[12] said. "Agency-University relationships should be a natural result of a clear realization that there is a real and true interdependence between the two programs."

Perhaps a review of the attempts to elucidate the controversial roles and functions of the rehabilitation counselor as a base for the development of pertinent educational curriculum will bring into focus the new dimension of the challenge of training for the seventies. An historical look at the approach-avoidance movement toward professional identification in rehabilitation counseling over the past fifteen years could serve to throw into perspective the new professionalism which is the second dimension with which the seventies must cope.

REVIEW OF THE CONTROVERSIAL ROLES AND FUNCTIONS OF THE REHABILITATION COUNSELOR

From the beginning, the training of rehabilitation counselors has been a controversial subject. Primarily the debate seems to be rooted in the unresolved problem of rehabilitation counselor roles and functions. Two points of view were set forth in the early days of the organization. Many saw the role as one of a coordinator; others thought the functions described that of a counselor.

Two early representative voices advocating the realistic identification of this worker as a coordinator might be selected to be Anderson,[1] a university coordinator, and Johnston,[8] an agency representative. Perhaps the most prolific and urgent voice representing the professional counselor point-of-view at that time could be said to be Patterson,[18] also a university coordinator.

In 1956, Patterson presented a paper "Counselor or Coordinator?" at the Fourth Annual Institute for Rehabilitation Personnel at Southern Illinois University. After summarizing the conflicting concepts, he offered four alternatives for the training of rehabilitation counselors.

> One would be to consider the counselor as primarily a coordinator, and develop a training program which includes a sampling—a smattering—of knowledges from a broad area, including legal aspects of public assistance and social welfare programs, detailed medical information, administration of social welfare benefits and programs, public relation information, and social casework procedures, as well as some limited acquaintance with counseling. . . . A second approach would be to try to train an individual for both functions, for counseling and coordinating . . . which appears to be impossible in the time available. A third alternative is to concentrate on the training of competent counselors in the time available. . . . A fourth alternative. . . . Perhaps instead of thinking in terms of either counselors *or* coordinators, we should be thinking in terms of counselors and coordinators. . . . [pp. 14-15].

If the rehabilitation worker was to be a coordinator, certain relevant training would be indicated. If, on the other hand, the rehabilitation worker was to be a counselor, professional education would be required.

This debate led to still another disputation relevant to the basic academic foundation of the educational program. If the personnel in question were to assume the role of a coordinator, it would follow that skills in the areas of supervision, administration and research utilization would be mandatory. If the worker was to be a counselor, professional theory and supervised practice would be essential.

Hall and Warren[4] reported on a national conference held for the purpose of discussing content and philosophy of curriculum for rehabilitation counselor preparation. The preliminary consensus seemed to be that the curriculum should be multidisciplinary in nature, with emphasis on skills "peculiar to the handicapped."

When an analysis was made (drawing upon the limited practice from 1920 to 1956 when the 1954 law was implemented) of the various topics essential to the education of the rehabilitation counselor, or coordinator, the task seemed formidable indeed.

From the behavioral and social sciences, such subjects as psychology, sociology, anthropology and economics seemed relevant. In the field of education, the areas of special and vocational education appeared pertinent. From the health services, medicine, nursing, physical and occupational therapy, and speech and hearing therapies all seemed applicable.

In summary, it would seem that work roles and techniques were borrowed and integrated to form a pattern of approach to the training of this new specialist. The focus on the individual was borrowed from psychology and medicine. From social work came the emphasis on the importance of family and community group membership. Vocational evaluation was adapted from skills of vocational counseling and industrial psychology. From vocational education was derived training and placement skills. All of this, then, was to be superimposed upon and mediated through specific knowledge and concern for "physical, mental, emotional, and social disability" and the impact of that handicap on human behavior and function.[7] Even with adaption and integration this constituted a threatening array of techniques, skills and theories.

Inasmuch as three universities had established programs for the purpose of educating rehabilitation counselors on a private (as opposed to federally supported) basis prior to 1956, the curricula of these programs became models for discussion. Interestingly enough, each of the three had chosen different approaches. The New York University program (originating in 1941) was basically education. Ohio State (originating in 1944) chose a social work approach, and the Wayne State curriculum (originating in 1946) was founded on special education.

Since the first rehabilitation workers (following the 1920 act) were employed by the Veterans Administration, the first rehabilitation educators were drawn from professionals with training similar to those working for VA. They were usually psychologists or educators with basic training and philosophy in the area of counseling. Working curricula models were, therefore, already in existence.

So, the consensus of the 1956 National Conference would seem to be a fourfold one. First, that the program should be graduate in approach. Second, the core curriculum should be counseling, therefore, basically psychological in nature. Third, the course of study should be interdisciplinary rather than specific. Fourth, a time period of two years should be allocated in order to cover minimal levels of the comprehensive materials deemed essential.

The diversity of programs growing out of this National Conference indicates that with these four points consensus ended! A review of the course offerings of the universities involved reveal many differences in emphasis. This would be expected since each counselor educator responsible for such a program must implement the consensus in light of his own professional training and commitment, the skills and interest of his faculty, the academic requirements of his graduate school, and all these modified to meet the personnel needs of the consumer agencies at the local, state and national levels.

Still another unresolved argument centered around counselor preparation purpose: for present jobs or future positions. Agency administrators, suffering from pressures for personnel, tended to reinforce preparation for the immediate job. Counselor educators, caught in their dual responsibility to the universities and the students involved, leaned toward preparation for the positions projected to the future.[27]

In 1957, once again Patterson addressed himself to the timely problem of "The Counselor's Responsibility in Rehabilitation."

> To many people the rehabilitation counselor is a cross between a social worker and a psychologist . . . as a result of his uncertain status, the rehabilitation counselor is at present neither fish nor fowl but an unfortunate mixture . . . and will continue to suffer . . . because of the ill-defined nature of his position, with consequent differences of opinion and disagreements regarding his duties and functions [p. 7].

Patterson then developed two alternative descriptions of the counselor's functions. The first delineated the rehabilitation counselor as an eligibility determiner, appraiser of client job potential, vocational plan developer, plan implementation agent and (where indicated) a referral agent. He then questions:

> One might ask: What is the client doing all this time? Too often he is literally doing nothing, except what he is told to do by the counselor [p. 11].

The second characterization of the rehabilitation counselor sketched the role of a *professional counselor* working toward a goal of independence on the part of the client. The ingredients of this approach Patterson depicts as involved with such intangibles as counselor attitudes, understanding and recognition of unique differences among clients. Through the relationship made possible by the qualities outlined above the counselor's goal then became the development of responsibility and independence on the part of the client.

Patterson then leaves us with this pointed query.

> Which of the two descriptions of the counselor's functions, do you think, is most likely to result in the development of responsibility, of social and occupational independence, in the client? How long will it be before we can say—that rehabilitation counseling believes that if he (the client) is given sufficient understanding and help in making each step toward recovery, (he) may be able to make his own vocational plan [p. 11].

Both advocates were able to make pertinent points in favor of their respective claims. That decade (the fifties) ended with no definitive answer to the debate. Most of those involved in the controversy took the stand that this new occupation was just emerging, and only the passage of time could bring resolution of the discussion. So, they looked to the sixties!

DEVELOPMENTS DURING THE SIXTIES

In the early years of the sixties, again Patterson seemed to dominate the scene in the literature. Although he continued to advocate professional identification, as a scholar he meticulously reported both sides of the coin (coordinator and counselor) as he reviewed the changing trends in rehabilitation counseling.

In 1961, Patterson addressed himself to "Trends in Vocational Rehabilitation Counseling." At this point he recounts four emerging trends significant to the evolving functions of the rehabilitation counselor.

The first trend sketched was that of increased specialization in rehabilitation counseling. This particularism could have to do with a specialty within the rehabilitation process (such as placement counselor, intake counselor, et cetera) or it could take the form of counseling a particular group of clients (that is, the emotionally disturbed, the blind, et cetera).

The second direction outlined was that of the increasing variability of the situation in which the rehabilitation counselor worked. By 1961, rehabilitation counselors were employed not only in the general agencies and the commissions for the blind but in mental hospitals, rehabilitation centers, alcoholic clinics and so forth. This development brought into focus the "need to define and redefine duties and functions" of the rehabilitation counselor.

The third trend related directly to the second in that it portrayed a movement *away* from the older more rigid definition of what a rehabilitation counselor should do and *toward* a more flexible and experimental look at the roles and functions *required* to perform in the various settings.

Trend number four pertained to an evolution toward professionalism of rehabilitation counseling.

From the coordinator's point-of-view, Super, in 1964, pointed out that despite some gradual upgrading and clarification of professional roles in rehabilitation counseling, many in the field still maintained that *dissemination of information* was the major role of that specialization. Basically, the question was, and is, Shall we educate for a profession or train for a trade?

This question led to strife again. As Martin[10] pointed out:

> The university should *not* be the place to *train* an individual in the conduct of a trade or profession, but rather to *prepare* the individual for a lifetime of scholarship in the trade or profession. Trades and professions are learned by experience in the outside world. The University must provide an attitude of inquiry and an environment conducive to the study of man and his universe. Here the problem-solving methods of study, intuitive and conscious, are applied to the interactions of man and the universe [p. 5].*

This position reactivates the question of professionalism in the context of training. Back in 1954, Towle made the point:

> The function of a profession in society, and the demands implicit in the practice, determine the objectives of education for that profession.

---
*Italicizing for emphasis by Cobb.

The responsibilities which its practitioners must assume designate the content of knowledge and skill to be attained [p. 4].

Is the university the proper place to train rehabilitation counselors? Is the field a profession? If so, the profession should be instrumental in determining content of the curriculum and the university is the proper location for the program. By the mid-sixties, these questions had still not been solved. Counselor roles and functions in rehabilitation were still developing. Professionalism was emerging but had not arrived. So, many agency administrators, out of sheer necessity as well as honest conviction, continued to espouse the pragmatic view of training personnel to fill gaping vacancies. Many counselor educators continued to defend the professional approach, out of the same honest conviction as well as pressures brought by standards of university functioning. For, paraphrasing Martin,[10] it is not the usual role of the university to prepare for other than at profession levels.

Some experts in the field looked upon these differences in role expectations and perceptions of training with alarm and admonished the counselor educators to "realign present curricula with the realities of agency practice."[14]

Others, with equal concern, held that agency conceptions and practices should be modified to include a more professional future for the rehabilitation counselor. For the purpose of decision-making in the context of education of the rehabilitation counselor, the question was not only should the educational efforts adjust to agency reality but should greater emphasis on counseling be instigated within the agency? The problem also involved a decision for specialized versus generalized training. In addition it led to a still more tantalizing inquiry: Should this decision be determined by the agency administrators, by the university educators or should it be a compromise effort?

To further complicate this already complex and controversial topic of education of the rehabilitation counselor, a national movement toward utilization of support personnel to supplement the efforts of the counselor appeared on the scene in the last half of the sixties. Short-term emergency training in empathy, geniuneness and warmth was advocated by Truax[28] and others[3] as sufficient for effective counseling of rehabilitation clients in many situations. Undergraduate training[6] had been initiated in Pennsylvania in the early sixties and now had spread to a number of universities throughout the country. Graduates from these programs had proved to be effective workers in areas of rehabilitation. So, to the quandary as to directions, philosophy and content of the graduate curricula for rehabilitation counselors had been added the problem of undergraduate possibilities through the training of support personnel. This addition, of course, lent greater confusion to the already clouded area of rehabilitation counseling roles and functions.

The second half of the sixties was marked by a research approach to the problem. By 1966, wide-scale organized research on the roles and functions of the rehabilitation counselor started appearing in the literature. That year, after conducting a comprehensive and vigorous research project involving a large population, Muthard, Miller and Barillas[14] reported their inability to get wide agreement on measures of successful counseling performance, pointing out a lack of consensus on professional roles.

In 1969, one of the most extensive and exhaustive investigations of this controversial topic was published.[13] This research was designed to "provide basic information regarding the work of the rehabilitation counselor." It included sections on the perceptions of counselors, supervisors, administrators and other professional rehabilitation workers of the rehabilitation counselor and implications of the rehabilitation counselors role, perceptions held by rehabilitation counselor educators and vocational rehabilitation administrators for the preparation of counselors (p. 3).

There was revealed an encouraging congruence between job categories reported by counselors, administrators and counselor educators. The eight categories of job responsibility reaching consensus were the following:

1. Placement
2. Affective counseling
3. Group counseling and teaching
4. Vocational counseling
5. Medical referral

6. Eligibility and case finding
7. Test administration
8. Test interpretation

This itemization could be considered as a basic pattern structure of the perceptions of the counselor's responsibility in rehabilitation; however, this listing of agreed upon activities represented only four fifths of the perceived inventory of tasks, which indicates that even in 1969 the rehabilitation counselor's job was still not thoroughly standardized.

Despite the concurrence on eight categories of responsibilities of the rehabilitation counselor reported in this study, there were differences in emphasis placed on the tasks by the rehabilitation counselors and the administrators.

The counselors seemed to place priority on counseling, rehabilitation planning and collaboration with other agencies. Administrators and supervisors reported greater emphasis on placement, affective counseling and referral. This discrepancy in deemed importance could be responsible for the "role strain" reported by some counselors in the field. The counselor educators' profile of emphasis was very similar to that reported by the counselors themselves, particularly the trained counselors. This would be expected since the educational programs eschewed by the counselor educators should reflect their analysis of task importance and, inasmuch as students usually reflect, to some degree, the orientation of the programs from which they come.

It is interesting to note that the analysis of counseling time spent in each of the categories had not changed materially since the 1956–1967 decade. It is also engaging to observe the difference in emphasis on certain tasks made by agencies. Whereas the counselors in the rehabilitation facilities reported greater importance on counseling per se than the blind or general agencies, these agencies indicated greater weight placed on activities involving occupational information and test information than the facilities personnel deemed worthwhile. The agency for the blind reported more emphasis on job placement than did the general agency or the facilities. These agency differences are not great enough to justify specialty programs of counselor education, but the information could be highly relevant to counselor placement.

Just as there were discrepancies in the perceived importance of certain counselor responsibility in rehabilitation, there also seemed to be a lack of agreement in the evaluated levels of education required for specific tasks. The counselors reported the desirability of graduate education (master's level) to do affective counseling, group procedures and test interpretation. They thought medical referral and vocational counseling could be accomplished by an individual with less academic education with specific on-the-job training. Counselors in the facilities placed higher focus on graduate education than did the counselors in the agencies *per se*.

No report was found indicating rehabilitation administrator's evaluation of educational levels for certain counselor activities, but it is generally agreed that although they favor graduate educational attainment, they must deliver services to more clients than can be served by adequately trained professionals. Therefore, they must utilize employees with lesser training. This group (agency administration) has shown ingenuity and creativity in experimentation and demonstration of the effectiveness of the undergraduate, on-the-job trained employee.

Despite some continued divergence in roles and functions ascribed to the rehabilitation counselor by the counselors themselves and the rehabilitation agency representatives, a decided trend toward congruence is evident. Much of the seeming disparity could be due *not* to basic philosophical differences, *but* to the hard facts related to the unending and ever-increasing burden of services to be rendered by the agencies and the inadequate supply of professionally trained counselors produced each year. It is most encouraging to observe that there was congruence "between what rehabilitation counselor educators *think* should be changed in the rehabilitation counselor's job and what rehabilitation leaders *expect* to change by 1980."[13]

Of this study, McAlees[11] said that it accomplished three tasks pertinent to the reevaluation of roles and functions of the rehabilitation counselor:

1. Identification with greater precision of the components, of profession performance in rehabilitation counseling, i.e., functions actually performed;
2. Developed methods by which this performance may be measured, with a degree of reliability and validity that exceeds those of techniques presently used;
3. Has helped identify the variables which may influence differential rates of achievement of individual counselors [p. 23].

Of the disparity of perceived roles, McAlees said:

> It was also interesting to note that the roles and functions of the rehabilitation counselor are seen from at least three unique vantage points: (1) the counselor, (2) the supervisor-administrator and (3) the educator, and that these varying perceptions could possibly mitigate against truly effective cooperative efforts between agencies—educational institutions—and counselors. It is evident that decisions regarding roles, functions and educational preparation will require increasingly close cooperation and collaboration between agencies and educational institutions. Lack of agreement about *future* roles is an area definitely in need of further study and consideration.

He concluded by stating:

> Since rehabilitation counseling involves the exercise of judgment based on sets of principles and concepts which allow for effective appraisal, programming and outcomes in the individual's unique situation rather than a simple routine application of techniques, this (study) should assist in our efforts to develop and refine the profession of rehabilitation counseling [p. 24].

Samler,[22] in a provocative series of papers designed to explore the changing challenge of the professional counselor, asked a question pertinent to rehabilitation counselor educators, "How, therefore, are counselors trained?" His answer indicates his decision that the counselor "must emerge basically as a psychological worker" but that this is no longer sufficient expertise. Holbert and Miller[5] state that the hoped for product of training is

> not simply a technician skilled in employment of a variety of techniques—although he certainly must be that. . . . He must be an open and flexible person possessed of a great amount of self-awareness and self-knowledge, sensitive and attuned to receiving and communicating vital messages with other persons [p. 29].

Therefore the training program

> should provide the kind of atmosphere which will allow a cultural

concept of the healthy person to emerge as a person who lives effectively with himself and others [p. 30].

Although most counselor training programs offer such an opportunity for self-exploration within the supervised practice operation, by the last of the sixties many had added well-planned group and individual activities to ensure this personal growth throughout the program.

So ends the sixties still on a note of question and controversy. Russell Nixon, in 1969, summarized the parameters of the challenge remaining as that decade closed:

> Vocational rehabilitation is called on to change—or perhaps it is better said to add to—its arsenal of services. While preserving the quality of its case-by-case, multi-service care, vocational rehabilitation must now move into an area where the usual psychological tests do not apply—indeed they may be perverse—when the usual physical therapy and some aspects of counseling will not apply. It now becomes necessary to go beyond attention to "individual pathology and personal failure" or handicap into consideration of social and political factors [p. 17].

Not only was the sixties unable to formalize the roles and functions of the rehabilitation counselor, that decade witnessed a whirlwind of expansion into a diversity of new service categories to the point that roles, functions, specializations, technique and skills essential to the performance of the task of the rehabilitation counselor had multiplied the complexity of the solution of the controversy.

The goals for training of the rehabilitation counselor remained unclear. There was still the question, Are we training counselors, coordinators, a combination, or both? Still unanswered was the query, Are we training for a profession or are we doing vestibule training for a specific job? Upon the answers to these questions should rest the content and approach of the educational curriculum.

Added questions related to the times in which we live (the population explosion, the knowledge explosion, technological revolution and social turmoil) brought new responsibilities to the rehabilitation counselor and added new dimensions to the training challenge faced by rehabilitation counselor educators.

These new dimensions focus around challenges in manpower utilization in the new era and the call for a new professionalism to meet the needs of the diversified clientele served.

In terms of educational programs, policies and philosophy these new dimensions may well necessitate a revamping of program offering and a reevaluation of goals for training. Graduate schools have served as the focal points for education of rehabilitation counselors throughout the sixties. Signs of change indicate that the "academic setting is no longer sacred as the locus for the development of professional skills. Agencies may take on aspects of academia through practice of in-service training conducted by university faculty."[25]

HISTORY OF THE MOVEMENT OF REHABILITATION COUNSELING TOWARD PROFESSIONALISM

From the time of the inception of the rehabilitation counseling program (1954–1955), the desirability of becoming part of an ongoing profession or developing a new professionalism has been present in the minds of all who were, and are, involved. The controversy on this issue seems not "to be or not to be" a profession, as much as it is to decide whether it should be part of the profession of counseling psychology, vocational counseling, and so forth, or to become a new profession.

Agreements seemed to have been reached, in the first decade of the life of the program, that to be a professional would give the counselor greater social status, a better income, more dependable tenure, greater control of duties and more authority as a leader.[17] It was also pointed out that the success of this quest for professionalism rested upon the nature of the work of the counselor and the manner in which he accomplished that work.

Obermann[17] summarized the personal characteristics of a professional individual as being (a) competent, (b) effective, (c) facilitative (of the work of other professions), (d) an individual of integrity and (e) skilled in the art of communication.

Although the personal characteristics are demanding, there has never seemed to be a question raised as to the qualifications of the rehabilitation counselor in this area. As a group, rehabilitation counselors have been recognized as devoted, ethical and effective in their work. They have always occupied a role of "coordinator" of services and in that role have been responsible for the facilitation of the work of an interdisciplinary team for the benefit of the clients served. Although much remains to be accomplished, the rehabilitation counselor has proven his effectiveness in communication of rehabilitation tenets among professionals on the team and the clients served and has done a creditable job in communication with the public.

Academic and/or professional qualifications have been criticized, weighed and found wanting from time to time. Krantzler[9] declared that "even to ask What is a Rehabilitation Counselor? is to become enmeshed in metaphysical quicksand." He pointed out that there is a lack of evidence of the existence of a "unique body of knowledge and skills essential to rehabilitation counseling." He also criticized the "standards" of selection and employment of the rehabilitation counselor, reminding that "Graduate education is not mandatory for employment: indeed, some indications exist that undergraduate education and on-the-job training may be preferred. Thus, there is no thrust to upgrade the Rehabilitation Counseling field professionally." He also indicated the absence of "certification or other form of legal recognition" and the lack of a "single, powerful organization with which Rehabilitation Counselors identify."

Krantzler[9] also set forth a number of items in the area of professional behavior in which he deemed the field of rehabilitation counseling lacking. Paraphrasing somewhat for brevity, these points include the following:

1. Lack of job independence or opportunity to act creatively; since they act as employees instructed as to what to do rather than as experts with professional standing.

2. Enjoy little respect as professionals from other professions and display minimal evidence of "concerted involvement" in professional growth and self-development.

3. Salaries are lower than other professionals with similar responsibilities.

If these criteria are applied to the rehabilitation counselor and

The Challenge of New Dimensions in Rehabilitation 141

his work, it must be recognized that to date rehabilitation counseling is not a "profession." Although progress is being made toward the establishment of a "unique body of knowledge, based upon scientific principles" that relate specifically to rehabilitation counseling, it is still not a substantial offering.

Certainly in the beginning there was no single professional organization with which the rehabilitation counselor could identify. In the outset this was a problem of absence of such an organization. At present the quandary is not the absence of a suitable professional organization but *which* professional organization. During the sixties a plethora of professional organizations came into existence as divisions of numerous national associations. The National Rehabilitation Counseling Association (NRCA) is a division of the National Rehabilitation Association (NRA) and offers an opportunity for professional affiliation. On the other hand, the American Rehabilitation Counseling Association (ARCA) is a component of the American Personnel and Guidance Association (APGA) and invites professional membership. The American Psychological Association (APA) also extends the hand of professional identification through the Rehabilitation Counseling Association (RCA) and Division 22, Psychology of Disability. Complication now arises because members of the rehabilitation counseling group vacillate between a desire to identify as a part of one (and which one) of the established professions represented, or to "hold-out" and develop a separate professional identity.*

Barber[2] defined an "emerging profession" thus:

> The emerging or marginal profession is an occupation which is not so clearly high or so low on both of the first two attributes of professionalism—generalized knowledge and community orientation—that its status is clearly defined by itself and others. . . . Its members are not homogeneous with respect to the amount of knowledge and community orientation they possess. . . . It is the elite of an emerging profession that takes the lead in pushing for the advancement of professionalism in its occupational group and in claiming public recognition of its new status. . . . The leaders of an emerging profession will have to engage in some conflict with elements both inside and outside their

---
*Counselor educators now also have choice between affiliating with the Council of Rehabilitation Counselor Educators (CRCE) of NRA, or with the Association of Counselor Educators and Supervisors (ACES) of APGA.

occupational group ... they may meet with some opposition from the less professional members within the group ... and they may themselves be branded as "encroachers" on other established and professional specialties [p. 671].

Even Krantzler[9] concedes that:

> The Rehabilitation Counselor is an "emerging" professional ... he can either resign himself to the status of being simply a white-collar employee; or he can accept the professional challenge and strive to remake his image by improving himself and his profession. It is a fact of life that nobody hands anyone power on a silver platter. Professionalism implies power over one's own working destiny. The only way Rehabilitation Counselors will obtain that power is through their own active participation in the kinds of activities that make professionalism possible. There is no easier answer [pp. 8-9].

Jacques[7] joins Krantzler in asserting that the counselor himself is the key to professionalism of the field. She points out that:

> Traditional structure of authority (in rehabilitation) has effectively prevented the development of autonomous professionals who could give primary attention to client needs. ... Effective professional control with counselors assuming responsibility for their own autonomy, and therefore able to represent the best interests of the clients, is needed to balance organizational power ... the counselor will not be effective—as a full professional, nor develop into an agent of social change or renewal, until his professional identity as the client's trusted advocate is clear to himself, his client, his peers, and his employing agency [p. 54].

Another concept inherent in professionalism is not only the acceptance of the rehabilitation counselor as professional among professionals but also an acceptance of support personnel or "new careerists" on the part of the professional counselor and other rehabilitation personnel.

In its fifteen years of existence, rehabilitation counseling, like the girl in the cigarette advertisement, has "come a long, long way!"[23] Educational requirements have improved, salaries have increased, ethical codes of behavior have been developed, professional organizations with which to identify are available, respect from the community served is evidenced by the clamoring for services, and it enjoys unusually fine financial resources.

In short, we have what it takes to make vocational rehabilitation a

The Challenge of New Dimensions in Rehabilitation 143

dynamic and driving force in our country in the 1970's IF. . . . If we have leadership that's progressive, open-minded, and far-sighted [p. 4].

Krantzler[9] sums it up and places the responsibility for leadership squarely on the shoulders of the counselor . . . specifically the graduate of the rehabilitation counselor training programs.

> The current era is one of profound social change characterized by an increasing demand for greater participation in decision-making processes by those affected by the decisions or responsible for implementing them. In a sense we are witnessing a revolt against the alienating factors of our society. The new entrants from the graduate schools to the Rehabilitation Counseling field are products of this era. Within the next few years they will play a prominent role in their agencies and organizations. Will they respond to conditions in the same apathetic way as their predecessors? Perhaps it is later than many agencies and graduate schools think [p. 9].

Jacques[7] declares that:

> Out of all the turmoil engendered in attempts to find professional identification coupled with the social changes of our time may come a new professionalism.
>
> A clear recognition that the past and present methods of delivering services to people have been ineffective seems to permeate the entire professional world. From the ground swell of concern expressed by all areas of the helping professions, should emerge a personal and social renewal process as the basis of all future planning and delivery of services. . . .
>
> Perhaps renewed cooperation in joint problem-solving tasks, the recognition that knowledge must be connected to operational programs and the awareness of the ever present need to change in response to the human situation may provide the directions for a new counseling professionalism.

Jacques points out, however, that "four priority issues need concerted attention and implementation so that a new professionalism directed toward human and social renewal may be achieved."

1. The counselor with professional autonomy, collaborating with clients as helper and as advocate in problem solving tasks.
2. The fractionated professional areas of counseling with the other helping professions joining together collaboratively, rather than competing for isolated professional areas and interests.
3. Counseling and the helping professions extending theory and practice beyond the psychology of primarily the middle class American

to include the culture and sociology of other classes, races and nationalities.

4. Team counseling requiring practitioners with expertise at various levels of training and backgrounds of life experience to focus on the multiple problems of clients [pp. 53-54].

Newman[15] reiterates Jacques' suggestion that a new professionalism is imminent. He states:

> Maximizing the potential for each handicapped person implies a broader conception of professional tasks than personal counseling and seeking out appropriate resources on behalf of clients. It implies a responsibility to analyze the extent, organization, and quality of community institutional arrangements and resources for meeting the basic needs of our handicapped citizens.
>
> To my knowledge, we do not yet train people nor have we begun to conceptualize the knowledge base or job requirements for new challenges which face us in this new area of community development for handicapped people.
>
> We must recognize the shortcomings of our present reliance on the professional and face up to what John Gardner calls "professionalism" or "credentialism". . . .
>
> Beyond this, rehabilitation workers should be taking the lead in facilitating better communication and working relationships among all human service career fields. This could begin with consultation and collaborating with other professional manpower systems [p. 48].

In the beginning, the major opposition to the concept of "coordinator" as compared with the "counselor" role was that professionalism lay by way of the counseling route. Ironically enough Sussman, Haug and Joynes,[25] speaking of training the rehabilitation counselor for the realities of practice as they exist in the field, reverse that decision and declare:

> Finally, the rehabilitation counselor is most likely to find professional autonomy in relation to the coordinating aspect of his work. . . . If the rehabilitation counselor seeks professionalism as a means to assume leadership of the rehabilitation team, and to exercise power on behalf of his client, then it is a mistake for him to focus upon psychology as the basis of his professional expertise. Leadership and power may be expected to accrue in larger measure to the coordinator . . . the practitioner whose esoteric knowledge is sociological as well as psychological, who emphasizes the system as well as the psyche, and who possesses the skill and the autonomy requisite to operate within it [p. 13].

NEW DIMENSIONS OF THE CHALLENGE FOR THE SEVENTIES

So we have come the full circle of a decade and a half and enter the seventies faced with the crucial challenge of unresolved controversy over roles and functions of rehabilitation counselors. The question of professionalism still approaches and recedes and now takes on the look of a new professionalism reflecting the challenge of the seventies. The second dimension of change to be reckoned with this decade is that of new structures and utilizations of manpower.

Newman[15] epitomizes this challenge. He states that with the expansion and extension of services offered by rehabilitation must come drastic changes in the systems of delivery of those services. This, he thinks, calls for a change in the structure and utilization of manpower. This effort should bring the services closer to the diversity of clientele served. He envisions such innovations as "mobile rehabilitation teams, indigenous case-finders, etc." This new manpower system he perceives as enhancing the "ability to attract increased numbers of service personnel" and the "kind of individuals best able to understand and communicate with the kind of client receiving our services."

Newman then defined the rehabilitation counselor as a "model rehabilitation generalist . . . called upon to perform an extraordinarily varied range of functions." After a masterful delineation of this "broad range of functions," he adds:

> We are now forced to question whether it is reasonable or economical to expect one kind of staff person to perform so many different kinds of duties and possess so many different kinds of skills [p. 45].

He states that although an honest effort has been made to "restrict full professional status to those practitioners with master's degrees . . ."

> The evidence surrounding the rehabilitation manpower crisis forces a reappraisal of our position. It is clear, for example, that in spite of our efforts, most rehabilitation counselor positions in public rehabilitation agencies are filled by persons who do not possess graduate degrees.* Our expanding role in new social welfare legislation related to

---

*Jacques[7] states that in 1968 approximately 600 master's level graduates were employed in state and federal agencies, as compared to a total of 6000 rehabilitation counselors employed in the United States.

the vocational rehabilitation program places new kinds of demands on our staff and points out a need for a qualitative enrichment. Other social welfare programs have demonstrated that less well academically trained indigenous personnel can be effective in providing social services. How slowly we have accepted this approach in rehabilitation [p. 46]!

Three alternative solutions to this manpower dilemma are then presented. Paraphrasing Newman for brevity, the following alternatives are suggested:

1. Reduce the time requirement for the master's degree.
2. Increase financial support to graduate schools in an effort to produce more counselors at the professional level.
3. Develop a systematic plan for differential utilization of personnel.

Inasmuch as counselor educators seem to agree that a two-year graduate program is mandatory to professional mastery of the rehabilitation counselor curriculum, the first alternative did not seem feasible to Newman. In light of recent and expected budget cuts, the second suggestion did not appear plausible. The third, therefore, seemed to him the realistic solution to the challenge. This alternative would provide several levels of personnel trained to supplement and enhance the contribution of each (a new kind of rehabilitation team).

This concept projects a three-level staffing pattern.[15] In descending order the personnel occupying these levels would be known as rehabilitation counselor, rehabilitation casemanager and rehabilitation aide. He declares:

In rehabilitation, we need a manpower system that provides a structure into which employees with different academic and social backgrounds may be fitted. Our system should provide for a progression into positions of greater responsibility for employees who have demonstrated unusual ability, regardless of their formal degrees or credentials. Our system should reward attainment of education, but should nonetheless place a special value on achievement of techniques relevant to the field of rehabilitation. It should provide for a training continuum from the lowest entrance level in the hierarchy to the highest levels of employment, and should include formalized training programs spaced at intervals along the progression. It should provide a means to utilize available manpower effectively. Our system should fill the gap between the professional and subprofessional levels [p. 46].

Newman continues:

> The key aspect of this system is that through experience and provision of an agency staff development program, the aide can eventually achieve the case-manager status. The case-manager similarly may have the opportunity to become a rehabilitation counselor [p. 47].

Looking ahead, Newman thinks that:

> A three-level rehabilitation team provides one opportunity for enriching agency potentials at the same time that high professional standards are maintained. There will always be a basic demand for highly trained professionals in the rehabilitation field [p. 47].

To the counselor educators and to agency administrators this training of manpower challenge is a provocative one. If the challenge is to be met, it calls for a close collaborative effort on the part of both. This new dimension of training calls for continuation and enrichment of the existing graduate programs. It also implies a continuum of cooperative training covering emergency, short-term preparation of aides and probably case managers. It demands continuing education efforts as well, in order to make possible progressive movement on the career ladder.

Research for the purpose of identification of tasks and responsibilities at each of the three levels is mandatory. Concerted effort is necessary to then develop content and approaches for each step on the ladder. Together the agencies and the universities can meet this challenge. Perhaps at long last, the seventies will see the end of the controversy over rehabilitation counselor roles and functions! With this solution maybe this decade will witness a clarification of professional goals for the education of rehabilitation counselors.

As we commit ourselves to the sobering task of developing these two new dimensions of the training challenge for the seventies, let us remember the admonition of our distinguished leader through the fifties and sixties, Mary E. Switzer.[26] She cautions:

> The horizons ahead where rehabilitation can be cutting edges of progress are broad and golden. There is no limit to the groups of people who can be helped and served by this program. The limit lies only in the need for knowledge to deal with the unsolved problems. We are still lacking an organized approach in many areas, which we must have before we can follow the road so successfully cleared by the rehabilitation leaders of the past. . . .

The challenge of the future will be to maintain the dual characteristic of rehabilitation as we have known it, for they are the essential ingredients of its success. First, the personal, committed, devoted relationship of the counselor to the person being served; and, second, the services be directed to the goal of work. Unless these two characteristics are preserved, the essential quality of rehabilitation will be lost. . . . Despite the destructiveness of war and deprivation, the chaos of civic revolt and protest, the violence of natural disasters, rehabilitation has consistently emerged over the years as the force that heals. Rehabilitation joins men and nations together, that they may begin again and move closer toward shared dreams of freedom and opportunity. . . .

May it continue to bring even more hope to the millions to whom life means so little without *hope* [pp. 49-50].

REFERENCES

1. Anderson, R.: Rehabilitation counselor as a counselor. *J Rehab*, 24:4-5, 1958.
2. Barber, B.: Some problems in the sociology of the professions. *Daedalus*, 92:669-688, 1963.
3. Griswold, P.: The Detroit DVR responds to the inner city challenge. *Rehab Rec*, 1969, p. 33-37.
4. Hall, J. H., and Warren, S. L. (Eds.): Rehabilitation counselor preparation report of the Charlottesville Workshop. Washington, D.C., 1956.
5. Holbert, W. M., and Miller, J. H.: Traditional versus experimental model for counselor education. *J Appl Rehab Counseling, 1 (3):* 21-30, 1970.
6. Hylbert, K. W.: Experiment at Penn State: Bachelor of rehabilitation. *J Rehab, 29 (2)*:23-24, 1963.
7. Jacques, M. E.: Rehabilitation counseling: Scope and services. *Guidance Monograph Series*, 1970, Series 5.
8. Johnston, L. T.: Rehabilitation counselor as a coordinator. *J Rehab*, 1958.
9. Krantzler, M.: Is rehabilitation counseling a profession? *J Appl Rehab Counseling, 1 (1)*:3-9, 1970.
10. Martin, S. P.: The role of the university in professional education. *Studies in Rehabilitation Counselor Training, 3*:1-5, 1964.
11. McAlees, D. C.: Rehabilitation counselor roles and functions. *The Profession, Functions, Roles & Practices of the Rehabilitation Counselor*, 1969, p. 21-25.
12. Moriarty, E. J.: Agency-university communication, coordination & cooperation in pre-service training. *Studies in Rehabilitation Counselor Training, 3*:6-10, 1964.

13. Muthard, J. E., Dumas, N. S., and Salomone, P. R.: *The Profession, Functions Roles and Practices of the Rehabilitation Counselor.* Jacksonville (Fla.), Convention Press, 1969.
14. Muthard, J. E., Miller, L. A., and Barillas, M.: A time study of vocational rehabilitation counselors. *Rehab Counseling Bull, 9:*53-60, 1965.
15. Newman, E.: Changing rehabilitation manpower utilization. *J Rehab, 36 (5):*45-48, 1970.
16. Nixon, R. A.: Rehabilitation-human reinforcement in a troubled world. *J Rehab, 35:*14-17, 1969.
17. Obermann, C. E.: The rehabilitation counselor as a professional person. *J Rehab Counseling, 28:*37-38, 1962.
18. Patterson, C. H.: Counselor or coordinator? *J Rehab, 23 (3):*13-15, 1957. (Presented at Southern Illinois University in 1956.)
19. Patterson, C. H.: The counselor's responsibility in rehabilitation. *J Rehab, 24(1):*7-8, 11, 1958.
20. Patterson, C. H.: Trends in vocational rehabilitation counseling. *Rehab Counseling Bull, 5:*59-67, 1962.
21. Patterson, C. H.: University and agency contributions to professional education. In *Agency-University Communication, Coordination, and Cooperation in Rehabilitation Counselor Education.* Studies in Rehabilitation Counselor Training, No. 3, 1964.
22. Samler, J.: The counselor in our time. *Rehab Counseling Bull, 11* (3-SP), 1968.
23. Smith, D. R.: The rehabilitation counselor as an infighter. *J Appl Rehab Counseling, 1(3):*3-5, 1970.
24. Super, D. E., and Thompson, A. S. (Eds.): *The Professional Preparation of Counseling Psychologists.* New York, Columbia University, 1964.
25. Sussman, M. E., Haug, M. R., and Joynes, V. A.: The modern model of rehabilitation counselor roles. *J Appl Rehab Counseling, 1 (3):* 6-14, 1970.
26. Switzer, M. E.: The cutting edge of rehabilitation. *J Rehab, 36(5):*48-50, 1970.
27. Towle, C.: *The Learner in Education for the Professions.* Chicago, University of Chicago, 1954.
28. Truax, C. B.: The effects of supportive personnel as counselor-aides in vocational rehabilitation. *NRCA Prof Bull, 8 (4),* 1968.
29. Truax, C. B.: The training of nonprofessional personnel in therapeutic interpersonal relationships. *Amer J Public Health, 57:*1778-1789, 1967.
30. White, T. K.: The golden years of vocational rehabilitation (The editor's view). *J Appl Rehab Counseling, 1(3),* 1970.

6

The Professional Status of the Rehabilitation Counselor

W. Alfred McCauley

Introduction
Some Historical Perspectives
Further Perspectives
A Look at the Forces Impinging on Professionalization
A Basis for Conflict in Rehabilitation Counseling
Aspects of Professionalization in Current Practice
Elements in Professionalization
Summary
References

REHABILITATION counseling is an "emerging" profession. Its roots in practice go further back, however, than the title, "rehabilitation counselor" or "vocational rehabilitation counselor," which was selected by a show of hands among state agency administrators in the 1946 Conference on Rehabilitation of the Tuberculous.

When the director of the Wisconsin rehabilitation program, William F. Faulkes, raised the question of qualifications and training of this rehabilitation worker whom they had just named, no agreement appeared among those conferees attending that meeting. Neither was there general agreement on the definition of *rehabilitation* as related by Obermann.[7] Today some still would argue whether there is an adequate definition of rehabilitation. There are also those who claim that we still have no agreement on the qualifications and training of the rehabilitation counselor. The historical situation set out above does not imply that there were no aspects of practice that represented "professionalization" and that practice had no framework in which it was carried out, no matter how adequate or inadequate our definitions.

The current status of the rehabilitation counselor has aspects of professionalization; it also has aspects of little professionalization, depending upon whose perceptions of status dominate the argument about the matter. There is still controversy as to what he is and does. Content of his training has no uniformity in design, except in limited aspects. The nature of his practice varies somewhat from setting to setting. His job title in relation to his knowledge and skills and where he practices varies also. How then can we speak of his professional status?

The manner in which I deal with the scope of this subject is my own point of view and much of it comes from my perceptions of the development of practice. My wide variety of experiences as a rehabilitation counselor, an educator of rehabilitation counselors, an administrative person within the state-federal programs of rehabilitation and as an executive of the largest organization of rehabilitation counselors contribute as the basis of my perceptions. The frame of reference in which I treat the subject draws upon the contributions of a number of others however.

INTRODUCTION

Vollmer and Mills[12] have provided the frame which seems most nearly adequate for handling this subject. They use five terms which they suggest as leading to more preciseness for discussion: *professionalization, professionalism, professionals, professional groups* and *professions*.

They define *professionalization* as "the dynamic process whereby many occupations can be observed to change certain crucial characteristics in the direction of a profession, even though not very far in this direction." Professionalization is evolutionary in its development.

Profession is a term to "be applied only to an abstract model of occupational organization—an ideal type that would result if any occupational group became completely professionalized." This form of occupational organization is always one of *becoming*.

Cogan[2] sees definitions of profession from a number of frames of reference: the "dictionary and legal definitions," the "arbitrary and applied definitions," the "definitions expressed in terms of power and prestige," the "profession as a formal association" and definitions relative to "techniques of internal regulation."

Cogan suggests this definition of profession as tentative and for our purpose in this manuscript:

> A profession is a vocation whose practice is founded upon an understanding of the theoretical structure of some department of learning or science, and upon the abilities accompanying such understanding. This understanding and these abilities are applied to the vital practical affairs of man. The practices of the professional are modified by knowledge of a generalized nature and by the accumulated wisdom and experience of mankind, which serve to correct the errors of specialism. The profession, serving the vital needs of man, considers its first ethical imperative to be alturistic service to the client [p. 49].

Vollmer and Mills use, *professionalism* as a term "to refer to an *ideology* and associated activities that can be found in many and diverse occupational groups where members aspire to professional status" and with which Strauss[11] associates four "values": "expertise," "autonomy," "commitment" and "responsibility."

Professional groups is a term used "to refer to associations of colleagues in an occupational context where we observe that a relatively high degree of professionalization has taken place."

Professionals is a term used to describe "those who are considered by their colleagues to be members of professional groups."

There are many forces that affect the interrelationships of the above terms and affect the work activities as they relate to "rehabilitation" and "rehabilitation counseling." These forces and activities operate both to enhance and retard the process of professionalization.

SOME HISTORICAL PERSPECTIVES

At the time that the 1946 Conference on Rehabilitation of the Tuberculous and the administrators of divisions of vocational rehabilitation in the states decided to use the job title, "rehabilitation counselor," for those employees in their agencies who were

The Professional Status of the Rehabilitation Counselor   153

agents of the divisions and represented their agency's services to disabled persons. There were some fifteen job titles assigned to such personnel across the country. My own title at that time in such a public agency was "rehabilitation representative." Other such job titles were "rehabilitation agent," "rehabilitation coordinator" (still used by one public agency), "rehabilitation supervisor," et cetera. This proliferation of job titles and the expanding programs after the passage of Public Law 113, Seventy-eighth Congress, in 1943, and the inevitable bureaucratization that was to affect the work activities forecasted the need for a more uniform job title to the heads of these programs.

Most of these administrators came from backgrounds in educational system administration and operated agencies administratively anchored in departments of education in their states. The federal administration was anchored in the Federal Board of Vocational Education in the Office of Education until 1943, when the Office of Vocational Rehabilitation was established by the Federal Security Administrator. By 1946 the vocational counseling movement and, to some degree, the school guidance movement had led to the establishment of job titles, "counselors," in state departments of education job classification and certification schemes. Quite expectedly, the administrators "by a show of hands" adopted this job title as the preferred title to be made more uniform in the job classification systems in their own administrative structures. By 1949 nearly every state rehabilitation agency had adopted "rehabilitation counselor" as title for the worker serving disabled people as agents of this program.

Little real analysis of the role as related to "rehabilitation," the modifier, or to the noun, "counselor," appeared in kinds of activities, the range of activities, skills and knowledges demanded, or what constituted professionalization in practice at that time.

In 1927, H. B. Cummings of the Vocational Rehabilitation Service, Federal Board of Vocational Education, in the Proceedings of the Fourth National Conference on Vocational Rehabilitation of the Disabled Civilian held in Memphis, discussed the trends developing in the state-federal program. Obermann[7] reports that Cummings noted that "the programs for civilians were as varied as the number of states offering them," that there was "a growing emphasis on *quality* of rehabilitation and less emphasis on *quantity*." He noted also "a more careful selection of cases for rehabilitation." Cummings continued, "Good business suggests that funds be expended in such a way as to yield the greatest return to the State. Obviously, this is accomplished by rendering service to that group of disabled persons who can be rehabilitated in a comparatively short time, who will earn a living, and, more, when rehabilitated, will remain rehabilitated when once so considered by the State."

Elsewhere in the Proceedings, according to Obermann, Mr. Cummings thought that "he could see the beginnings of a better definition of the work of the rehabilitation specialist. That definition is still developing today."

In the 1928 Milwaukee Conference on Rehabilitation, Dr. A. H. Edgerton, a specialist in counseling from the University of Wisconsin, led the discussion on vocational counseling[7] and said:

> The growing demands of unbiased guidance to aid young disabled as well as disabled adults in adopting their individual aptitudes to appropriate studies and occupations imply the need for basing methods of counseling on scientifically determined evidence whenever possible. Facts rather than opinions are required in order that counseling services may help the individual to diagnose his interests and capabilities and to make his own vocational decision and adjustments.
>
> Although common sense is important, the counselor will be dependent at all times on his knowledge of facts and principles in each case. Mere opinion must give way to facts secured through trustworthy investigation . . . sensitiveness to problems relating to effective counseling, rather than reliance upon mechanical devices or psychological tests alone, should characterize the work of the counselor.

These observations revealed the vision and anticipated the problems that remain basic to both administration and practice in rehabilitation today. The term *counselor* was introduced by the educator, not the administrator. The economic emphasis as the basic justification for rehabilitation was played up in all the early reporting on program achievements and still remains the essential rationale for justifying rehabilitative services for adults today. Even at that time, however, there were those in and out of Congress who supported concepts of social, economic and cultural gains that could derive from offering every individual opportunities to develop and participate to the fullest extent of his capabilities regardless of how disabled he might be. On the other hand, certain issuances (Federal Board of Vocational Education, Bulletin #148) from within the Board of Vocational Education administering the federal program in 1930, reflected some lack of perception of the disabled person as having dignity and self-esteem and having rights and privileges usually accorded to others, including the privilege to dissent from plans being made for him in the rehabilitation process. The client seemed to have to be deserving if he were to be served.

In the above Bulletin #148, the desired worker qualifications were characterized as "broad-gauged, open-minded agent who is willing to try out a new idea is the man who will contribute most to the development of this program." The program focus during its first twenty-three years was heavy on training with even gradual reduction of state funding for medical and other supportive services which were not funded by federal funds. The focus on training was also an outcome of the educationally oriented leaders and the base of administration in the federal and most state agencies in offices or state departments of education.

In congressional hearings the shift of public priorities with involvement in World War II, the need for an increased manpower pool for civilian production to support the military effort, and the articulate and enlightened presentations and rationalizations for a broader program of services for serving the disabled individual, paid off in the passage of Public Law 113 and provided the breakthrough for vocational rehabilitation programs to have resources to broadly serve the disabled. Still, both the law and the regulations for administering it in the federal and state partnership made disabled persons meet a financial means test which was a carryover of a charitable connotation from earlier days. Programs were still focused to enhance the economy rather than the individual in their essential rationale. Their "agents" arranged or provided minimal services to enable the selected individual to enter employment.

The further expansion of the law to provide: (a) a wider scope of financing; (b) services to those suffering severe disabilities; (c) extension of the program to reach greater numbers of disabled persons; (d) the construction and expansion of rehabilitation facilities; (e) elimination of architectural barriers that stood in the way of effective rehabilitation with the disabled; (f) expansion of the training of rehabilitation workers; and (g) establishment of research and demonstration to enhance knowledge about the impact of disability and suggest improved skills for better serving the disabled person—all this had roots further back in the experience of administrators and rehabilitation workers over the years.

The history of the movement is exciting; many have contributed to its making. Some have left their mark for progress or retardation. Depression and war created climates that influenced progress of the movement. Political philosophies in a strong federal base for administration, as well as conflicts in the internal structural basis of administration, required strong outside organizations of interested citizen groups, vested interest groups and their lobbying with Congress to bring change when internal politics in administration could not do so. All these factors had impact upon the professionalization of practice in rehabilitation counseling. However, a closer look reveals how the decisions made have had impact upon the directions of professionalization of practice.

FURTHER PERSPECTIVES

"Counseling" became the purported content of practice, primarily out of conceptualizations and formulations by administrators of public rehabilitation agencies without empirical studies to furnish the data for a more appropriate title for the rehabilitation worker they had named "rehabilitation counselor."

As far back as 1921, when vocational education was the primary force that shaped the philosophy for rehabilitation of the disabled, the services "trained around" disability. Yet there were those who recognized the need for improving physical functioning. There were those who recognized rehabilitation as a very complex and specialized personal service that would differ for each disabled person. Those sensitive in administration emphasized the importance of sound counseling and of reconstruction or physical restoration before training should begin or run concurrent with it. There was, even then, recognition that the individual rehabilitation worker (called agent then) must see the problem of disability as involving the whole family. Yet the practices of today, in far too many situations, have not adequately incorporated this concept and the supporting knowledge and skills for involving the whole family in resolving problems with the disabled person.

What have been the forces that have brought rehabilitation counseling to the professionalization of practice that it has today? There are many that can be reviewed, some mentioned, and others better articulated. From these we can see that practice is being professionalized, that there is striving for professionalism (ideology) but not yet agreement about it and that the practice is not yet a profession in the light of definitions set out earlier. What forces have impeded and enhanced professionalization?

Certainly *bureaucratization* has affected the work activities since most rehabilitation workers are employees of bureaucratic enterprises. Certainly, also, *socialization* which encompasses background education and specific job training with its purported skills and values has been a factor. Now more recently, *acculturation* is becoming more intimately related to work in the rehabilitation field as values, norms and social behaviors of workers identify more with an ethos among practitioners.

What are the evidences that "expertise," "autonomy," "commitment" and "responsibility" are the values in professionalism now manifested in the growth toward professionalization of practice in rehabilitation counseling?

A LOOK AT THE FORCES IMPINGING ON PROFESSIONALIZATION

The economic bias that has been the basis for all the typical cliches that justify rehabilitation services, and which translates all administrative and service practices and expenditures into numbers of disabled persons successfully rehabilitated, has deep roots in American society and the vocational rehabilitation movement.

It has influenced from earliest days the acceptance of disabled persons into the rehabilitation system, the directions of movement of the disabled person through it if he complied with the demands in the rehabilitative process and was able to hold employment (too often any kind of employment) when he eventually exited from the system.

The reinforcers for practitioner performance relating to his behaviors in this process were extrinsic rewards furnished by the system for numbers of "cases closed rehabilitated," the size of the case load handled, the quality of record keeping, the movement of cases through the various and categorized steps of the rehabilitation process, and so forth.

Contributions to many of the disabled persons who were introduced into the system and process, which may have had positive outcomes for the individual but never quite took him into remunerative or gainfully employed status, did not count in the reward system. Thus, the bureaucratization with the explicit and implicit boundaries for practice left great leeway for manipulation of the intake process to select referrals that best fit the practitioner's perceptions of potential successful movement to outcomes that bring rewards from the system. Knowledge of what best suits the system's operational processes, and skills to select referrals and move them through the system, is often the higher priority focus for in-service training. Thus, the focus of training, from the system's management point of view, should be upon regulations, eligibility, the fit of client problems within these frames and rationales that allow the appropriate referral to get involved in the rehabilitative process and have successful outcome as measured in a "case rehabilitated."

The impact of management's view of "qualified personnel" may even go so far as to have management claim special privilege in the selection of who shall prepare to work in the system as professionals. These are but a few of the examples of the characteristics of bureaucratization as it relates to professionalization.

W. Richard Scott[12] has set out a

> . . .detailed description of the differences between bureaucratic and professional models of organization and four areas of role conflict

associated with these differences: (1) the professional's resistance to bureaucratic rules; (2) the professional's rejection of bureaucratic standards; (3) the professional's resistance to bureaucratic supervision; and (4) the professional's conditional loyalty to the bureaucracy.

Scott says that when professionals are employed in bureaucratic organizations there are two important theoretical problems that may be distinguished.

> First, professionals participate in two systems—the profession and the organization—and their dual membership places important restrictions on the organization's attempt to deploy them in a rational manner with respect to its own goals. Second, the profession and the bureaucracy rest on fundamentally different principles of organization, and these divergent principles generate conflicts between professionals and their employers in certain specific areas.

The work of a rehabilitation practitioner is a complicated job. If he has all the basic skills required for doing the work and has incorporated into his practice the norms and standards which will govern his performance and all others in like class have these same skills, each can perform the task independently of his colleagues. Each will apply the internalized standards to both his own work and that of his colleagues so that their performance is controlled by external surveillance. The primary control is that which each worker applies to it.

On the other hand, when activities are divided so that some workers perform certain ones and others perform different ones, and norms and standards are not internalized so that some system of rules must guide how the work will be done, some workers must be given the roles of interpreting and following through on the rules. Those who supervise must coordinate the efforts of the many to assure accomplishment of the task. Professionalization of rehabilitation counseling must take many twists and turns when practitioners cannot always differentiate clearly among the forces operating toward which goals under the above circumstances.

A BASIS FOR CONFLICT IN REHABILITATION COUNSELING

In 1954, when the passage of Public Law 565 provided for the federal funding of higher education programs for rehabilitation practitioners, there was conflict in the higher levels of administration as to where such training should be located, the structure or curriculum within universities with which the practice should be identified and the essential content of the curriculum. Some felt that since "rehabilitation counseling" had no image in "professional" practice (it got this designation as a job title "by a show of hands in 1946, remember!), and since "counseling" was the primary content of skill (and this decision was made without empirical data to back up such an assumption), therefore, the curriculum for purposes of acceptance by universities, as well as to give it some prestige, should be anchored in schools of social work or psychology or educational psychology or draw heavily on the content in such training. On the other hand, no real guidelines were laid down as to curriculum content in its broadest spectrum. The curriculum should be at graduate level, it was agreed.

As a result of this total situation, state agency administrators levered in some states to have the curricula set up in independent departments in cooperative schools; others allowed certain departments of psychology or social administration to take the initiative and organize the curricula along departmental lines as departmental heads perceived the need for curriculum content for training rehabilitation counselors. Many schools brought in counseling and clinical psychologists from the Veterans Administration and other rehabilitative institutional settings to guide the curriculum set with a bias toward psychological counseling. This hodgepodge without many similarities, except that behavioral science content must be a core element, was allowed to settle down into the task of training the "rehabilitation counselor" with primary emphasis on "counseling" skills.

Later the complaints began to arise from the rehabilitation agency administrators that graduates were not always good employees because they "knew nothing about vocational rehabilitation counseling" when the emphasis was on "rehabilitation," rather than on "counseling."

Discussion between administrators and educators have gradually brought about some curriculum changes in some schools but the conflict still exists to the extent that some agency administrators refuse to employ graduates of some curricula, preferring to hire their own staff and provide in-service training to turn them into the "professionals" they desire. For a number of years no more than half of university graduates in "rehabilitation counseling" have taken employment in public and private rehabilitation agencies, although some schools have a high rate of graduates taking employment in such agencies, while other schools have a much lower rate. Could there be conflict in role perceptions?

One wonders what the nature of training would be today if the show of hands in 1946 had given a rehabilitation practitioner a different title! One wonders how many universities would go on training rehabilitation practitioners if federal subsidies for teaching and stipends for students after fifteen years were to be suddenly suspended or phased out over a few years! Would there be a sufficient identity with a new social service professionalism to motivate universities to continue training? Would there be motivation among rehabilitation administrators to employ the graduates of these universities, unless the agencies could have more control over student selection and curriculum content? Would the outcomes add to the professionalization of practice? Can agencies and educators reach agreement so that the conflicts can be resolved in training practitioners who will move together with all forces to professionalization of practice? Do we need a new common basis and rationale for practice anchored in an applied science; a reorganization of knowledge systems, based upon a new perspective of the needs of disabled people from a survival frame of reference in today's complex world, perhaps even an ecological frame of reference as stated by Alvin D. Puth?[9] His conceptualizations on research policy has much for consideration in the practice of rehabilitation counseling.[10]

Can we design and carry out empirical research based on client needs and an appropriate process for relieving them and from this data reorganize knowledge and practice and perhaps find even a job title more appropriate than *rehabilitation counselor?* Can we test how special aspects of client needs are not being met by current professions, determine the overlap and unique aspects of their contributions and find a new profession to fill the gaps instead of seeking to become the all-encompassing practitioners that some would have us strive for?

These are questions and issues that lie at the heart of professionalizing an appropriate practice.

ASPECTS OF PROFESSIONALIZATION IN CURRENT PRACTICE

If professionalization is a *dynamic* process, then we must look into the dynamics for its evolutionary character. There were rehabilitative procedures and facilities functioning in American society over a hundred years before the rehabilitation counselor got his job title. There were certain knowledges about disabled persons and their needs before that time. There were certain values and underlying rationales for rendering services to disabled people before that time also.

On the other hand, there was not agreement on what constituted rehabilitation and its underlying rationale except primarily in an economic frame of reference. Nor was there agreement on the essential characteristics of practice by those who carried out functions within agencies offering rehabilitation services.

Standards for hiring rehabilitation workers in 1945 or 1946 varied among state and private rehabilitation agencies just as they do today. Salaries varied just as they do today. Work loads varied just as they do today. Workers came heavily from backgrounds in education as teachers or guidance or administrative personnel in education systems for reasons already set out elsewhere. They had baccalaureate or master's degrees in most states at that time and they also had experience in dealing with people—children and youth and their families. They had experience in dealing with some community agencies that related to children's and their families' problems.

With in-service training under supervision (I had four days under a supervisor in the hills of West Virginia before being on my own) and later short courses about disability and some of its concommitants, these rehabilitation workers *did* help many disabled persons back into the mainstream of living. In other words, there was a certain position of professionalization on the continuum of changing characteristics crucial in moving in the direction of a profession.

There were knowledges and skills yet to be developed; there were rehabilitative resources yet to be planned and constructed. There were cooperative relations with others who could and did assist in the task, such as physicians social workers, community agency personnel, employers, educators and a wide range of "helping-others" involved in the total task, whose skills and knowledges likewise were to be expanded such as my own. Certain "expertise," "autonomy," "commitment" and "responsibility" characterized my own and others practices in the rehabilitation process as it progressed at that time. A personal experience will illustrate.

We were serving very few paraplegics then because even the physicians had not learned much about the medical successes with this disabled group coming from experiences of World War II. Paraplegics from coal mine accidents had been referred to me by the Workmen's Compensation Commission in my state after they had exhausted all benefits under that program and were about to be sent home, more likely with decubitus ulcers than not, because physicians and nurses had not learned the best care techniques. Were medicine and nursing any less professionalized because of such ignorance? Was my practice any less professional as a rehabilitation worker when I visited such a referral in a remote shack on some coal company's property and looked down upon ulcers as large as saucers and later looked into the face of a pleading wife who was doing her best to take care of her man and say to her, "I'm sorry, but there is nothing that I nor my program can do at this time to help your husband?" Perhaps all of us could have contributed to professionalization of medicine and rehabilitation counseling if we had raised our problems by asking sharp questions of our respective fields as to why these problems could not be handled! In 1945 there were few places that were available to render such assistance to such a case, even if agency policy would have condoned the necessary expenditures. We didn't do much to seek change!

However, by 1949, I learned more about paraplegia in reading and talking with returned veterans and accepted my first case, a nurse whose back was broken in a car wreck on a slippery night. My administrator later chided me for accepting the case and for investing as much money in the case as I did. After a long struggle in a fairly new rehabilitation center where staff was also learning about paraplegia, she learned the skills and self-care that later allowed her to return to nursing in a limited capacity, working from her wheelchair. She is now supervisor of nurses in a nursing home. By 1948 I had moved further along the continuum of professionalization of my practice and so did every other rehabilitation worker who was committed to growth and development of his skills.

I entered graduate study in 1949 and completed my master's degree, majoring in guidance and with substantial credits in social work, to broaden my knowledge and skills. Out of my maturity and experience, I was able to ask questions that professors could not answer and sent me seeking further in reading and querying new resources. Were they less professionalized because of their ignorance or I more professionalized because of my knowledge and experience? Perhaps they should have helped me ask sharper questions and suggested in what places!

In this same interim, rehabilitation resources were being developed, old programs received new directions or new dimensions, and rehabilitation techniques were improved. New concerns were raised by new interest groups coming into the arena of disablement, such as the United Mine Workers of America, the Liberty Mutual Insurance Company, new organizations for certain disability groups, social security and others. Such groups began to challenge the limited scope of traditional agency services and practices in rehabilitation.

The criteria of eligibility and lower thresholds of feasibility, a term used so much by rehabilitation workers in administrative assignment for the selection of cases with which they were willing to work, were applied in the decade of the fifties. New knowledge and skills were gained in training, research in medicine and other aspects of rehabilitation and with increased development of rehabilitation facilities and federal and state financing. The patterns of development and expansion varied from state to state, however, depending much upon administrative leadership, state financial inputs of matching federal funds and a climate for innovation. The Federal Government with a great deal of influence of private lobbying interests was able to liberalize financing and expand program elements in support of improved services to disabled persons, still primarily from a rationale for fitting such persons to contribute economically. All of this contributed to moving rehabilitation counseling practice further along the continuum to increase professionalization, especially for those rehabilitation workers who were willing to grow through every opportunity for training, new experiences and willingness to work with new disability groups not previously very prevalent in case loads, such as the mentally retarded, the mentally ill, the more seriously physically disabled, the hard-core welfare client, et cetera. Of course, there were many practitioners who stopped on the continuum of professionalization at various points because they felt they knew what best rehabilitation practice was or that nothing new could be learned in advanced training. There were some who got master's degrees and have since taken very little training in continuing education with or without additional graduate credit. They, too, have stopped on the continuum toward professionalization of practice. Such workers have failed to realize that knowledge in rehabilitation and demands for services to increased disabled populations and new target groups makes this a rapidly changing field. *Just to stand still is to go backwards in rehabilitation today in relation to needed knowledge and skills.*

It can be said for rehabilitation practitioners that most have become concerned with professionalization and want to exhibit characteristics of growth in that process. However, there is yet much movement to be made.

ELEMENTS IN PROFESSIONALIZATION

According to Gross:[4]

As any occupation approaches professional status, there occur important internal structural changes and changes in the relation of practitioners to society at large. A useful way of discussing these changes is by reference to criteria of professionalization: the unstandardized product, degree of personality involvement of the professional, wide knowledge of a specialized technique, sense of obligation, sense of group identity and significance of service to society.

Ernest Greenwood[3] says that:

> ...after a careful canvass of sociological literature on occupations [he] has been able to distill five elements, upon which there appears to be consensus among students of the subject, as constituting the distinguishing attributes of a profession. Succinctly put, all professions seem to possess: (1) a systematic theory, (2) authority, (3) community sanction, (4) ethical codes and (5) a culture.

If we attempt to relate these attributes to rehabilitation counseling and within the framework of Cogan's definition of a profession set out earlier, there may be grave doubts as to whether our practice yet has all these attributes even though we can identify evidence of some. For example, the skills characterized in a profession emanate from knowledge organized into an internally consistent system, a *body of theory,* consisting of abstract propositions that generally describe that or those phenomena which is the profession's primary interest. Mastery of skill requires a mastery of theory underlying that skill. Training, then, must involve preoccupation with systematic theory to a considerable degree. Under such circumstances, preparation for the profession must be both an intellectual and a practical experience. Theoretical knowledge is much more difficult to master than operational routines and therefore requires more training from the service or operational setting toward the formal educational setting (university) as the function of theory becomes more important to application of skills.

In the rehabilitation counseling field, there is little or no theory based upon empirical and systematic research as a basis for formulations and rationality for what we do, particularly as it relates to giving us the knowledge about the meaning of disability, the meaning of rehabilitation and the meaning of processes that are carried out. We still hold on to traditional definitions, based on early 1900 attitudes, economic primacy of objectives and a work ethic that becomes harder and harder to justify in the current context in which work is done and has meaning in our society. Rather we should be eager and ready to discard any portion of the system with a formulation demonstrated by research to be more valid.

A spirit of rationality stimulates self-criticism and theoretical controversy. It is time for a researcher-theoretician to emerge in rehabilitation counseling and help us search for and develop theoretical systematization even if we have to find a new job title and reconstruction of application of knowledge and skill out of new possible formulations. Even a reorganization of knowledge may be necessary for appropriate formulations.

The current status of professionalization of our practice has not yet attained this attribute. Even though professionalism in our society is being challenged, it is not upon this attribute of a systematic body of theory that the challenge is focused. The humanitarianism in today's society may offer us some new climate for research in rehabilitation. At this time, however, the theoretical base for rehabilitation counseling has not crystallized to the extent that it can furnish support for autonomous practice.

If we follow Greenwood's distinguishing attributes further and look at *professional authority,* here we find some interesting speculations for rehabilitation practitioners and professionalization.

We call those who receive our services "clients." This puts a label upon them with negative connotations as compared to our own status in relation to them, which gives us the positive image. They are supposedly ignorant of theoretical background and the character of their needs and the frame of reference for meeting them, as the professional perceives them. Therefore, the client must submit to the authority and monopoly of professional judgment of the practitioner. However, the professional's *authority function* should be confined to those areas of expertise in which he is educated and skilled if he is to abide by operational ethics in his service. Talcott Parsons[8] calls this quality *functional specificity* and it has many implications for the client-rehabilitation counselor relationship, among them being: "(1) one cannot prescribe guides for facets of the client's life where the professional's theoretical competence does not apply, and (2) one cannot exploit the client for purposes of personal gratification."

Another extension of authority by the professional group is in seeking and obtaining *social sanction*. Control over training curricula by an accreditation process; over admission to the profession by certification and licensure for screening those qualified to practice; over privileged communication and an immunity from community judgment on technical matters relating to the profession—all are extensions of authority within the profession and sought with community sanction.

Rehabilitation counseling has not yet spelled out its unique *functional specificity* nor its areas of expertise. Yet the field is seeking social sanction in certification and licensure in some places (California). Some practitioners question whether the practice is ready for these courses of action, while others hold that the forces that operate to keep the practice under the control of service systems slow the process toward professionalization and keep the members of professional groups from exercising control over much of their own work destiny, aspirations and opportunities for crystallizing an identity in professional practice. Rehabilitation practitioners are working side by side with those who have such professional identity; they make major judgments that affect courses of action in behaviors of other professionals in relation to client needs and yet do not have comparable identity and status that goes with such responsibility.

The service ideal, a base of technical competence and autonomy in practice as basic conditions in professionalization do have some visibility in rehabilitation counseling practice, even in state and private agency structures, but it is sometimes difficult for practitioners in these systems to understand the degree of their manifestation.[6] However, these are the very elements that must be demonstrated as the basis for any legal sanction or regulation such as certification or licensure.

> Certification is the milder of the two concepts in respect to its ramification upon professional practice. It generally includes a statement of the profession's goals, a definition of practice in very general terms, a set of qualifications for acceptance, a statement on the standards of practice and procedures for examinations and disciplinary actions. As a legal regulation, certification puts fewer constraints upon practice

says Johnson,[5] compared to licensure.

Has rehabilitation counseling answered the question as to why it is in business to the satisfaction of all those who practice it and of society? Formulations are not very explicit because an appropriate *raison d'etre* has not yet been agreed upon by all concerned parties. A glance at the introductory paragraph in an article by Anthony and Carkhuff[1] reveals little or no agreement upon roles and functions, orientation of training or areas of specialization. It acknowledges the limitations of research to find the basis of service. There are those that acknowledge that the *absolute* of productivity or work as the goal of rehabilitation outcomes with disabled people served in vocational rehabilitation programs is too limited. There are others who are equally certain that the goals of self-actualization and improved skills for survival of the disabled are too encompassing and not unique to rehabilitation counseling practice alone.

Like social work, the professionalization of rehabilitation counseling will only be as successful as its efforts in cooperating with other helping professions, so that disabled clients can attain optimal capacity for self-management and no longer need rehabilitation counseling services, except in extreme cases requiring continued follow-up. Because outcomes are the function of many contributions of many professions and systems of service in which the "counselor" may have been the primary facilitator, integrator, individualizer, expeditor, coordinator, crystallizer or some other such action agent, he cannot claim that his impact was primarily responsible for successful outcome. These behaviors, both in relation to developing client insights, motivation, sustained participation in a rehabilitative process and growth in self-actualization, cannot be claimed to be the unique contribution of rehabilitation counseling or the outcome of counseling by such a practitioner alone.

What is the base of real technical competence in rehabilitation counseling? The rehabilitation practitioner does use and puts into operation a great deal of material and information contributed by other disciplines (often without much training in the frame of reference from whence they come) in addition to his own contributions. The community and all its institutions are in his arena of action when such systems, their manipulation, or change, are necessary to help the disabled person reach his goals. Not only is he a change agent in use of his relationships with his client for greater client insights and clarification of alternatives for courses of action open to him, but also he is a change agent in social systems to accommodate and enhance his client's self-actualization. These elements in practice are not unique to the rehabilitation counselor, however. Social work has great vitality in these processes.

It can be said that rehabilitation counseling practice does have (a) values, but such cannot be legalized in licensure; (b) a growing body of knowledge and skills, but is not ready with a rational base founded upon empirical evidence, however, and, thus, cannot be licensed upon this basis, although organizational certification might be feasible upon such a limited base as we have; (c) the helping relationship that operates over a wide spectrum with the client and others, but licensure would likely limit the scope of relationship involvement in the rehabilitation process, although certification may not; (d) a conscious use of self as a change agent but skills in this realm are functions of growth and education and should not be regulated by licensure; and (e) an outcome or goal orientation as the focus of practice rather than a clinical therapeutic approach, but this cannot be regulated by licensure. So we can speculate that the practice can embrace organizational certification *only* at this time, not licensure, and thereby attain some community sanction.

Autonomy in practice, the competence to engage in self-regulated practice, implies that one must work in accord with norms of the profession by strict adherence to a code of ethics, agreed upon by all who are to practice as rehabilitation counselors. Efforts to date to have practitioners contribute to the development of such a code and thereby identify with it and apply sanctions against those who violate it have been disappointing. Armchair codes are easily come by but those developed out of the critical incidents in the daily practice of rehabilitation counselors are more difficult to develop and adopt. Why?

Some suggest that practitioners in this field do not yet have a sufficient professional identity, commitment to high quality practice, a theory or *raison d'etre* for their practice which they can translate into a rationale requiring a professionalized pattern of behavior in serving the disabled. Others say that such behavior cannot be expected when practitioners identify with or adopt the goals of the structure in which they work as primary over the goals of clients whom they service. In other words, it is not always clear "for whom they work," the client or the agency.

Since rehabilitation counselors work primarily in bureaucracies, these structures "often play a co-operative role in respect to the practitioners' adherence to professional norms" as related by Johnson.[5] Since most practitioners in this field work in agency structures and under supervision, it is doubtful if full autonomous activity can be sanctioned and thereby hangs the block to legal regulation in licensure.

Certification within guidelines agreed upon by both the National Rehabilitation Counseling Association and the American Rehabilitation Counseling Association and implemented nationally could be made consistent with the state of the practice only when there can be agreement reached upon the body of skills and knowledges requisite for this field of practice and training is geared to provide them.

There is not yet a "culture" that sustains this practice. Standards for employment are dictated by the administrative structures in which practitioners are employed. Recruitment to the field, both for employment and training, has no supporting rationale or active structural participation. Much of the rationale for recruitment is based upon assumptions and generalizations both by fellow practitioners and administrative personnel. These generalizations operate somewhat in this fashion: "I have found that coaches in high schools work well with youth, and a few that I have hired worked out very well, therefore, coaches make good rehabilitation counselors." Similar rationales go for ministers, teachers, personnel men and others. There is even evidence that indigenous aides are employed because they are ex-alcoholics or ex–something-else, ergo, they can work best with alcoholics. Unfortunately, this is too much the kind of rationalization that goes on in recruitment in many agencies today. Of course, there are more enlightened techniques used by more enlightened practitioners and administrators, but it is this wide range of recruitment and employment practices that has brought many people into rehabilitation counseling practice without sufficiently organized in-service training plans or advanced training opportunities to help them develop the kind of identity and growth that moves them along the continuum toward professionalization of practice.

The culture of a profession includes its values, its norms, its symbols. Rehabilitation counseling has some characteristics of a culture but these are not well developed or identified. Most agree that rehabilitation counseling is a social good and that community welfare would be impaired without it. Practitioners generally hold that they are wiser about service-related matters than the laity or their clients. They believe that they should have professional authority and have the force of a group value.

Some rehabilitation counselors manifest some of the norms of a professional group. There are some role definitions. There are some who follow the prescribed processes for seeking admission to the profession and professional organizations or for advancement in the hierarchical structures for practice. There are proper ways for accepting referrals, receiving them or dismissing them, of questioning and working with them, of continuing with them or rejecting them. There are many evidences of behavioral norms relating to a variety of situations, most often within a service agency structure.

Then, there are the symbols of the profession as a part of the "culture." These include the certificates, the insignias, some history, the journal, the organization's heroes, sometimes its villains, its stereotypes of the good client or poor client, the professional and *ad infinitum*.

Then, of course, there is the career concept, the professional attitude toward work, not a means to an end but an end in itself. The professional receives the intrinsic rewards as primary and monetary gain, secondarily. A total personal involvement exists, the "shop talk" permeates social discourse, and the profession becomes a whole social environment. These are the cultural characteristics of professionalization. Rehabilitation counseling has many of these characteristics of its culture.

SUMMARY

Where, then, is rehabilitation counseling on the road to professionalization?

It has some characteristics in practice that justify calling it an "emerging" profession. Efforts are being made to identify its uniquenesses, its *raison d'etre*, its standards of practice. There is effort to develop a code of ethics and to attain some community sanction through at least a certification process, even if limited or sanctioned within the professional organization's structure alone. There is evidence of some characteristics of a culture to which practitioners are striving to add or contribute.

On the other hand, there still is the challenge for development of systematic theory which at this time is still somewhat nebulous except that which emanates primarily from an economic justification and this is too shifty to hold as an anchor for professionalization. A great deal of effort, research, conceptualization and formulations have yet to be done in this area. The National Rehabilitation Association as a primary citizen interest group and the two professional associations, the National Rehabilitation Counseling Association and the American Rehabilitation Counseling Association, are prime organizations for assuming some of these responsibilities for developing new formulations. Their members, through their membership support and involvement, can contribute to this effort. Less than half of all known rehabilitation counselors belong to the latter two organizations, however.

Authority as an attribute is still bound heavily in regulatory and legal structure for a majority of practitioners, although within such structures there is great maneuverability in mobilizing total resources for clients. The limits are often imposed more by the practitioner's own limited vision than inadequate underlying systematic theory and knowledge and skill and by the other limits imposed upon him. Demands placed upon him by the work structure leave little time for reflection, introspection or developmental opportunities for broadening his vision, however.

At any rate, it is a stimulating field of practice to enter, to help to shape and from which to derive satisfactions when one assumes the attitude "that not to be sure is the best road to learning" and growing toward professionalization. Rehabilitation counseling is a challenging career upon which to embark. Continuous searching for new knowledge and skills moves the practice further toward professionalization. That professionalization does not come from the efforts of one practitioner working alone, however. It comes from a sense of need for helping all practitioners in rehabilitation counseling to move together toward professionalization.

REFERENCES

1. Anthony, W. A., and Carkhuff, R. R.: Effects of training on rehabilitation counseling trainee functioning. *Rehab Counseling Bull*, Vol. 13, No. 4, June 1970.
2. Cogan, Morris L.: Toward a definition of profession. *Harvard Educational Review*, Vol. 23, Winter 1953.
3. Greenwood, Ernest: Attributes of a profession. *Social Work*, Vol. 11, No. 3, July 1957.
4. Gross, Edward: *Work and Society*. New York, Thomas Y. Crowell Co., 1958.
5. Johnson, Donald E.: Legal regulation of the social work profession. *Social Casework*, Vol. 51, No. 9, November 1970.
6. McCauley, W. Alfred: The power, practice and problems of rehabilitation counseling, *NRCA Professional Bulletin*, Vol. 8, No. 3, May 1967.
7. Obermann, C. Esco: *A History of Vocational Rehabilitation in America*. Minneapolis, T. S. Dennison and Company, Inc., 1965.
8. Parsons, Talcott: The professions and social structure. *Social Forces*, Vol. 17, May 1939.
9. Puth, Alvin D.: Rehabilitation Counselor—T.H.E. Therapeutic Human Ecologist. *NRCA Professional Bulletin*, Vol. X, No. 1, January 1969.
10. Puth, Alvin D.: Key considerations in developing basic NRA policy on scientific rehabilitation research. *J Rehab*, Vol. 36, No. 6, November-December 1970.
11. Strauss, George: Professionalism and occupational association. *Industrial Relations*, Vol. 11, No. 3, May 1963.
12. Vollmer, Howard M., and Mills, Donald L. (Ed.): *Professionalization*. Englewood Cliffs, Prentice-Hall, Inc., 1966.

PART THREE

THE REHABILITATION PROCESS

Case Finding
Work Evaluation: An Overview
Techniques of Counseling in the Rehabilitation Process
Selective Training
Vocational Placement

7

Case Finding

John M. Cobun

General Consideration for Adequate Referral Systems
Sources of Referral
Additional Case-Finding Techniques
References

A LTHOUGH CASE FINDING has been considered to be a technical part of the casework process, the development of case-finding techniques has been generally either overlooked or considered to be of a minor significance. The purpose of this chapter will be to indicate that case finding is of prime importance since all subsequent parts of the casework process depend upon the location and initiation of services for persons who can be helped most by vocational rehabilitation.

In the early days of vocational rehabilitation in the United States, the development of case-finding techniques was not a particular problem. Prior to the passage of the 1965 Amendments to the Vocational Rehabilitation Act, Public Law 333, vocational rehabilitation was generally considered to be the privilege of a select few rather than a legal right of all who met the criteria for eligibility. It had been accepted, at least unofficially, that state rehabilitation programs were serving only a small percentage of the citizens who should be eligible for services. State agencies were grossly understaffed with rehabilitation counselors. In many instances, a counselor was responsible for a large territory and was practically autonomous in his selection of cases and in the determination of their eligibility for services. The general pattern was that he was employed by the state agency, assigned to a territory or a particular type of case load, provided a certain amount of case service funds with which to purchase needed services and oriented to the work of the rehabilitation counselor by actually performing on the job. In most instances, he received more referrals than he could adequately process, so it was quite expedient to accept only those persons who were most insistent or who showed the greatest potential for being rehabilitated in a short period of time. Unfortunately, unless the counselor was very conscientious and properly grounded in the philosophy of vocational rehabilitation, persons who were most in need of services were often screened out and never became a part of the actual case load. The rationale for these actions was that, after all, why should the counselor spend time and energy in the development of referral sources when through his normal activities he was able to locate more cases than he could adequately serve? For the most part, the client who was rejected for service had little or no recourse concerning the counselor's decision.

The passage of the 1965 Amendments to the Vocational Rehabilitation Act did much to affect the case-finding responsibilities of state vocational rehabilitation agencies. As previously noted, with the passage of this piece of legislation, vocational rehabilitation services became the right of every citizen rather than the privilege of a few. Considerable emphasis was placed on the necessity for the development of plans whereby each state would assume the responsibility for seeing that all handicapped persons who were eligible for, and who could profit from, vocational rehabilitation services would be receiving such services by 1975. Along with many other changes in the structure of the state programs, this necessitated the development of a more sophisticated plan for locating handicapped persons. No longer would the rehabilitation worker be able to make arbitrary decisions concerning eligibility for service. The handicapped person who was rejected for service would be notified in writing of the decision and would have the right of appeal of the decision through a specifically designated appeal process.

GENERAL CONSIDERATION FOR ADEQUATE REFERRAL SYSTEMS

It seems unnecessary to say that before a person can benefit from vocational rehabilitation services he must be first made aware of the fact that such services are available. The rehabilitation worker must realize that the success of his efforts will be in direct proportion to the number and type of individuals who are referred to him for service. Without the proper input of clients who could profit from the efforts of the rehabilitation agency, the counselor's efforts to serve his referral population are doomed to failure. In addition to the fact that state and federal regulations stipulate that each citizen is entitled to know about available vocational rehabilitation services, it is simply good practice to assist in the dissemination of this information so that the program may be conducted most effectively. Much time and effort will be saved in the processing of referrals if persons who are applying for service are made aware of the nature and purposes of the program prior to their filing an application.

The method of development of referral systems is determined to a large extent by the setting in which the agency representative is working. The counselor who is assigned to a rural area and has the sole responsibility for the provision of services within that area will operate in a somewhat different manner than will the person who is working in a more urban area. It is quite possible that the rural counselor will know on a first-name basis many of the persons who are employed by other governmental agencies who are potential referral sources within his territory. He will often be affiliated with a religious group and one or more service organizations and will thus have the opportunity to come in contact with persons who will know of potential candidates for vocational rehabilitation. Although the range of placement possibilities may be somewhat limited due to the number of industries within this type of territory, the counselor has the advantage of knowing personally many of the employers and thus will be in a position not only to make effective placements but also to receive referrals of persons who are injured in industrial accidents or who are generally known as part of the community. He is usually able to develop more clear-cut vocational plans for handicapped persons because of a knowledge of specific placement possibilities following the completion of these plans.

The counselor employed in the urban setting will find himself in an entirely different situation. He will be one of a number of persons employed by the agency to work in a given territory. His assignment may be for a specific location or to work with a particular project or a specific disability category. He will be encountering other agencies who have a number of persons employed, and it thus becomes more difficult for him to develop the personal approach as employed by the rural counselor. He is unable to develop a more sophisticated system of referral. In most instances, cases will be assigned to him with no effort being required on his part.

Guidelines for effective case finding which are usually discussed seem to be more applicable to the situation experienced by the rural counselor than for the person working in the urban setting. It is generally considered to be good practice to make the referral process as simple as possible for the person who is referring the individual to the agency and for the person who is being referred. Although official referral forms may be developed, the completion of such forms should not be a requirement required before a person may become known to the agency. Individuals and agencies should be encouraged to make referrals in the most convenient manner whether it be by the agency's forms or by personal or telephone contact.

The agency should strive toward the development of an open-door policy so that persons may walk in at any time and apply for service. This principle works quite well when the office is dealing with only a small number of applicants, but it becomes more difficult when larger numbers of persons are being considered. Without a systematic method of handling "walk-ins," counselors can become completely engulfed with referrals to the point that they are incapable of providing adequate services. Many urban offices find it necessary to assign one or more persons as intake counselors to process all referrals coming to the agency and then assign cases to certain counselors according to territories or other types

Case Finding 181

of work assignments. This method of control makes for a more equitable case load for all counselors working within the assigned area. Modifications of this system can be made to handle the situation whereby a person or agency may make a referral with the specific request that the case be handled by a particular counselor. One potential drawback to intake counselor method of assigning cases is that if all referrals are to be distributed among all counselors, the individual counselor may cease to exert efforts to develop good referrals since he can see no immediate reward for doing so. The agency as a whole has the responsibility for public relations by maintaining contact with individuals and other agencies within the community. Persons in charge should assign each counselor the responsibility for maintaining contact with certain agencies so that no one agency will be contacted by many persons while other agencies get few contacts.

One of the prime considerations in the development of a case-finding system should be that all referrals will be processed as quickly as possible. This is necessary not only for the maintenance of interest on the part of the client but also to encourage additional referrals from the referral source. Nothing will cause the referral process to break down more rapidly than will the development of the feeling that referrals are made to the agency and that nothing happens to them. The person receiving the referral should report back immediately to the referring agency indicating not only that the referral has been received but also what action can be anticipated. This is particularly true for reporting back to persons who have not made previous referrals and also for individuals who are not attached to agencies and who are not generally thought of as being required to make referrals. As an example, if a physician is making a referral, and particularly if he is to continue to be involved in the treatment of the individual, he will be interested in knowing what action is taken by the rehabilitation agency on behalf of his patient. The best method to assure additional referrals from a desirable source is to make certain that a good job is done with the first referral made to the agency. This involves not only properly serving the client but also letting the referral source know what action has been taken.

As a general rule, vocational rehabilitation agencies should develop procedures whereby referrals will occur early in the period of disability. This is particularly true in the case of industrial accidents and other traumatically induced disabilities. Perhaps a distinction should be made here between the acceptance of the referral and the actual contact of the client by the counselor. In certain instances, it is possible that the counselor can make contact with the client at too early a date. Particularly with cases such as traumatic blindness, paraplegia and quadraplegia, if contacted too soon, the client may not be able to psychologically accept the physical limitations which will ultimately be imposed upon him. In these instances, the counselor may wish to note the referral and then contact the family or the physician to let them know that he will be available to begin working with the disabled individual when it is considered to be the proper time. Should the counselor insist on moving ahead and contacting the client before he is psychologically ready to accept his limitations, it is possible that damage could be done to the relationship with the client that the counselor would be unable to overcome at a later date. The important thing to consider is that the counselor should be ready and available to the client at the earliest feasible time in the period of disability.

The development of referral sources and good case load management are quite closely related. Counselors who are working with a general case load should exert efforts to develop referrals from all agencies who are serving the handicapped within their territory, or who generally would be in a position to know of potential clients. He should attempt to receive a well-balanced variety of disabilities so that he does not become too active with any one disability category. If the counselor is not constantly aware of good case load management practices, it is quite easy for him to develop the practice of getting more cases from agencies where he is better known or of disability categories with which he is most familiar at the expense of overlooking agencies or disability categories which should be receiving services. Constant efforts must be made to develop systems whereby referrals will be arriving on a continuous basis rather than on a hit-and-miss situation.

SOURCES OF REFERRAL

The sources through which disabled persons may become known to state agencies may be classified as primary sources, secondary sources or tertiary sources. Primary sources are usually those which perform some direct service for disabled persons early in the history of disablement. These include physicians, hospitals, schools, workmen's compensation commissions, state or local health departments and so forth. It is these sources which are generally considered to be most valuable to the program and it is upon them that the greatest amount of effort should be made since it is usually with the clients referred by them that agencies are able to do their best work. This is true for a number of reasons. It is important to reach cases as early in the history of disability as possible in order to minimize the demoralizing effect of the idleness and hopelessness which almost invariably results from long-standing disabilities. Also, as previously noted, rehabilitation can always be accomplished much more easily in the early stages of disability before habits of idleness and dependency have been formed and while the client retains certain skills and abilities as have not been directly affected by the disability. Another reason for the emphasis on working with primary sources of referral is that it is economically desirable to outfit them for remunerative employment with as little delay as possible.

Secondary sources are those which provide some service to the disabled person after the period of convalescence, usually when the client has some definite plan for his future. Examples of this type of source are state employment services, public and private welfare agencies, sheltered workshops and veteran's associations. It can readily be seen that although secondary sources provide a large number of referrals, some of which are good prospects for rehabilitation, these are frequently cases of comparatively long standing and the services which can be rendered to them are sometimes limited.

Tertiary services are those which provide only incidental services to the disabled, or in some cases none at all, or which come in contact with persons who might benefit from vocational rehabilitation services. Examples of such sources might be private trade and business schools, artificial limb companies and interested individuals. While many excellent referrals may come from these sources, it must be remembered that they may not be familiar with the policies and standards of the rehabilitation agency and may often refer persons for whom no service can be performed. Thus, much effort may be expended in the processing of referrals which will not become active cases with vocational rehabilitation. This is not intended to minimize the importance of this type of referral source, but merely to emphasize the need of the rehabilitation worker for close continuous cooperation with persons and agencies who can refer clients at the time when their need can be recognized most readily and their potentiality utilized most effectively.

Most state agencies are organizationally designed into the levels of state headquarters, district or regional level, and the local level at which the counselor operates. As with any other part of the program, in the development of referral sources each level of operation has its own unique responsibility. It is the responsibility of the state office to establish and maintain cooperative written relationships with other agencies and organizations on a statewide basis. This provides the overall guidelines and organization under which the regional and local level personnel can operate. The state office should be also responsible for general statewide publicity such as that provided by the Governor's Committee to Promote Employment of the Handicapped. It will be responsible for the preparation of pamphlets and printed material for publicity and general public relations activities throughout the state.

At the regional level, emphasis should be placed on the development of policies and procedures for the development of referral services on a more concentrated level then would be done on the state level. Specific attention should be given to agencies and individuals who are present on a regional but not on a state basis, with the person in charge of the district or regional office providing the impetus for these activities.

It is at the local level where the primary responsibility lies for

Case Finding   185

the development of referral sources. Only the person who operates within the local office can know about the peculiar situations which must be considered for the effective development of methods of referral within his own area, and no amount of activity from the two higher levels can effectively do the job. It is the counselor who must resort to regular visits to referral agencies, the acceptance and proper processing of referrals and the reporting back to the referral agencies on the disposition of the cases. It is he who must conduct the public relations activities on a personal basis since he will be ultimately working with the disabled individuals.

ADDITIONAL CASE-FINDING TECHNIQUES

In the early days of the vocational rehabilitation program, it was generally believed that all that was necessary to reach the handicapped population was to develop referrals on a "come-and-get-it" basis. By this we mean that it was commonly accepted that if the general population knew about the agency, the services which were available and where the office was located, persons in need of these services would rush to the doors of the agency requesting such services. We now know that these assumptions are simply not true. People often will not contact the agency on their own, and in such instances, vocational rehabilitation workers must develop special techniques for locating these persons.

The early vocational rehabilitation worker was typically a white, middle-class, male of early middle age who operated the program as if all of his clients were of the same background. He found it difficult to relate to individuals who came from other socioeconomic backgrounds and, therefore, the preponderance of cases served were those who generally came from the same type background as that of the counselor. Today, considerable effort is being made to reach persons from lower socioeconomic levels who are probably more in need of service than are the persons who were formerly being served. Numerous studies have shown that these persons often do not respond to the simple information techniques which vocational rehabilitation agencies have used in the past. Many of these referrals have been exposed to so many government agencies that it is impossible for them to understand that vocational rehabilitation is not just another social agency. It is extremely difficult for them to realize that they will be treated as individuals and that one person will be available to assist them in looking at their problems and in developing an individual plan for overcoming many of these problems which are caused by lack of employment. There are additional reasons found concerning why persons will not contact the agency. They often confuse it with public welfare and because of personal pride do not wish to apply. They do not fully understand what the agency is "all about" and are afraid that they will be required to undergo certain physical restoration procedures; they often believe they will be required to repay any cost involved in the rehabilitation process or, in many instances, because of their current way of life which has been brought about by long periods of frustration, they are simply not motivated to the point where they will assume a positive role in the solving of their economic problems.

A number of approaches have been tried to develop referrals in addition to the classical one of requiring the client to initiate the request for service. One approach is to utilize the success stories of individuals who have been successfully rehabilitated to demonstrate to potential clients that the rehabilitation process does work. As an example, for a number of years the State of Maryland conducted a public service television program called "Comeback," in which successfully rehabilitated clients appeared and told their story of vocational rehabilitation. This success story may be done through the mass media or it may be utilized on a more local, personal basis.

In the last several years, much effort has been put forth to advertise vocational rehabilitation services through mass media. Examples of such are television station spot announcements and advertisements in newspapers sponsored by organizations such as the President's Committee to Promote Employment of the Handicapped or by private employers. It can be seen readily that this approach has certain limitations because of the fact that the people who should be receiving the message are the least likely to have access to the media being used.

A rather unique approach has been developed by a number of state agencies to reach certain groups of generally inaccessible potential clients such as drug addicts, alcoholics and the socially disadvantaged. This approach calls for the employment of nonprofessionals as indigenous workers or case aides to assist the counselor in not only locating persons but also in providing services to these individuals once they have been located. This approach has been particularly successful in some ghetto areas of the large cities where the typical professional rehabilitation worker is not accepted in the home area and is totally unable to speak the language of the client. In these instances, the case aide will be hired from the local home area, will assist the agency by explaining the program to the local citizens to get them in touch with the agency and will further assist the process by acting as an intermediary between the professional counselor and the client.

It may be summarized that none of these methods for getting potential clients to the agency will work satisfactorily in all cases. In some instances, the client initiative method will be all that is required. In others, when the population either will not initiate the action or cannot do so, it is the responsibility of the rehabilitation worker to locate and urge the individual to avail himself of the services of the agency. It is only in this way that the rehabilitation program can say that it is adequately fulfilling the vocational needs of the handicapped citizens of the community.

REFERENCES

1. McGowan, J. F., and Porter, T. L. (Eds.): *An Introduction to the Vocational Rehabilitation Process.* Washington, D.C., U.S. Department of Health, Education and Welfare, 1967.
2. Thomason, B., and Barrett, A. M. (Eds.): *Casework Performance in Vocational Rehabilitation.* Washington, D.C., U.S. Department of Health, Education and Welfare, 1959.
3. Rusalim, H., and Baxt, R.: *Delivering Rehabilitation Services.* Washington, D.C., U.S. Department of Health, Education and Welfare, 1969.
4. *Report of the National Citizens Advisory Committee on Vocational Rehabilitation.* Washington, D.C., U.S. Department of Health, Education and Welfare, 1968.

8

Work Evaluation: An Overview

Paul R. Hoffman

Definitions
Historical Background
Theory of Work Evaluation
Educational Qualifications for Work Evaluators
Methodologies of Work Evaluation
Factors Evaluated
Utilization of Work Evaluation
Responsibilities of Rehabilitation Counselor and Work Evaluator
Work Evaluation Today and Tomorrow
Summary
References

W ORK EVALUATION has become a positive force in helping to assess the vocational strengths and weaknesses of the handicapped and disadvantaged and to develop a plan to assist them in obtaining a more meaningful and rewarding place in society. Although work evaluation has not proved to be a panacea that helps us towards adequate assessment and development of adequate plans in all cases where we previously failed, it has become an important technique that has helped us where before we were failing.

DEFINITIONS

There are a number of terms in this field which are ill-defined and, unfortunately, cause considerable confusion at this time. These are the terms of *prevocational evaluation, vocational evaluation, work evaluation* and *work adjustment*.

The term *prevocational evaluation* means different things to different people. To some professionals, it means the evaluation of such factors as activities of daily living, social development and basic educational abilities. These are characteristics which an individual must have before he can even consider preparing for a vocation or being evaluated for a vocation. The term *vocational evaluation* came into vogue in the fifties; however, then it was utilized more in relation to the evaluation of aptitudes, potentials and abilities, the type of evaluation we now refer to as work evaluation. The author's preference would be to limit the term *prevocational evaluation* to the former concept.

Vocational evaluation for some has been defined as evaluation for pertinent medical, psychological, vocational, educational, cultural, social and environmental factors. For others, it has been defined as a more limited endeavor—that is, the evaluation of an individual's vocational strengths and weaknesses through the utilization of work, real or simulated. Work evaluation is never defined as the broad concept that was mentioned for vocational evaluation but as evaluation of vocational strengths and weaknesses of the handicapped and disadvantaged through the utilization of some specific methodologies, mainly the utilization of work, real or simulated.

Work adjustment, a treatment process utilizing work or aspects of work to modify behavior, is also at times defined as an evaluation process. It is not an evaluation process but is, as the words indicate, an adjustment or treatment process. While evaluation does take place during work adjustment, the objectives of the evaluation are different from that of the work evaluation process. In work evaluation, the objectives are to assess the vocational strengths and weaknesses as related to developing a vocational plan. In work adjustment, the objectives are to determine the success or failure of the adjustment plan and to determine when to terminate the work adjustment process. Prevocational, vocational and work evaluation are assessment processes, and work adjustment is a treatment process.

Confusion does exist in the field in relation to these terms, and there is a need for standardization. In this chapter, it will be necessary to use the terms *work evaluation* and *vocational evalua-*

tion interchangeably. In relation to the author's own thoughts and reference to some sources, the term *work evaluation* is used. In reference to some other sources, the term *vocational evaluation* is used. The process being referred to is the assessment of vocational strengths and weaknesses through the utilization of work, real or simulated, for the purpose of developing a vocational plan of action.

HISTORICAL BACKGROUND

Work evaluation is not new, although it has been gathering considerable momentum in the last few years. Morton Bregman,[1] in a speech entitled "The Use and Misuse of Vocational Evaluation in the Counseling Process," noted that in World War I, the Portvillez School in Belgium believed a disabled soldier could be helped to select an appropriate trade training program only by trying out in several trade classes. By this method of evaluation, the soldier could select a course in which he was interested and in which he had showed a potential. Mr. Bregman further noted the development of the scientific job analysis and the early work of Munsterberg, one of the pioneers in the field of psychological testing. When confronted with the problem of developing a test to select streetcar operators for the Boston Railroad Company, Munsterberg built a model streetcar on which he was able to try out prospective operators.

Psychometric testing became a force in this country during the 1900's. Of special importance to the field of work evaluation were job performance tests developed by the military during the Second World War. For example, the United States Air Force developed the two-hand coordination test as part of the Air Force Classification Test Battery and, to help select pilots, the complex coordinator test which required a person who has never flown a plane to operate a stick and rudder bar on an instrument on which he had to follow a pattern flashed before him.

There is a situational or simulated approach to testing in which the client is placed in an actual work situation. This technique has been the mainstay of work evaluation in the sheltered workshop movement, where it had developed to the greatest extent. Situational evaluation in a sheltered workshop mainly takes the form of placing a client on the production line in the workshop. The situational technique was utilized in a different setting in a planned, applied manner by the Office of Strategic Services during World War II, when they set up problem-solving situations in which groups of men were placed in actual conditions with resource materials available but not specified. The personnel in the groups were forced to solve a problem in a "live situation."

In the mid-thirties, the Institute for the Crippled and Disabled (ICD) in New York City instigated what was known as a Guidance Testing Class. This became the forerunner of some of the work undertaken by ICD. After passage of Public Law 565 in 1954, the Institute undertook a five-year project with the United Cerebral Palsy Association of New York City, the New York Division of Vocational Rehabilitation and the New York Employment Service to explore improved techniques of determining the potential of the cerebral palsied. The five-year project led to separate facilities adapted to the needs of the group. Next, the Institute for the Crippled and Disabled obtained a five-year Research and Demonstration (R & D) project from the Vocational Rehabilitation Administration and developed the TOWER System. TOWER is an acronym for the words, *Testing, Orientation and Work Evaluation in Rehabilitation*.

Another important facility in the history of the development of work samples is the Vocational Guidance and Rehabilitation Service of Cleveland, Ohio. During the years 1959-1964, they undertook research in obtaining and using job samples. Resulting from this project was the R & D report entitled *Obtaining and Using Actual Job Samples in a Work Evaluation Program,* which was under the direction of Robert Overs. This project also received support from the then Vocational Rehabilitation Administration.

A recent and valuable work was the research undertaken by the Jewish Employment and Vocational Service of Philadelphia in 1968, through a grant from the Manpower Administration. This had led to important findings concerning the validity of the technique of work evaluation and the development of a series of work samples. The history of the development of this battery of work samples dates back to the thirties when the Jewish Employment and Vocational Service of Philadelphia began to search for a way to adequately assess Jewish immigrants to this country. A severe language barrier hampered assessment by the standard methods.

Until recent times, there has been a paucity of literature on work evaluation. One of the early articles, by Henry Redkey,[13] was entitled "The Function and Value of a Pre-Vocational Unit in a Rehabilitation Center." Walter Neff[12] wrote an article, "Problems of Work Evaluation," that has become a classic in the field and is often quoted and referred to. Another major paper and first attempt at a theory was written by William Gellman.[4] This paper, "The Principles of Vocational Evaluation," was presented at a workshop at Stout State University in 1967 and was published in 1968 in *Rehabilitation Literature*. Pertinent information to assist in organizing and operating a work evaluation program can be found in a 1966 publication of the Vocational Rehabilitation Administration (now Rehabilitation Services Administration) entitled *Guidelines for Organization and Operation of Vocational Evaluation Units: A Training Guide*. Literature in this area is on the increase in recent times. An annotated bibliography on work evaluation has been published and is kept up to date by the Materials Development Center of Stout State University.

Until recent times, the only training programs for those performing in the field of work evaluation were short-term institutes. The Institute for the Crippled and Disabled in New York City is well known for six-week programs on work evaluation, utilizing the TOWER system. Auburn University in Alabama was the first university to undertake regular short-term training for personnel in this field. The program in Sheltered Workshop Administration at the University of Wisconsin held some one-week training programs in work evaluation.

As the field of work evaluation developed, a body of knowledge accumulated, and the role of the evaluator was defined. It became apparent that short-term programs were not sufficient to train a "qualified work evaluator." Through a pilot study funded by the Vocational Rehabilitation Administration, professional training at the graduate level for work evaluators was established. Stout State University, University of Arizona and Auburn University established graduate training programs for work evaluators in the order listed.

A national center for the collection, development and dissemination of materials on work evaluation and work adjustment has been established by the Research and Demonstration Division of the Social and Rehabilitation Services, Department of Health, Education and Welfare. This is the Materials Development Center of Stout State University, through which information and materials on work evaluation and work adjustment are made available to professional workers in the field of vocational rehabilitation.

In 1965 the American Association of Work Evaluators was founded in the state of Georgia. Soon the organization drew the interest of people from other states. In 1966, at the annual conference of the National Rehabilitation Association (NRA) in Denver, a group of interested persons gathered to discuss the development of an organization within the NRA framework for people in work evaluation. From that conference, an *ad hoc* committee was formed to investigate the development of a work evaluation division of NRA. From this committee, the Vocational Evaluation and Work Adjustment Association was formed, and it became an official division of the National Rehabilitation Association at the annual conference in New Orleans in 1968.

THEORY ON WORK EVALUATION

There is no single comprehensive theory for the field of work evaluation. The field has borrowed from a number of sources. It has borrowed from the field theorist psychologists who pose that the behavior of individuals cannot be understood until the individual's environment, his perception of that environment and the resulting interaction with the environment are understood. Kurt Lewin stated this in his formula in which behavior is a function of the person plus his environment. Another psychologist, Henry

Murray, emphasized both the needs within the individual and the pressures from his environment and the vectors resulting from these two interacting forces.

Donald Fiske[3] indicated that the performance of any task is a complex function of the individual's capacity to carry out the task, the appropriateness of direction of his effort and the effort itself. Combining this and ideas from the field theorist, the author has stated in a paper presented first at a conference in Texas that performance is a function of an individual's capacities, his efforts and the appropriateness of his efforts plus the effect of his environment.

William Gellman[4] notes that vocational evaluation is ahistorical—that is, it is concerned not with the past but with the present and with future prediction. The theory he sets forth denotes four correlates between the theoretical and the empirical aspects of vocational evaluation. The first correlate is that of the work sector, the field in which productivity or work tasks take place, and it is characterized by achievement-oriented behavior using acquired behavioral patterns and skills to obtain an economic objective. The second correlate is that of work personality, a characteristic pattern of work activity displayed by an individual in a work situation. The third correlate states that work personality is developmental and is acquired during growth. His fourth correlate states that each culture uses different types of work personalities as ego models for training, selecting and rewarding people who are or will become productive. He notes that vocational evaluation is a means of determining the stage and the type of work personality in an individual. It is impractical to review this entire article at this time, but it should be noted that Dr. Gellman goes on to discuss goals, processes, techniques and principles.

Gordon Krantz[8] examined two models currently being utilized for the basis of work evaluation and finds them lacking. He notes that one model is based upon clinical psychology and is mainly concerned with such factors as defensive mechanisms, impulse control and gratification of needs. The second model he has labeled "Homespun-Eclectic Theory." He notes that such factors as mechanical aptitude, grooming and relating to supervisors are the bases for the work evaluation programs. Mr. Krantz prefers to utilize a model based upon the theory of employability and suggests using the methodology of critical incident technique to observe the kind of employment problems currently experienced by the population for which the program is designed. Having defined these problems, the evaluator is then to describe them in terms of the client behavior. Description is in positive terms, such as seeking work with a specific minimum frequency, appropriate interview behavior, rate of production appropriate to the job setting or adequately traveling in the community. Assessment then consists of looking for the specific behaviors or lack of the specific behaviors.

Julian Nadolsky[11] notes that both vocational evaluation and existential analysis are developments resulting directly from a dissatisfaction with traditional approaches that have been utilized to understand man's behavior. In both there is an attempt to obtain a more total self-comprehension by the individual through somewhat unstructured and individually oriented programs and procedures. Existentialism may be "viewed as a period or epic of individual supremacy where the emphasis is upon analyzing the subject-object relationship and the endeavor is to understand the emerging or becoming of a total human being through such relationships" (p. 22). Vocational evaluation is defined as a "process which attempts to *assess* and *predict* work behavior primarily through a variety of subject-object assessment techniques and procedures" (p. 23). In Mr. Nadolsky's framework, existential philosophy is applicable to work evaluation technology.

Unfortunately, little, if any, research has been done in relation to theoretical factors. Rehabilitation facilities have developed their particular work evaluation programs for a variety of reasons, but theoretical reasons have not been one of them. Sheltered workshops have tended to make a virtue out of the so-called real work situations and have not attempted to go beyond these techniques. Rehabilitation centers without subcontracts or other forms of production have developed and defended work samples as offering a wide range of test situations and as giving the opportunity for developing tests in graded levels and other innovations. Neither type of facility has, for the most part, developed a work evaluation program on the basis of theoretical factors.

At this stage of development, work evaluation borrows heavily from other fields of endeavor for theoretical foundations and is eclectic in nature. The research undertaken by the Jewish Employment and Vocational Service of Philadelphia, mentioned earlier, has resulted in data supporting the work evaluation process, but further research and study are needed. Also needed is a careful examination of the objectives to be obtained when establishing work evaluation units, in order to decide on the methodology to use.

EDUCATIONAL QUALIFICATIONS FOR WORK EVALUATORS

Not too long ago, the common belief of personnel in rehabilitation facilities throughout the country was that a good evaluator was an individual who had worked in industry or business. Little concern was given to educational qualifications. When the pilot study for initiating the first graduate program in the field of work evaluation was undertaken, considerable opposition was met as to the need for high-level training programs. A few thought that a graduate program was needed, a few more felt that a program at the undergraduate level would be best, but the majority seemed to feel that if any training was needed, a short-term program would suffice. This feeling is not nearly as prevalent today, and it is now quite common to sample opinion that reflects favorably towards the need for a good training program for work evaluators. Rehabilitation facilities are discovering this need every day as they attempt to set up work evaluation departments and hire personnel. The individual being hired who lacks training for the job, discovers it fast. Every training program in existence today and every well-established work evaluation program receive many letters requesting all known information on work evaluation. These letters are efforts to obtain help in setting up a work evaluation program and are most often from individuals who are hired as developers and administrators of work evaluation departments but who lack the appropriate knowledge and skills.

A questionnaire study of the type of information that should be provided in training work evaluators was conducted in 1966 by Stout State University. Two hundred and fifty questionnaires were sent to rehabilitation facilities in the United States with work evaluation units. A total of 189 questionnaries, or 75.6 percent, were returned. The results indicated that information was needed, first of all, on procedures of work evaluation. Further, information was needed on work methods and job sampling, the vocational rehabilitation process, medical and psychosocial aspects of disability, report writing, counseling theory as it applies to working with individuals directly on the floor of the rehabilitation facility, principles of communication, occupational information and analysis, cost quality and contract procurement procedures, psychological testing, community resources, and information about the world of work.

At two short-term training workshops for work evaluators at Stout State University, job analysis was conducted by the attending work evaluators on themselves. The evaluators were from a variety of work evaluation programs and different parts of the country. Based on a sample of thirty-three, which is recognized as being grossly inadequate in number, it is noted that thirty-six separate factors were listed as knowledges and skills required in the field of work evaluation. Among the more often mentioned factors were accuracy; manual dexterity; knowledge of machines, tools and shop equipment; counseling and interviewing skills; supervisory skills; teaching and training skills; organizational ability; interpersonal relations skills; communication skills; research principles; methodology and statistics; job analysis; and manpower needs. Some of the less often quoted factors were such things as time-and-motion study, production management, personality theory, developmental psychology and learning theory.

Seventeen separate duties were identified by the thirty-three work evaluators. The items checked by more than half the evaluators in rank order from first to last were the following: report writing and record keeping; staffing and coordination; work sample administration, scoring and interpretation; behavioral assessment; training and teaching; work sample development; and psychometric testing. The other items listed, but by less than half the group in continuing rank order, were the following: counseling; supervision of clients; supervision of employees; behavior modification; group work; and case management or client programming. It is repeated that this study is not quoted as a valid study of the duties of work evaluators due to the limited sample and the bias of the sample, but it does point up some of the duties, knowledges and skills required as seen by practicing work evaluators.

Karl Egerman, in research undertaken while he was director of the Research and Training Center in Vocational Rehabilitation at Johnstown, Pennsylvania, reports on duties of evaluators. This study was also biased; the names of the persons sampled were obtained from the National Rehabilitation Association as best they could identify work evaluators in those days. This was not a true sampling of work evaluators throughout the country, and the sample was heavily influenced by personnel from the southeastern region of the United States, but the study does have considerable value. It indicated that work evaluators were engaging in the following: attending and participating in scheduled staff meetings; observing clients at work; helping clients adjust to the work environment; writing reports; administering work samples or other performance measures; developing recommendations for training and placement; teaching clients good work habits; interviewing people who knew the clients; interviewing clients' families; lecturing periodically on vocational evaluation procedures; and supervising the workshops in vocational evaluation and prevocational training.

In essence, the job of the work evaluator is complex and comprehensive. The day when a work evaluation unit can be set up by an untrained individual has passed or should have passed. When possible, it would be desirable, in obtaining administrators for work evaluation departments, to hire an individual specifically trained for his field—that is, someone who has a master's degree from one of the training programs in the field of work evaluation. Such personnel are in short supply, however, and will be for a considerable amount of time. In lieu of this, it is recommended that facilities turn to allied professional training to obtain administrators for their units. Allied fields would be rehabilitation counseling, psychology, industrial arts and occupational therapy. Each of these fields has certain limitations for personnel entering work evaluation, and it would be best for persons trained in one of these fields to have experience in work evaluation prior to being hired as administrators.

Pertaining to secondary personnel in work evaluation programs, people with master's degree would be desirable, but due to the shortage and upward mobility of people with master's degrees and the expense involved to hire them, it is necessary to turn to lesser trained persons. Rehabilitation facilities must then carefully select the type of people they will utilize in secondary positions. If separate departments are set up in the work evaluation units, such as mechanics and clerical, then personnel with educational backgrounds in these particular fields may be obtained, but it will be necessary to provide them with extensive in-service training on the many subtleties that go into evaluation.

METHODOLOGIES OF WORK EVALUATION

Job Analysis

Walter Neff[12] writing in the *Personnel and Guidance Journal*, as quoted earlier, listed job analysis as a methodology of work evaluation, along with psychometrics, work samples and situational testing.

Job analysis is a process of defining the significant worker traits and requirements, and the technical and environmental facts of a specific job. It is an important technique for the work evaluator to know. It can assist him to (a) identify job requirements and specific qualities required of workers for various jobs, (b) develop work samples and (c) do client evaluation. The job analysis formula of measuring what the worker does, how he does it, why he does it and the skill involved in doing it lends itself readily to evaluating the qualifications and abilities of a client placed on a job. However, it is rare that job analysis, when used, is used to evaluate a particular client. It is used more often as an adjunct technique to learn about the requirements of a job so as to help select clients who have the qualifications to succeed on the job or to lay the foundation for building a work sample. Once the traits required to do a job are known, it is possible to compare worker traits with the traits required by specific jobs. Perhaps this would be best referred to as *work-trait comparison* or *job-man analysis*.

Psychometric Testing

Psychometric testing is of value to work evaluation. It is quick, relatively inexpensive and objective. The range of psychometric testing is broad. There are tests for measuring intelligence, interests, aptitudes, dexterities, academic abilities and personality. There are tests pertaining to the field of clerical work, mechanical work, electronics, drafting, computer programming, business and many others. There are tests for people with high intelligence and much education and tests for persons with limited intelligence and poor education.

With proper use, psychometric tests have a place in work evaluation. Their use by work evaluation programs will depend upon the staffing pattern of a rehabilitation facility and the presence of psychologists and psychometrists. Tests have their severe limitations, and their very limitations are what led to the development of the work evaluation methodologies of work samples and situational work settings.

Work Samples

A work sample is a test that is an actual job or a simulated job. A work sample may be an actual job, administered and observed under standard conditions, or it may be a mock-up of a component of a job. It may be a job made up by the evaluator to resemble an actual job in industry or business and to measure traits important to successful employment.

There are a number of advantages to the work sample method of evaluation. One of the major advantages is that it tends to look like work and often holds the interest of clients as opposed to the psychological test. The client can objectively see how well he is or is not performing, and the work sample test often holds more meaning for him because of this factor. The work sample offers the evaluator the opportunity to observe actual work behavior, and an experienced evaluator can innovate work samples to meet the particular needs of a client. Language inadequacies, reading disabilities, speech impairments, educational deprivation and cultural differences are often less influential on work sample evaluation than evaluation through psychological tests. Work samples may be established in a large variety of areas in order to get a more comprehensive measure of client potential.

There are disadvantages to this method. It is expensive. The expense is that of the time and materials it takes to build, maintain and administer work samples and in the replacement of parts or supplies. Work samples are time-consuming on the part of the evaluator since most of them require the presence of an evaluator for timing and for observation of behavior. Work samples also have the disadvantage of requiring continual reconstruction and standardization.

The Situational Approach

Evaluating an individual who is placed on a job or jobs in the sheltered workshop has been referred to as the situational approach because it attempts to simulate actual working conditions. This approach has advantages. It offers work situations simulating work in which to conduct evaluations; wages are paid; work is performed with actual commodities destined for sale; foremen are present who set standards for quality and quantity of work; regular working hours are maintained; interpersonal relationship situations can be similar to those in business and industry; and in general, the overall situation more closely resembles that of industry and business than in a work sample facility. The author would point out, however, that the sheltered workshop is definitely not the same as industry or business for fairly obvious reasons.

There are limitations to this method of evaluation. Sheltered workshops are limited by the work contracts they have, and it is impossible to reproduce, within the confines of a workshop, the vast variety of types of employment or to measure for the many types of basic skills which go into different jobs. Another limitation is related to one of the advantages—the complexity of the situation of a worklike setting makes it difficult to separate the variables that are producing the effect.

Job Tryout

The utilization of work stations under actual work conditions is another technique of work evaluation. These may be work stations in institutions, rehabilitation facilities, schools or in business and industries.

Work stations within institutions, rehabilitation facilities or schools, such as in food services, laundry, maintenance, and buildings and grounds, may be utilized as an evaluative method. This method of evaluation also has certain advantages. It provides an opportunity to observe attitudes, motivation, initiative, ability to follow orders, work quality and quantity, and other factors pertinent to employment and vocational development, while still in the institution or other setting. The individual under observation may be observed under actual work conditions and can be placed in a role where he must meet standards and expectations close to that of normal workers. There are also limitations to this method of evaluation. Sometimes the situation is not a "real work situation" as too often in these settings, no wages or only token wages are paid. One of the major problems is obtaining cooperation of the regular work supervisors who at times do not wish this extra responsibility or who sometimes use such placements as a source of "cheap" help.

The other job tryout method is the use of work stations in business and industries. In these situations, wages are paid, usually by the business or industry offering the work station. In some situations a subsidy is given to the business or industry by the sponsoring program. The advantage here is similar to the above. The individual may be observed under actual work conditions. The major difficulty is obtaining the cooperation of employers, including not only the head of the business or industry or a department chief but also the immediate floor supervisor. Without the cooperation of the latter, the program will fail.

FACTORS EVALUATED

The process of work evaluation focuses upon two classifications of factors to be evaluated, *general employability factors* and *specific employability factors*.

General employability factors are those which an individual must possess in order to be generally employable. These include such factors as social development, grooming and hygiene, work personality, work habits, physical tolerance and performance rate. Examples of factors under work personality include relation to supervisors, relation to co-workers, frustration tolerance, and reaction to instructions and criticism. Work habits include such factors as attendance rate, punctuality, not leaving a work station inappropriately and safety consciousness. If these factors are acceptable, the individual is generally employable and may be evaluated for a specific vocational plan. If not, the individual will require either social development or referral to work adjustment for improvement of those factors found to be below the level of acceptability for general employment.

Specific employability factors include skills, aptitudes, dexterities, achievement, interests, intellectual level of functioning, personality factors and physical tolerance. These are factors pertinent to specific vocational development and employment. It will be noted that some of the factors are repeated from the list of those under general employability. There are personality factors, such as "reaction to supervisors" which are related to general employability and other factors related to specific jobs. As examples, it would be undesirable to recommend sales work to someone who prefers to be alone with minimum interaction with people or a position beyond one's physical tolerance.

UTILIZATION OF WORK EVALUATION

As indicated in the preceding section, the technique of work evaluation can and should reveal more about a client than merely skills and things he can do. The technique of work evaluation can provide information as to aptitudes, dexterities, skills, intellectual level of functioning, interests, work habits and personality factors.

The amount of information for the different categories will vary from client to client. For one client, considerable information as to personality factors will be obtained while for a second, very little. To the trained evaluator, however, work evaluation can produce a wealth of information.

The performance of a client on a work sample for business skills, handtool manipulative ability, power tools, assembly tools, and the like, will, of course, reveal information as to the client's skills, aptitudes and dexterities. Similar information can be obtained by observing him on various jobs in the sheltered workshop, but this kind of information comes best from work samples.

Intellectual level of functioning can be obtained by administration of intelligence tests and academic achievement tests (such as the Wide Range Achievement Test) and by careful observation of his behavior during the evaluation program. A client who can do a task from written instructions has a higher level of academic verbal ability than a client who requires that instructions be read, but the latter has a higher level of intellectual functioning than the client for whom the instructions must be demonstrated. Two clients may measure approximately the same on intelligence tests, but one may reveal a higher degree of functioning from the standpoint of learning ability. This can be observed in a work evaluation program in relation to the rate of learning exhibited on work samples. This factor can also be observed by the rate of learning exhibited on production tasks in a sheltered workshop. The way a client approaches a task can reveal the manner in which he tackles problems. In attempting to solve problems, an individual approach may be that of trial and error, concrete or abstract approach, and with plan and forethought or impulsivity.

The work evaluation program can also reveal information as to a client's interests, especially in a work sample department with a wide range of work evaluation tasks. One technique for measuring interest is to obtain the client's preferences and nonpreferences for the various tasks. A second procedure is to observe carefully his verbal and nonverbal reactions. Examples of the latter would be his facial expressions with various tasks or his performing below the expected level on a particular task.

It is to be expected that some clients will dislike all of the tasks of the evaluation program. This may be due to a number of reasons. The variety of tasks may be too limited to present the client with an area he likes. This would be especially true in a sheltered workshop with only a limited number of contracts. The client may be unable to correlate some or all of the tasks with specific jobs. The client may not be motivated towards working but may be seeking other gains, such as support by society.

Obtaining a client's reaction to the various tasks can reveal information other than interests. It can reveal a discrepancy between interests and ability. For example, a client may indicate that the task or tasks which appeal to him most are those above his ability level. On the other hand, those tasks which appeal most to the client may be ones below his level of ability. The results of the work evaluation can, at such times, become a valuable tool in counseling and working with the client.

Work evaluation offers the opportunity to observe the client under a variety of conditions and over a period of time. As such, it offers an excellent opportunity for the observation and evaluation of his personality. How does he react to authority figures? to male authority figures as opposed to female? to his successes and failures? to older persons? to persons his age? to younger persons? to frustrating situations? to difficult tasks? to the unexpected? to pressures created by time limitations? Is he dependent or independent, or does he manifest a mixture of dependency and independency according to the situation? Is he aggressive, passive or passive-aggressive? Is he a loner or gregarious?

Work evaluation, especially in the sheltered workshop situation, lends itself to the observation of work habits. Does he report on time? Does he waste time during assignments? Is he dependable? responsible? Is his grooming appropriate? Does he take care of equipment?

Not every individual serviced by the vocational rehabiltation process requires work evaluation. A client with at least average intelligence, a grade school education and with some appropriate motivation can usually be evaluated faster and more economically by standard procedures. There are many clients, however, for whom work evaluation should be used as an adjunct to standard procedures or as the preferred methodology. Some guidelines for such clients are as follows: (a) low intelligence, (b) poor education, (c) cultural background different from that upon which most psychological tests are standardized, (d) subcultural backgrounds, such as youth gangs, that create negative attitudes to standardized testing, (e) emotional or behavioral problems that interfere with standard assessment, (f) immaturity, (g) lack of adequate work experiences, (h) history of many low-level jobs, (i) aspirations which exceed or are below ability level, (j) handicapping conditions that prevent adequate assessment by standard procedures and (k) presence of basic questions not answered by other procedures.

The work evaluation process may now be utilized to determine eligibility for rehabilitation service. Public Law 89-333 authorized rehabilitation counselors to utilize work evaluation to assist them in making the determination as to "reasonable expectation for success" required before rendering rehabilitation services. From the above description of the work evaluation process, the potential of work evaluation for aiding the counselor in this decision should be obvious. The chance to observe a client under the conditions of work evaluation and for an extended period of time will result in information about a client not available through medical examination and standard psychological testing. When should a counselor use work evaluation for assisting in this decision? He should use it when there is a questionable doubt in his mind from other assessment techniques (interview, review of history, medical examination and psychological examination) as to the decision of "reasonable expectation for success."

RESPONSIBILITIES OF REHABILITATION COUNSELOR AND WORK EVALUATOR

The rehabilitation counselor has some definite responsibilities towards the work evaluation process. No counselor should send a client to a facility with a simple statement, "Please evaluate." The counselor should carefully state the specific questions he has in relation to the client. This will not prohibit the work evaluation department of a facility from evaluating beyond these questions, if such evaluation is called for and agreed upon by the counselor, but it will assist the work evaluation department in meeting the needs of the counselor. The counselor should also prepare the client for the process and not have him enter work evaluation with false conceptions and unanswered questions.

The counselor should provide the work evaluation program with information on the client. This will include pertinent information on medical and psychiatric data, psychological tests, family history, work record and educational attainment. Work evaluation is not a passive process that simply measures objective factors but takes on meaning dependent upon the background of the client. As indicated in the section, "Theory on Work Evaluation," work evaluation is ahistorical and concerned with the future, but an evaluator with the knowledge that a client has a third grade education, was a common laborer all his life or once held a high-level job can render more effective evaluation and interpretations. Since he needs to know if the client has a history of psychiatric or other problems, the evaluator usually has to spend time interviewing the client if this information is not supplied by the counselor.

The counselor should become familiar with the work evaluation program he uses and visit as often as time and distance permit. Visitation to work evaluation programs will familiarize the counselor with the process, enable him to determine which program is best suited for a particular client and establish effective communication with personnel of the work evaluation programs.

The work evaluator also has definite responsibilities. If a client is referred for a specific purpose, the evaluator should contact the counselor before pursuing a different track, if that seems desirable, unless arrangements are made ahead of time. The evaluator should keep the counselor abreast of developments for clients in evaluation for long periods of time. He should write reports in clear and concise language without a lot of professional jargon and should do more than just report facts. A series of facts about a client, while they may cover the essential findings, need to be integrated to render effective interpretation. The work evaluation report should answer the specific questions asked by a counselor or indicate why the evaluator is unable to answer those questions. The evaluator must remember that it is the counselor who is buying the services. At times, evaluators tend to act as if they were the ones mainly involved with the client and can do as they please. When effective communication is worked out between counselor and evaluator, there will be few problems.

WORK EVALUATION TODAY AND TOMORROW

In the recent past, utilization of the methodology of work evaluation was limited to rehabilitation centers, sheltered workshops and the clients served by these facilities. Today, work evaluation programs are found in these facilities, in institutions for the retarded, the mentally ill and the public offender, and in high schools with special education groups. The recent amendments to the Vocational Education Act earmarked 10 percent of the funds for the handicapped. Through this allocation, there will be further application of the methodologies of work evaluation serving the population covered by the act. Programs such as WIN (Work Incentive Program) submit their clients to work evaluation methodologies. The Manpower Development and Training Programs supported by the Department of Labor have begun either to refer clients to work evaluation units or use the technology themselves.

Work evaluation projects have been funded mainly by the Rehabilitation Services Administration of the U. S. Department of Health, Education and Welfare. They are now being supported by other federal agencies, such as the Department of Labor. It was the Department of Labor, through the Manpower Administration, that sponsored the Research and Demonstration project at the Jewish Employment and Vocational Service in Philadelphia.

Work evaluation has been utilized mainly with the handicapped and disadvantaged. This author sees the technology of work evaluation as having considerable relevance to those whom we do not consider disadvantaged or handicapped. There are large numbers of young people in our high schools and vocational schools who do not know what it is they want to pursue in life, and a comprehensive and well-developed work evaluation unit could offer much to help these young people made pertinent decisions. It is one thing to read about an occupation in a two- to four-page pamphlet put out by professional vocational guidance organizations and another to do the job. Written information is cold and sterile, and it is difficult to visualize what it is really like to undertake a particular type of work. Through the realities of work samples, however, an individual may determine exactly what potentials he has at the moment, what potentials he can develop through instructions of graduated work samples, and he can also get an actual feeling for the work involved. Through work samples, the young person can learn not only of his current level of ability but of his potential and his interest. This, combined with information from pamphlets and the counselor, could help him more readily select a suitable occupation in life.

SUMMARY

Work evaluation is a process of assessing vocational strengths and weaknesses through the utilization of work, real or simulated, for the purpose of developing the vocational plan of action. There is, unfortunately, considerable confusion in the field concerning terms pertaining to this process, and there is a need for standardization of terms.

Work evaluation is not a new process, although its development and utilization have accelerated in recent years. Theoretical principles have been borrowed from other disciplines, but in recent times theorists in the field have attempted to set down specific theoretical principles for work evaluation.

The process of work evaluation includes the techniques of psychometric tests, work samples, situational settings and job tryout. Job analysis is important as an adjunct technique to provide information for job-man matching and to assist in building work samples. Work evaluation focuses upon evaluation of general and specific employability factors and is used with persons for whom other standard assessment techniques have failed to generate a vocational plan of action. The process of work evaluation and the duties of the work evaluator have developed to the point of requiring professionally trained evaluators.

REFERENCES

1. Bregman, Morton H.: The use and misuse of vocational evaluation in the counseling process. *Some Recent Advances and Research in Vocational Evaluation.* Research and Training Center in Vocational Rehabilitation. Johnstown (Penn.); University of Pittsburgh, 1967.
2. Egerman, Karl, and Gilbert, James L.: The work evaluator. *J Rehab, 35 (No. 3)*:12-14, May-June 1969.
3. Fiske, Donald W.: Problems in measuring capacity and performance. *Proceedings of the Iowa Conference on Pre-Vocational Activities, Conference at the University of Iowa.* Iowa City, University of Iowa, 1960.
4. Gellman, William: The principles of vocational evaluation. *Vocational Evaluation Curriculum Development Workshop.* Stout State University, April, 1967, and *Rehab Lit, 29 (No. 4)*:98-103, April 1968.
5. Hoffman, Paul R.: Work Evaluation. A speech presented at the rehabilitation conference sponsored by the Texas Division of Vocational Rehabilitation, Houston, Texas, February 1969.
6. Institute for the Crippled and Disabled: *TOWER: Testing, Orientation and Work Evaluation in Rehabilitation.* New York, Institute for the Crippled and Disabled, 1967.
7. Jewish Employment and Vocational Service: *Work Samples: Signposts on the Road to Occupational Choice.* Final Report on Experimental and Demonstration Project, Contract No. 82-40-67-40, U.S. Department of Labor, Manpower Administration. Philadelphia, Jewish Employment and Vocational Service, 1968.
8. Krantz, Gordon: Theory Underlying Vocational Evaluation." Unpublished paper presented at Stout State University, 1968.
9. Lewin, Kurt: *A Dynamic Theory of Personality.* New York, McGraw-Hill Book Co., 1935.
10. Murray, Henry A.: *Explorations in Personality.* New York, Science Editions, Inc., 1962.
11. Nadolsky, Julian M.: The existential in vocational evaluation. *J Rehab, 35 (No. 3)*:22-24, May-June 1969.
12. Neff, Walter S.: Problems of work evaluation. *The Personnel and Guidance Journal, 44 (No. 7)*:682-688, March 1966.
13. Redkey, Henry: The function and value of a pre-vocational unit in a rehabilitation center. *Amer J Occup Ther, 11 (No. 1)*:20-24, January-February 1957.
14. Redkey, Henry, and White, Barbara: *The Pre-Vocational Unit in a Rehabilitation Center.* Washington, D.C., U. S. Department of Health, Education and Welfare, Office of Vocational Rehabilitation, 1956.
15. Vocational Guidance and Rehabilitation Services: *Final Report: Obtaining and Using Actual Job Samples in a Work Evaluation Program,*

Research and Demonstration Project RD-412, Department of Health, Education and Welfare, Vocational Rehabilitation Administration. Cleveland, (Ohio), Vocational Guidance and Rehabilitation Services, 1959-1964.
16. Vocational Rehabilitation Administration: *Guidelines for Organization and Operation of Vocational Evaluation Units: A Training Guide,* Rehabilitation Service Series Number 67-50. Washington, D.C., U. S. Department of Health, Education and Welfare, 1966.

9

Techniques of Counseling in the Rehabilitation Process

John G. Cull and John D. Hutchinson

Anatomy of the Counseling Session
Greeting
Opening the Interview
Body of the Interview
Closing the Interview
Summary

IN THE counseling literature there is an abundance of information on philosophy, theory, approaches, et cetera. However, for the new professional worker, little is written on techniques of counseling which helps to insure the success of the counseling relationship. Generally these techniques are gradually learned during many counseling sessions. When discussing these techniques with experienced counselors, it is obvious that many feel such techniques stem from common sense or that everyone knows about them. We beg to differ. We have found in working with new counselors that many who have a good academic grasp of counseling theories still have difficulties in counseling sessions because of a lack of knowledge about how to put the theory and philosophy to work in practice.

ANATOMY OF THE COUNSELING SESSION

Regardless of the theoretical approach a counselor uses, what follows in this chapter holds true. The chapter sections are vehicles by which the counselor's theoretical orientation are implemented. While there may be some minor shifts according to varying theoretical approaches, the basic value and usefulness of these techniques remain constant. In vocational rehabilitation counseling interview sessions fall into three general types. There are interviews in which the goal of the counselor is to provide information to the client; secondly, some sessions are scheduled for the client to provide information to the counselor; and thirdly, the bulk of the counseling contacts may be classified as problem-solving sessions.

In each of these types of counseling sessions integral parts of the session are the same. Generally in each counseling session regardless of type or purpose the period should be divided into the following parts: greeting, opening, body of the interview and closing. These parts naturally will be divided unequally, but the counselor should decide before each interview roughly how much time will be spent in each area.

GREETING

Counseling is a directed personal interaction between two individuals. In order to interact effectively, each individual must accept the other. A basis for a warm working relationship must be established. Without this relationship very little, if any, counseling will occur. Instead of counseling sessions, the counselor will engage in conversations with the client. The counselor will gain very little insight into the feelings, motivating forces and reasons for actions of the client. Without the development of this relationship, the counselor often will become frustrated. He will feel thwarted. The client will be obviously motivated to achieve in the vocational rehabilitation process, but somehow things just will not seem to click.

The development of this relationship or rapport is a major underlying goal of the early counseling sessions. While the interviews will be scheduled for other purposes (to explain the vocational rehabilitation program, to prepare the client for various evaluative procedures, to obtain basic information, et cetera), the counselor pays particular attention to the development of a working relationship with the client. During the first few sessions the counselor should become an individual who cares rather than the representative of an institution. A client can relate to another individual but cannot relate or interact with an institution or program or the representative of an institution or program. Therefore, at this point the counselor is recognizing the humanity of the client and is giving the client the opportunity to do the same with him.

While a concerted effort is required to develop this relationship, once developed little effort is required to continue it. However, some effort is required and this aspect (developing the relationship) of counseling should not be neglected. The remnant of the major effort to establish rapport is the greeting of the client. Each counseling session should be started with a personal greeting. The time spent on this part of the counseling interview is an inverse function of the warmth of the relationship established. After a strong, warm relationship has been established less time is required; however, the greeting never should be overlooked or omitted. We feel a counselor and client must have feelings of friendship for the counseling process to succeed. "Greeting" is the normal activity of friends prior to getting down to more serious business.

If the contacts between counselor and client are relatively frequent, the greeting might be minimal; however, if the counselor and client have not had recent contacts the counselor should spend more time on this aspect of the interview. This is obvious since it is natural that the longer the period between contacts, the greater the need for renewing the relationship which has been established.

OPENING THE INTERVIEW

After the greeting the counseling session is opened. The object of this next phase is to state the goals of this particular session. The counselor should give the client an evaluation of the progress being made in the rehabilitation process and tell him how the current interview fits into the process. For example:

> As you know up to this point we have been gathering some basic information to help us evaluate your abilities and develop a plan of

action. I have received some of the reports we requested. Today you and I will go over these reports. I will interpret them and next week we will start discussing our plan of action.

If the client does not know or understand the goals of the interview, he is forced to "second guess" the counselor. Each question posed has to be evaluated by the client. His response is directed at achieving his perception of the counselor's goal. If the statement of the goals of the interview is skipped and the counselor begins a counseling session with the question, How are things going in school? the answer almost invariably will be "fine," or some other noncommittal answer. Until the client figures out the purpose of this particular counseling session, his answers will remain relatively superficial and meaningless.

We have observed counseling sessions in which the counselor failed to clearly state the goals he wished the client to achieve. In the majority of these sessions the client's searching and simultaneous defensively fending off the counselor is quite obvious. The counselor realizes something is wrong, but he is unable to remedy the situation. We have seen some counseling interviews in which, after some time has passed the client discovered the goals of the counselor. After verifying his perception of the counselor's goals, the client proceeded to repeat the counselor's questions and change or amplify the answers he had given previously.

The answer to almost any question depends upon the reason for the question rather than solely upon the nature of the question. As in the previous example, if the client is asked, How are things going in school? Without discussing the purpose of the question, the answer will be a noncommittal "fine." This answer will change if prior to asking the question the counselor would say something like the following:

> Today I would like for us to discuss your progress in vocational training since— (a) I understand you need some additional help, *or* (b) I understand you are having some difficulty with some of the other students (or some of the instructors), *or* (c) I know of a possible job if you and your instructor feel you are 'ready,' *or* (d) I understand you have not been attending regularly, *or* (e) I understand you have lost some of your tools.

After discussing the role of a statement of goals in the counseling session, one wonders why so much attention has been paid to the topic in this chapter since it seems to be such an integral and necessary part of counseling, but it becomes a part of a counselor's technique only after he has gained some experience.

BODY OF THE INTERVIEW

In the body of the interview the goals which were just stated are achieved. There are several factors which determine the degree of success the counselor will enjoy. These factors generally fall into two categories, attitudes of the counselor and actions of the counselor. These will not be separated below since, as will be seen, the division is obvious.

Acceptance

One of the most important factors affecting the counseling session is the acceptance of the client by the counselor and the acceptance of the counselor by the client. This is an intangible phenomenon but as the counseling process proceeds it becomes evident. Acceptance is related to rapport but is distinct from it. If the counselor fails to accept the client or the client fails to accept the counselor, an emotional and often rational gap will develop in the relationship. While a warm relationship may exist between the two, without such an acceptance of each other the facility with which mutual counseling goals are achieved will be impaired.

Assurance of the Counselor

The self-assurance of the counselor will determine, to a great extent, the success of his counseling. If the counselor lacks self-assurance, it is difficult for the client to place his faith and trust in him. The rehabilitation counselor is making a major intervention in the client's life. This intervention may have lifelong ramifications for the client. When the client recognizes a lack of self-assurance on the part of the counselor, he will either reject rehabilitation services or enter into a program of services with less than complete committment. Either alternative will usually result in the case being "closed—not rehabilitated."

Perhaps the single most effective action a counselor can take to increase his self-assurance and increase the image of assurance he projects to the client is adequate preparation. Prior to each counseling session the counselor should review the case material he has obtained on the client along with what has been recorded in the progress notes. A counselor who has to ask the client what was discussed previously or planned in another session or who forgets events the client feels are of prime importance to his rehabilitation does not instill confidence.

Sincerity

The sincerity of the counselor is completely obvious to the client. Much to the surprise of many counselors even most of a counselor's mentally retarded clients are able to discern a lack of sincerity. Regardless of words or obvious actions to the contrary, lack of sincerity "shows through." The counselor should be aware of his actions and comments and evaluate them against the criterion of sincerity. A counselor who does not "level" with his client is courting a counseling failure. A counselor should rarely, if ever, react in a false manner with the client.

Professional Bearing

Even though the counselor establishes a warm working relationship with the client and both share and appreciate the realization of the individuality and humanity of the other, there is a difference between them. The client expects and demands the counselor recognize the difference. Not only does the client demand the recognition of the difference, he demands the difference be sharpened and maintained. The client needs and wants a professional person with whom he can effectively interact. He does not want nor need an equal.

Too often the counselor mistakenly interprets the admonishment to "establish rapport with the client" to mean "get on his level" or "develop a buddy relationship with him." The counselor should maintain his professional posture and be aware of the image he is projecting. Contrary to the beliefs held by many new counselors a deep rapport can be developed while maintaining this professional distance.

Accuracy of Information

It is surprising the number of times a counselor will give inaccurate or misleading information in an attempt to keep from having to admit not knowing something. Even with the best case preparation a counselor will have gaps of knowledge. He should have the self-assurance to admit not knowing a point. While this sounds superficial it is important to the counseling relationship. The counselor is not expected to know everything, but he is expected to develop a genuine relationship. As with the other qualities, a lack of genuineness or accuracy of responding will impair the counseling progress.

Verbal Communication

The voice is the prime vehicle for communicating in the counseling process; therefore, the voice plays a vital role in the success of a counseling program with a client. The amplitude of the counselor's voice should be appropriate. It should be maintained at conversational levels except when appropriately raised. Before raising the amplitude of his voice the counselor should have consciously determined it was necessary. Many new counselors and some more experienced counselors almost shout at blind persons. They feel if the client cannot see he cannot hear. Many counselors working with clients whose native language is one other than English tend to raise their voice when the client fails to understand a concept. Often this can be observed also with counselors of the mentally retarded. Rather than explain a concept in simpler terms the counselor feels he can overpower the barrier to communication by repeating his words louder and louder.

The counselor's voice is a professional tool much as the scalpel is a professional tool of the surgeon. As such the counselor should develop his voice and use it in a fashion which communicates most effectively. Not only should he be aware of the amplitude of his voice (loudness or softness), but he should pay heed to the speed with which he talks and the clarity and tone of his voice. He should speak in a well-regulated voice (not too fast) which is clear. He should be particularly concerned with his enunciation. We feel a new counselor can materially benefit from recording selected counseling sessions to evaluate among other things his voice.

Another aspect of verbal communication which must be evaluated for each client is the counselor's vocabulary level. While it is obviously detrimental to the counseling outcomes for a counselor to use a vocabulary which is pitched at a level much higher than the level the client is prepared for, it is equally detrimental for a counselor to use wording which is inappropriately too simple. Again, we have observed new counselors in sessions who felt that since the client was physically impaired he must be intellectually impaired. These counselors would attempt to communicate with an intellectually capable client in an insultingly simple fashion. Often the client will attempt to communicate his displeasure by the tone of his responses and more obviously by increasing the vocabulary level of his responses. It is a sensitive counselor who recognizes these cues and modifies his level of approach; however, in many instances the counselor's unconscious stereotype of the relationship between physical impairment and intellectual impairment is so strong that the cues given by the client are ineffectual.

As a part of verbal communication the counselor might choose to use levity. If the time is well chosen and the content of the response impeccable, lightness can be highly effective in a counseling interview. Regretably, these two conditions are not always met. While levity can be highly effective it also can become a devastating influence on the outcome of counseling sessions. A counselor would be wise to sparingly interject lightness into the counseling session. Levity misinterpreted by the client can effectively block the establishment of rapport. Generally, people in a dependent status in a relationship tend to have more ideas of self-reference than people playing a more independent role. Therefore, a client easily may feel a counselor is laughing at him rather than with him.

Nonverbal Communication

While the voice is the prime vehicle for communicating in the counseling session, it is not the only vehicle. Nonverbal communication has a very powerful influence on counseling outcomes. The old adage "actions speak louder than words" is very true in counseling. We communicate many of our feelings and attitudes by our nonverbal behavior. Boredom, lack of patience, disbelief and lack of interest come through all too clearly in our behavior regardless of our words.

One of the most important actions we can take to communicate interest, concern and awareness is to look at the client. Do not read a folder, a report or a letter when the client is talking with you. Maintain good eye contact. A counselor does not have to adopt an eyeball-to-eyeball posture to communicate interest, but he does have to look at the client. If you feel this is unimportant, turn around the next time a friend or colleague is excitedly describing an event to you. Pay particular attention to his level of excitement or motivation to relate the incident to you. Many counselors feel note taking during a counseling session is not damaging to the overall result of the interview. We disagree. We feel note taking and case recording should wait until after the client has left. It takes very little practice for a counselor to develop the ability to record the pertinent points of the interview after the close of the interview.

As a part of eye contact or looking at the client, give him your undivided attention. Nothing seems more fruitless than trying to communicate your feelings or aspirations with someone who is shuffling and stacking papers; playing with a pencil, keys, or coins; or constantly cleaning, reaming, filling and lighting a pipe. While you may be interested and attentive, your nonverbal behavior might not communicate your attention and interest.

A type of client contact with which the rehabilitation counselor should be aware is voice contact. Without realizing it, a counselor often can reject a client through a type of contact similar to that discussed above. In this case the counselor will ask others to respond for the client, such as a spouse, parent, sibling, attendant, or reader. Often a counselor will ask a sighted spouse to tell the blind client (who is present) he should go in for a general medical examination or ask the sighted spouse or parent about the client's reaction to an event when the client is completely capable of responding for himself. In restaurants one will repeatedly see a waitress approach a group in which there is a blind customer and ask, "What will he order?" This behavior occurs also among counselors and with a wider distribution of clients than blind persons. When this lack of contact occurs, many clients are infuriated.

Control of the Interview

The rehabilitation counselor must always control the interview. If the client controls the direction of the interview, counseling ceases. We observed a student in counseling once who turned over control of the interview to the client without realizing what he had done. After asking the client about his vocational plans, the client responded and asked the counselor about rehabilitation counseling (a totally inappropriate field for the client). After the counselor responded, the client continued to elicit responses from the counselor regarding his educational background, his motivation for entering rehabilitation counseling, his hobbies and his vocational plans. It was a beautiful counseling session but the roles were switched. The counselor was totally unaware of the dynamics of the interaction between the two. The client was in complete control of the interview and none of the counseling goals were accomplished.

This counselor listened to the client but did not hear him. In counseling there is a vast difference between listening and hearing. Hearing implies a greater degree of understanding of what is being said than listening implies. A counselor should not only listen to what is being said but should be keenly aware of what the client is communicating on a more basic meaningful level— what is he feeling and what is occurring in the counseling session. The counselor should try to understand not only what the client said but why he said it and what he is trying to accomplish.

In controlling the direction of the interview, the counselor also should control the pace of the interview. After setting the goals to be achieved, the counselor should have a relatively clear plan of direction and should pace the interview in such a manner as to achieve the stated goal or goals in the allotted time available. Often a client will gain control, not only of the direction of the interview but also of the pace of the interview. This is done by his going into too much detail in responding to a question or by bringing too much extraneous material into the responses. If the counselor fails to be aware of this type of behavior, he will find he achieves fewer and fewer of his counseling goals. Also he will discover he knows a considerable amount of facts about the client but has developed relatively little insight into the client's feelings.

A third type of control of the interview is that of the sequence of the interview. After the statement of the goals to be achieved, the interview should then proceed in a logical orderly fashion. This sequence should be outlined roughly (at least mentally) prior to meeting with the client.

If something has occurred with the client since the last contact which merits a change in the anticipated goals, the counselor should switch goals, but this switch should be conscious and discussed by the counselor and client. When the goals are not changed, the direction of the session should be obvious to both. If the counselor develops a hit-or-miss illogical sequence, he ends up confusing the client and wondering when he has fully accomplished the goals of the session.

The control of the interview is maintained, among other actions, by the type of questions the counselor asks. When closed questions are put to the client, generally he will answer in the shortest fashion possible. Closed questions do not elicit feelings or elaboration on the part of the client. The following are examples of closed questions:

> Do you like school?
> Where do you live?
> Do you get along well with employers?

Unless a counselor has a highly verbal client, the responses these questions elicit will be relatively useless. More productive questions would have been the following:

> Tell me your feelings about school.
> Tell me about your home and neighborhood.
> What are your feelings about employers and your relations with them?

Another type of nonproductive question counselors often ask

Techniques of Counseling in the Rehabilitation Process 223

is a leading question—one which has a predetermined answer because of the way it is phrased. For example:

You like school, don't you?
You get along well with employers, don't you?

Not only is the type of question important, but the clarity of the question also determines the quality of response. If the client only partially understands a question, he cannot respond to it as fully as the counselor would like. Therefore, care should be taken in phrasing the question or statement to insure it elicits the desired response. A part of the clarity aspect of questions is asking one question at a time. Often a counselor will ask several questions in one statement without realizing it. For example:

The last few weeks your attendance on the job has been poor, why? Aren't you interested in the job any longer? You have to work regularly to hold a job, what are you going to do?

When a counselor asks a question, he should be sure he has the answer before going on to the next question. First, he should be sure the client answered the question which was asked. Often in a counseling session the answer bears little or no resemblance to the question. The response should be evaluated and discussed or the question repeated. Secondly, the counselor should be patient and allow the client ample opportunity to respond fully before asking the next question or making the next statement.

Often a counselor will fire questions at a client and conduct an interview at too rapid a pace because of his uncomfortableness with silence. The counselor must develop a tolerance for silence. Silence in the counseling session does not imply counselor inadequacy. In order to thoroughly evaluate the client's responses, there are many times in which silence is the most appropriate event in an interview.

The last facet of interview control to be covered is the control of the depth of the counseling session. The depth of the interview is controlled by the focus of questions asked and statements made. The more the focus is on feelings of the client, the deeper the session will progress. In many instances the counselor needs to explore the feelings of the client; however, he should be aware of his professional limitations and as such not allow the counseling to proceed to a depth for which the counselor is not prepared professionally to work with. Conversely, if the counselor fails to elicit the feelings of the client their interaction remains on a too superficial level to be of value to the client.

There is a broad band in which vocational counseling is effective. If the counselor allows the sessions to become too deep they become less vocationally oriented and generally less productive. If the counselor does not take the interview to sufficient depth, he will remain on the conversational level and will discover his "counseling" is rather unproductive.

Atmosphere of the Interview

The client's participation is essential for the success of counseling and his participation is a function of the atmosphere the counselor creates. The counseling atmosphere proceeds on several levels at once. It may be supportive and permissive, authoritarian or threatening, and structured or unstructured. It may be cynical, exacting, warm or possessive. The counselor can best determine the atmosphere he creates by observing the type and quality of participation coming from the client. Also the counselor can get feedback from the client through his reaction to the counselor. Is the client guarded and defensive or is he comfortable and open in his interaction?

CLOSING THE INTERVIEW

The last part of the interview is the closing. Surprisingly, the new counselor often has trouble closing an interview. This is especially true if the client is quite verbal. A natural ending comes and the session continues. The counselor realizes he should terminate the interview but does not know how to go about the task. If he is lucky most of his interviews just naturally wind down and are terminated, not so much by him but more by a tacit mutual agreement. If the counselor has difficulty closing the interview he does not control the interview.

Closing the interview is relatively simple once a pattern is established in the counselor's mind. The pattern for each interview should consist of the greeting, the statement of goals, the body of the interview and the closing. The closing consists of a restatement of the goals, a brief review of what was discussed, a brief evaluation of the accomplishment of the goals, a generalized statement of what goals will most likely be accomplished in the next counseling session, an assignment of responsibility for accomplishing tasks before the next session and the assignment of a definite appointment or a statement of the conditions which must occur prior to the assignment of an appointment for the next session. An example of a closing in keeping with the example set in the section on opening the interview follows:

> Now Mr. Smith in the few minutes we have remaining let us look at what we have accomplished. We were to discuss the reports we have received on you. We have discussed your General Aptitude Test Battery scores, the results of the interest test you took and have evaluated your past jobs and hobbies in light of these scores. We have discussed your interest in a particular vocation. Next week, we will explore this vocation in some depth. Prior to our next meeting on Friday at 11:00, you go to the vocational training school and talk to Mr. Jones about this particular vocation and I will contact some employers in this field to obtain some information regarding current demands, entry salary range, and advancement potential.

This is a quite natural closing to a counseling session. Some counselors get to this point and then almost compulsively ask the client some related question. This results in confusion for the client (is the interview over or not) and frustration for the counselor (after having closed the interview how do you go about closing it again).

SUMMARY

There are some common sense techniques which may be used to help insure the success of the counseling session regardless of the theoretical approach or counseling philosophy one adopts. To be most meaningful and productive, the interview should be viewed as consisting of four parts—the greeting, the opening, the body of the interview and the closing.

The achievement of counseling goals is dependent upon several factors including the mutual acceptance of counselor and client, the assurance of the counselor and his professional bearing, the counselor's sincerity and the accuracy of the information he relates in the counseling interview, his verbal and nonverbal communication and the maintenance of control of the interview.

The closing of an interview is smoother if there is a summarization of the interview and a statement of goals for the next interview along with the assignment of responsibilities for tasks to be completed prior to the next contact.

10

Selective Training

George R. Jarrell

A Definition of Training
General Training Methods
Formal Training Methods
Informal Methods
Summary
References

THE VOCATIONAL REHABILITATION ACT, as amended in 1965 (Public Law 89-333), states its purpose as that of "assisting states in rehabilitating handicapped individuals so that they *may prepare for* and engage in gainful employment to the extent of their capabilities, thereby increasing not only their social and economic well-being but also the productive capacity of the Nation." When an individual is referred to the state vocational rehabilitation agency, it is usually due to his inability to obtain or continue gainful employment. Barriers to the individual's employment may include a physical or mental disability. The rehabilitation counselor has to determine whether or not such disabilities can be remediated or, if not, what other skills can possibly be developed which will allow the individual to be gainfully employed in spite of his disability. Consideration must be given to the disabled individual's employment history, vocational interests and abilities, educational background and social and economic environment before developing a rehabilitation plan. In many instances, the rehabilitation plan will involve training. The majority of rehabilitation counselors are proficient in arranging for and motivating the client to complete physical restoration services, fewer are as competent in planning and arranging for training services.

A DEFINITION OF TRAINING

Training is defined as the "state of being trained." This definition offers little clarification of the concept to rehabilitation counselors employed in diverse settings. Frequently the counselor is as confused about the meaning of the term *training* as he is about who should be trained and in what areas. Availability of training and the client's willingness to undergo training are frequently the only criteria used to make this important determination.

Work has been defined by Zytowski[3] as "an expenditure of energy." Occupations may be arranged on a continuum with those that require the expenditure of physical energy at one extreme to those that require the expenditure of mental energy at the other, recognizing the fact that few occupations require exclusive expenditures of either. All too frequently only those occupations requiring physical output are considered legitimate training areas by rehabilitation counselors.

Training for the individual whose disability has resulted in a diminution of his ability to expend physical energy should be in an occupation with primary emphasis on the expenditure of mental energy. Likewise, for the individual whose impairment has resulted in a diminution in the individual's capacity to expend mental energy, the training emphasis should be physical output.

Vocational training is defined by Hamilton[1] as that kind of experience which equips a person with skills to do something for which someone will hire him. If rehabilitation counselors restrict their concept of training only to vocational training, the possibility of having to re-rehabilitate many clients is greatly increased. A well-planned coordinated approach to training based upon a comprehensive evaluation of social, economic, medical, educational and psychological factors is the best assurance of successful rehabilitation. Shabby, inappropriate or incomplete training may make possible the realization of the clients eventual vocational adjustment. According to Hamilton[1] this is true regardless of the extent or quality of the other services.

What is training in the rehabilitation process? How does the counselor determine who shall be trained? How do the counselor and the client arrive at the area or type of training? These are but a few of the questions all rehabilitation counselors must be prepared to answer if the disabled person is to successfully achieve the goal of vocational adjustment.

Evaluation of the client's readiness for employment is necessary in order to determine what he might be able to do and what he would like to do. Many rehabilitation counselors utilize the expressed interests of the client as a starting point in the determination of a vocational training area. This interest may be based on definite information concerning a particular job and its suitability as an employment objective, or it may be based on reasons which are superficial and in no way indicative of whether or not the work would be appropriate for the client. From the very beginning of the rehabilitation process, the counselor begins to make assessments in each of the following:

1. Useful skills possessed by the client which would allow him to obtain and hold a job.

2. The client's ability to function as a member of a group in any area of employment.

3. Areas in which the client's skills might be improved by training.[2]

Clients who have no work experience, this includes young clients and some who have been institutionalized for a long period, may require and be able to profit from personal adjustment and prevocational training. These are two distinct and different types of training and provision of one does not preclude the need for the other. The need for personal adjustment or prevocational training prior to formal vocational training is not likely to be recognized by the client. This determination should be made by the counselor as the result of the evaluation process and through counseling help the client to understand this need. In differing circumstances one type of training might be prevocational to one individual, personal adjustment training to another.

Like so many other areas of knowledge in rehabilitation, the categories into which we divide training for the purposes of discussion are not separate and distinct. For example, personal adjustment training is an integral component of any formalized vocational training program.

GENERAL TRAINING METHODS

Rehabilitation training may be said to include four broad classifications:

1. Personal adjustment training
2. Prevocational training
3. Compensatory skill training
4. Vocational training

Training may be needed within a single classification or in any combination of classifications. The potentialities of rehabilitation training can be realized only when appropriate to the needs of the client which have been identified as the result of a thorough evaluation. To be effective, training must be individualized for each client if it is to serve the function of preparing the client to enter the labor market and provide marketable skills.

Personal Adjustment Training

Hamilton[1] feels personal adjustment training can be used to assist in the development of habits, attitudes, insight and skills. This type of training can develop greater understanding of the demands of the workaday world, especially where the client has never before had paid employment. Attitudes compatible with the demands of the world of work, a sense of responsibility for one's own behavior, personal and work habits acceptable to the world of work, the ability to get along with others and the ability to take criticism as well as praise—these are all necessary if the client with a marketable skill is to obtain and hold employment. The actual activities followed under such training may be immediately or only remotely related to the employment objective.

Prevocational Training

Prevocational training is background and supplementary training which complements or facilitates the acquisition of knowledge and skills required by an occupation.[1] In general, prevocational training covers such background as is essential or complementary to knowledge of an occupation or skill in practicing it. In a prevocational program, the client is not trained to perform a particular job or for a specific vocational position. Instead he is encouraged to explore and find out what latent skills he has, in addition to determining those skills in which he can develop a ready proficiency. Prevocational training may therefore be an integral component of the evaluation process and conducted prior to the writing of the rehabilitation plan. Through meeting educational deficiencies, prevocational training makes possible the client's use of an existing skill. Teaching a person to read and complete an application for employment is a case in point. In this instance it is difficult to draw a rigid line with reference to whether or not the activity is academic or vocational. Self-reliance necessitates both the development of work skills and the assurance of their use.

Compensatory Skill Training

Lip reading, speech training, gait training and mobility training for the blind are illustrative of training in very specific skills which may be needed if the client is to enter and receive maximum benefit from a formalized training program or to reenter the competitive labor market.

Vocational Training

Vocational training imparts the knowledge and skills necessary for performance. It is differentiated from other types of rehabilitation training in that it provides specific occupational knowledge and skills required within the occupation.

Some private rehabilitation agencies maintain their own vocational shops. Tax-supported rehabilitation agencies purchase vocational training services for their clients from established facilities, just as they purchase medical service from established hospitals. In general, there are two ways of gaining vocational skills.[1]

FORMAL TRAINING METHODS

Public and private colleges and universities, trade and vocational schools, technical schools, apprenticeships and correspondence schools are the institutions which employ formal methods of developing employment skills. Formal methods of providing training are preferred by rehabilitation counselors because they require a minimum of counselor supervision. The institutions usually have stringent requirements in terms of class attendance and performance along with ongoing supervision of the client.

In increasing frequency, rehabilitation clients are being trained in four-year universities, both public and private. The long training period required is somewhat offset by the almost certain possibility of the client's obtaining employment. The wide diversity of courses offers the rehabilitation client a second chance at vocational exploration and in some institutions there is latitude for movement within the last two years. Graduate schools in large universities are also being used to train a few clients who became disabled after graduation from a four-year institution.

Junior colleges in many states are excellent resources. Many junior colleges provide training in the technical areas in addition to traditional offerings. A number of states have excellent junior college systems, with an institution within commuting distance for every resident. These offer an economical way to provide training for those clients who could not succeed in a four-year university.

The type of trade school found in many communities specializes within specific occupational categories such as automobile ignition, machine tool drafting, plumbing and watch repair. They are particularly desirable for occupational advancement in instances where disability requires that a skilled worker transfer to an occupation in which his former skills can be utilized. In general, this type of training experience is supplemental either to other training or to an existing skill. Usually the completion of a trade school provides only minimal requirements for employment in non-entry occupations. The disadvantages of this type of trade school lie in the fact that skills which it teaches are not readily transferable. Further, the value of the skills it teaches may be particularly limited by changing conditions of employment.

Approved apprenticeship programs are available in many of the occupational areas which are taught in trade or vocational schools. Whether or not the client should enroll in a trade school or apprenticeship program will depend on factors such as the client's age, educational attainment and the availability of apprenticeship training within the community. Apprenticeship programs of vocational training refer to learning under formal supervision usually while on a job. This method is particularly suited to those types of persons who cannot profit greatly from classroom situations. More importantly, this device makes possible training in many skilled trades for which school facilities are not available. Ordinarily, arrangements of this type come under careful scrutiny in labor union contracts; however, labor is usually cognizant of the needs of the disabled individual and willing to make special provisions for his entrance into apprenticeship programs. In addition to the difficulty in getting qualified clients enrolled in apprenticeship programs they usually require three to five years of training creating some reluctance on the part of many counselors to enroll a number of clients in these programs.

Correspondence study if chosen with discrimination, can be effective and sometimes is the only training resource available. However, the selection of correspondence study must be considered with an eye to the ethics of the school, the relevance of the material and the potentiality of the student. Correspondence study is most effective when it is considered as supplemental material. Frequently rehabilitation clients do not have the persistence to complete such courses without supervision. Of course, circumstances may alter any of these observations. Decisions of this type must be made for each client individually. For example, the oiler in the powerhouse who wishes to advance himself to the job of electrician may study with profit from correspondence courses. He has practical laboratory facilities in his daily work where he can observe others and discuss the practical application of his lessons with them.

Correspondence courses are also useful to make up academic

deficiencies. The young girl who wishes office and secretarial training can make up deficiencies in English. The would-be machinist can prepare himself for shop arithmetic through this source. It may be done with a minimum of interruption of other obligations, thus allowing for continuance on a present job. Correspondence courses have other values. In the case of the client with the preconceived job objective which is not based on a valid appraisal of himself or a realistic conception of his chosen occupation, the use of a simple correspondence course may serve as prevocational training or exploration.

The diversity and range of correspondence courses offer rehabilitation counselors in a variety of institutional settings the opportunity to provide training for their institutionalized clients. The self-discipline and perseverance required in all types of independent study can be therapeutic. Indirectly many correspondence courses serve as a source of occupational information and provide the initial preparation on which additional vocational training can be completed when the client leaves the institution. The counselor who is employed in a rehabilitation facility can easily monitor his client's progress in completing correspondence training which may be a difficult task when the client returns to his home community. For this reason self-study through correspondence courses may have more pragmatic value in an institutional setting.

INFORMAL METHODS

Formal training may not be available in the community in which the client lives. Sending him out of town to a training school may be neither possible nor necessary. Rather than limit the training opportunities to those available in a formal sense, an informal training program may be arranged within the community. Probably the best type of informal training is obtained by purchasing the services of a skilled worker to act as a trainer. This is referred to as on-the-job training. The small businessman such as the florist, radio repairman and small appliance repairman are examples. On-the-job training programs are readily adaptable to the individual and to local limitations. The same necessity for the quality of training must be observed and this requires frequent visits to the cooperating business to monitor the client's progress. Each counselor will have to develop the resources available in a particular community for provision of on-the-job training. The development of adequate training facilities is a mark of the successful rehabilitation counselor.

SUMMARY

Vocational training cannot be considered independently of other factors in the rehabilitation process. The most severely handicapped individual is the disabled person who must compete in the unskilled labor market. A well-planned training program for many of our disabled clients is the best insurance of quality rehabilitation. The rehabilitation counselor who hastens to plan for disabled clients without consideration for training is the first to question whether or not the services he provides warrant the attention of a well-trained rehabilitation counselor.

REFERENCES

1. Hamilton, K. W.: *Counseling the Handicapped in the Rehabilitation Process*, New York, the Ronald Press, 1950.
2. Lane, P. A., Soares, L. M., and Silverstone, L. S.: *Vocational Rehabilitation: A Therapeutic Pre-vocational Skill Training Program*, Bridgeport (Conn.), Antoniak Printing, 1970.
3. Zytowski, D. G.: *Vocational Behavior*, New York, Holt, Rinehart & Winston, 1968.

11

Vocational Placement

Richard E. Hardy

A Science of Vocational Behavior
Client-Centered Placement
Developing an Employment Program
Five Questions Counselors Must Be Able to Answer
Some Guidelines and Tools in Locating Employment Opportunities
Professional Placement
Getting the Client Ready for Employment
Eight Common Misconceptions About Vocational Placement
Job Analysis
Relating Psychological Data to Job Analysis Information in Vocational Placement
Follow-up After Placement
Summary
References

O NE OF THE MOST substantial contributions a rehabilitation counselor can make which affects his client's overall mental and physical adjustment is the placement of the individual on a job that is well suited to his abilities and interests. Vocational placement is underrated by many rehabilitation counselors and others who do not understand the full effects of its outcome. Helping the client find employment is often relegated to scanning newspaper want ads in search of opportunities or responding to a call from an employer who happens to have a job available. Certainly, occupational opportunities can be located through these means; however, the matching of the individual and the job is a complicated process which requires careful study and evaluation through interrelating all casework data on the individual with all information that can be secured relating to job requirements and job setting.

A SCIENCE OF VOCATIONAL BEHAVIOR

Lofquist and Davis[9] discussed a "science of vocational behavior" which they see as essentially vocational psychology. Whether one agrees or not that the "science of vocational behavior" is actually vocational psychology, the necessity for the full development of vocational behavior study as a science cannot be overstressed. The substantial growth during recent years of interest in the Vocational Evaluation and Work Adjustment Division of the National Rehabilitation Association and the subsequent publication of the *Vocational Evaluation and Work Adjustment Bulletin* have done a great deal to stimulate thinking and research on vocational behavior and practical problems of the individual and groups in the world of work. Certainly, in the future, vocational adjustment studies and work evaluation will take an even more prominent place in the rehabilitation counselor's work and in rehabilitation counselor education within university settings.

Above all, the rehabilitation counselor must be able to understand the "work personality" of his client. The "work personality profile" consists of such factors as vocational and avocational interests, abilities, needs, work habits, psychological maturity and interaction with on-the-job factors including job hierarchies, communication and health factors.

The rehabilitation counselor interested in developing expertise in placement should become familiar with available research on work adjustment. Studies done in vocational rehabilitation at the University of Minnesota[19] since 1957 offer a great deal of useful information.

CLIENT-CENTERED PLACEMENT

Rehabilitationists have heard much about "client-centered counseling" over the years. Because placement is an important part of the rehabilitation process, counselors should think of "client-centered placement." Job placement is a major client service which has helped rehabilitation agencies in getting substantial amounts of federal and state funds for program operations. The goal of work is one of the unique characteristics of rehabilitation. The placement of individuals on jobs through which they can find methods to maintain themselves is the concept which has allowed rehabilitation counseling to gain in stature as a social service profession with a substantial contribution to make to the individual and to society. In fact, most laymen would probably say that the location of appropriate jobs for clients is the main function of the rehabilitation counselor. It is interesting that rehabilitation counselors downplay the importance of placement in their jobs when they describe their activities to their friends and colleagues. Counselors might reflect more seriously upon their placement responsibilities if clients were thought of as consumers of their services and were given an opportunity to actually evaluate the jobs which they have obtained with the help of the counselor.

In fact, the use of the phrase "PLACE in employment" is one which misleads the rehabilitation counselor trainee and others concerning the method which should be used. The client and counselor must work together in order for the client to reach a decision concerning the type of job he wishes to have. After this decision is made and the rehabilitation counselor helps the client secure information about various jobs that exist in the geographical area where he wants to be employed, the client himself should take some initiative whenever possible to get employment with the assistance of the counselor. Once a feasible job is located, the client should be given the opportunity to evaluate it as the source of his future livelihood.

Quite often, when considering placement, the counselor is confronted with the dilemma of determining to whom he owes basic loyalty—the client or the employer—that is, should he be protective of the client when dealing with an employer or protective of the employer. How much of the client's problems and disability should the counselor relate to the employer? Should he obscure the client's disability in discussions with the employer?

If the professional relationship was bilateral and concerned only the client and counselor the answer to the dilemma would be immediately obvious; however, the relationship is trilateral.

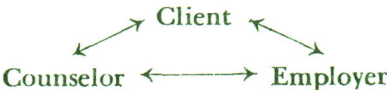

As such, the counselor owes equal professional responsibility to both the client and prospective employer. Therefore, the counselor should communicate with the employer in a basic, forthright manner. The counselor is professionally obligated to be honest in his dealings with the employer.

If the counselor fails to be completely honest and forthright with the employer, he not only jeopardizes his professional relationship with this employer thereby obviating any possibility of placing clients in this area in the future, but he also takes a great chance of jeopardizing the client-employer relationship later when the employer becomes more aware of the client's attributes which the counselor chose to hide or misrepresent. Consequently, I feel rather strongly that the counselor should discuss with the client what he is planning to relate to the employer. If the client refuses to allow the counselor to discuss his assets, liabilities and disability with the employer, the counselor should modify his role in the placement process. His role should be one of providing placement information to the client, but he should not enter actively into the placement process with the client.

There are two limits to this interchange between the counselor and employer relative to the client:

1. The counselor and employer should discuss thoroughly those aspects and only those aspects of the client's background which have a direct relation with the job.

2. The counselor should communicate with the employer on a level at which both are comfortable in the exchange of information.

Quite often a counselor approaches a prospective employer regarding a specific client and as the conversation progresses the counselor finds himself relating information which, while highly pertinent in the rehabilitation process, has little to do with the client as an employee. In each instance in which the counselor makes an employer contact for placement purposes, the counselor should have summarized previously all material in the case folder which is directly related to the client's proficiency in a particular position—both his assets and liabilities. After reviewing this summary the counselor should refrain from relating any other information he may have derived from counseling sessions, training evaluations or diagnostic workups. A mark of professionalism is the ability to communicate the essential factors relating to the client and still respect the client's fundamental right to confidentiality of case material.

The second limitation to communication between the counselor and employer requires the counselor to assess the sophistication of the employer and communicate with him on that level. As a general rule the counselor should avoid using terminology which, though descriptive, is highly laden with emotional connotations. The most effective approach the counselor can take in discussing the client's assets and liabilities is to describe behavior rather than categorizing it with diagnostic labels. For example: This person experienced learning difficulties in the academic areas rather early and is slow in learning new procedures. He is ineffective in dealing with abstract concepts and carrying out complex, oral instructions and should not be placed in a situation requiring independent judgments in changing conditions; however, he is very adept in performing concrete tasks and is capable of making routine, repetitive judgments. This description means more to the employer than the term "mental retardate."

DEVELOPING AN EMPLOYMENT PROGRAM

Counselors who are involved with placement should be familiar with information offered in the publication, *Workers Worth Their Hire* (American Mutual Insurance Alliance),[1] which is available through the President's Committee on Employment of the Physically Handicapped. Myths concerning employment of the handicapped are disspelled by information given in this publication. Counselors will find that discussions of the excellent record of handicapped persons in such areas as safety, absenteeism, production and motivation to work are of considerable help to them in their discussions with employers, union leaders and work supervisors. The counselor should be certain that he not only talks about these factors with top agency employment officials but also that he manages, at the appropriate time, to mention these subjects to supervisors within the work area. The degree of acceptance which supervisors give to handicapped clients is often highly influential in not only helping them "get off to a good start" but also in maintaining their work at a level commensurate with the supervisor's expectations.

Some rehabilitation counselors have felt that the counselor should not have a specific client in mind when talking with an employer, but that he should sell the concept of hiring the handicapped to the employer and later get into the work setting in order to locate the types of jobs which would be available to handicapped individuals. This concept can be extremely useful and can help open many doors to handicapped employees; however, after convincing the employer of the value of hiring handicapped persons, the counselor often will be asked to refer a prospective employee immediately if a particular opening exists in the work setting. If a counselor is unable to meet this request, his public relations and sales program can be substantially damaged in terms of future placements with the employer.

Each rehabilitation counselor should constantly evaluate his efforts in placement to make certain that he is moving clients toward jobs in line with their overall adjustment and ability. One of the key sources of learning about job opportunities for any client is often the client's past experiences and previous job responsibilities. In many cases, clients will wish to return to the type of employment held prior to the onset of the employment handicap. In fact, many former employers will feel a responsibility for injured employees and wish again to offer them employment after they have received rehabilitation services. The client will offer many insights about himself to the counselor who then has the responsibility to match abilities, needs and interests of the client with requirements and offerings of the job. One of the primary sources, then, of information about types of employment for the client is the client himself. This information can be gained by a study of his background and from interest inventories and interviews with him and his family.

The counselor will also wish to use the services of the state employment agency which maintains local offices throughout the United States. Many prospective employers inform the employment service of job openings. This agency also offers counseling, placement and evaluation services for handicapped job applicants. The Vocational Rehabilitation Act, Public Law 89-565, stipulates that the vocational rehabilitation state plan shall "provide for entering into cooperative agreements with the system of public employment offices in the state and the maximum utilization of the job placement and employment counseling services and other services and facilities of such offices."

FIVE QUESTIONS COUNSELORS MUST BE ABLE TO ANSWER

Of course, many different problem areas can arise when the counselor is discussing hiring handicapped workers with an employer. Questions range from, How will the person get to the place of employment? to What will he do in case of fire? Incidentally, these two questions usually can be answered with the same responses which any employee would give—in the first case, "By bus or car" and in the second, "Get the hell out like everyone else."

The first basic question which usually arises is that of increased insurance rates if handicapped workers are employed. This is most often an honest employer reaction to the question concerning employment of handicapped workers. Insurance rates would rise if individuals were employed in an agency which tended to have more accidents; however, handicapped workers have been proven to be as safe in the performance of their duties as other workers. In fact, some handicapped persons such as the blind have actually shown better records of safety than nonhandicapped workers. American Mutual Insurance Alliance[1] has published materials relevant to the fact that handicapped workers are as safe or safer than nonhandicapped workers. The counselor should have this information readily available and indicate to the prospective employer that indeed workmen's compensation insurance rates are determined, in part, according to the relative hazards of the work done by the industry in question. Yearly rates also are determined according to the industry's record of accidents and insurance claims. These are good reasons for hiring handicapped workers. If an employer persists in believing that his insurance rates will increase, the counselor should ask him to contact his insurance agent or read again his insurance contract.

A second question which often arises is this: Why should I hire a handicapped individual when I can employ "normal" persons whom I can count on for employment without difficulty? The counselor will have to answer this question according to his own philosophy and training. Some helpful responses might include the following:

1. Ask why he should not employ individuals whose employment records have been proven and who are well known and highly recommended by rehabilitation employment specialists.

2. Describe the medical, social and psychiatric evaluations completed on all clients (not being specific or violating confidentiality). In other words, why not hire an individual who comes to the employer, in a sense, "certified" as ready for employment?

3. Remind him that by doing so he is actually supporting what he, as a taxpayer, has already invested some money in—an employment program for the handicapped which has proven to be highly successful.

Another question which frequently is raised in employment interviews concerns the firing or dismissal of the employee and the employer's reluctance to treat the rehabilitant in the same manner he would treat other employees. The counselor again will have to rely on his own resources; however, an analogy may be helpful here.

Indicate that if you, as a salesman, were selling refrigerators and the employer bought one which later malfunctioned, you would stand by your product and attempt to get it in good working order. The counselor could briefly discuss follow-up procedures with the employer at this time. He might also indicate that once the handicapped employee has worked for the employer for a time, the employer will feel that he is a fully functioning, well-adjusted employee who should be treated just as all other employees are. Assure the employer of your confidence in the client.

A fourth question which counselors must be ready to answer concerns architectural barriers and physical limitations of the work setting. Counselors should be frank in their responses to questions concerning limitations of the client and restrictions imposed by the work setting. The counselor should be the first to indicate that certain jobs are infeasible for many of his clients. He should be certain to get across to the employer that he is not going to place a client on an unsafe job or on a job which he cannot handle.

A fifth question which often arises concerning employment of the handicapped is that of the "second injury" which might result in total disability and effect the workman's compensation payments made by the employer. In a vast majority of states and the District of Columbia and Puerto Rico, "second injury" funds or equivalent arrangements have been established. In these localities, the employer is responsible only for the last injury and the employee is compensated for the disability which results from combined injuries.

SOME GUIDELINES AND TOOLS IN LOCATING EMPLOYMENT OPPORTUNITIES

1. The counselor should be aware of industrial developments within the area that he serves and in adjacent areas.

2. The three volumes of the *Dictionary of Occupational Titles*[17] offer a wealth of useful information for rehabilitation counselors. Much emphasis is given to descriptions of physical and personality requirements for various jobs. In addition, these volumes can help expand the counselor's concepts about various types of jobs which are related to the general interest area of the rehabilitation client.

3. Employers with whom former clients have been placed can be important sources of information.

4. Previously rehabilitated clients can offer many sound ideas about existing employment opportunities.

5. Local Chambers of Commerce usually provide an industrial index which lists types of work available in most communities. Counselors also should coordinate their efforts with those of the state employment service since the mutual sharing of job information can be valuable to both employment service counselors and rehabilitation counselors.

6. When placing persons on jobs in rural areas, the worker should consider enlisting the support of local community leaders such as doctors, city councilmen, postmasters and religious leaders as well as Rotary, Kiwanis, Ruritan and other civic groups.

7. If the counselor is interested in assisting individuals in becoming small business managers and operators, he should get in touch with the Small Business Administration office serving his local area.

PROFESSIONAL PLACEMENT

In rehabilitation jargon, "professional placement" generally means developing client employment opportunities which require at least a college education. Bauman and Yoder[2] offer excellent coverage of this area of placement as it pertains to work for the blind. Professional placement is "facilitative" work for the counselor. The counselor can help his client in terms of giving advice and information; however, he must be certain not to take the place of the client in securing actual jobs. The client must be ready to meet without the counselor with the employer to discuss his professional qualifications for work. When he has a particular problem, the counselor should be able to assist him with information which could be helpful during the employer interview. For example, he should be coached on how to present himself most favorably. The counselor might help his client develop a resume or portfolio which would outline his training and give examples of any previous work done in the job field in which he wants employment. Other procedures usually followed in placement may or may not be appropriate according to the judgment of the counselor.

A worker in charge of professional placement may want to organize precollege orientation groups for clients. It will be necessary also for the counselor who is dealing with persons in training to inform them about services available while they are in training and away from their home area. If, for instance, clients are attending college, the rehabilitation counselor should help them become acquainted with college counseling center services at the institution they attend.[5]

Effective professional placement requires long-range planning on the part of both counselor and client. Two years before placement (in training cases) is not too early for the client to begin planning with his counselor in order to solve problems related to his securing the type of employment he wants. The counselor will need to prepare by knowing who the prospective employers are and the requirements of the job.

GETTING THE CLIENT READY FOR EMPLOYMENT

Planning for placement does not begin once the client has had vocational training and is ready "skill wise" for employment, but when the counselor first reads the client's rehabilitation referral form. The rehabilitation worker must constantly learn about his client in order to effectively help him secure the type of employment he needs. Jeffrey[8] has developed a job readiness test which helps in the evaluation of job preparedness of clients. While the total instrument is not applicable to all rehabilitation clients, certain questions are quite helpful with most rehabilitation clients.

Role playing is an excellent method to use in preparing a client for employment interviews. After going through a mock interview which includes a variety of questions, the counselor can give suggestions concerning how the client might improve the impression he makes with the employer. In role playing, it is helpful for the counselor as well as the client to play the role of the employer. Once this is tried, counselors will immediately realize the usefulness of this procedure. The client should realize that getting a job is not an easy task and that he, to the best of his ability, should participate in the job-securing aspects of placement. In some cases, it is an indicator of effective rehabilitation procedures when the client is able to, in fact, "get his own job," assuming of course that he is ready for employment. The ability with which the client will be able to do this will vary with his motivation and the severity of his social, mental or physical handicap.

The rehabilitation counselor must stress "training" as a partial answer to many of the problems of the handicapped worker. Overtraining a worker for a job which will affect his personal and family adjustment for many years to come is seldom done. In each case, the counselor must take an individual approach to helping his client. In the case of those who are educationally or socially retarded, various remedial programs may be necessary before actual work training programs can begin. In each case, the counselor must exercise considerable judgment concerning what his client needs in order to be totally ready for employment.

On-the-job training can be a very effective arrangement for client training. In many of these cases, the state rehabilitation agency will make "tuition" payments to the employer-trainer in order that the rehabilitation counselor may get the employer interested in training a client and evaluating his work. It may be necessary for the counselor to help the employer arrange the appropriate payment schedule for the client since he is not a trained employee and would not receive an amount equal to a regularly salaried employee.

Bridges[3] offered four major factors which are involved in successful employment of handicapped workers. These remain as highly important considerations for the counselor:

1. The worker should have the ability to accomplish the task efficiently—that is, to be able to meet the physical demands of the job.

2. The worker should not be a hazard to himself.

3. The worker must not jeopardize the safety of others.

4. The job should not aggravate the disability or handicap of the worker.

EIGHT COMMON MISCONCEPTIONS ABOUT VOCATIONAL PLACEMENT

1. Because placement occurs toward the end of the rehabilitation process, the counselor's responsibility to the client diminishes.

2. Placement is an activity which requires no counselor training and is a matter of matching an available client with an available job.

3. Client location of his job or "self-placement" cannot be effective rehabilitation work.

4. When a client is ready for vocational placement, the information in his case folder is no longer of value to his counselor since the client has been, in a sense, readied for employment.

5. Follow-up after placement always can be handled easily by phone or mail communications with the employer or client.

6. Labor market trends and job information and analysis are the responsibilities of placement specialists and employment service counselors, not of general rehabilitation counselors.

7. An employer will notify the counselor and the rehabilitation agency when he is dissatisfied with a client placement.

8. An employer will automatically call upon the rehabilitation agency to furnish him with additional employees when he needs them.

Rehabilitation counselors should be certain that their clients understand that it is not necessarily bad to be turned down for a job. Counselors should understand that experience has shown that nine or ten employer contacts often must be made before the counselor makes a placement.

JOB ANALYSIS

Every rehabilitation counselor should be thoroughly familiar with the techniques of job analysis for use in selective placement. The rehabilitation counselor has to be able to match the prospective worker's social, mental and physical qualifications with requirements of the job. Factors such as judgment, initiative, alertness and general health and capability must always be taken into consideration as well as the individual's social and economic background.

Job analysis should answer certain questions concerning the job. *What* does the worker do in terms of physical and mental effort that go into the work situation? How is the work done? In other words, does this job involve the use of equipment and mathematics, or does it require travel. *Why* does the worker perform the job? This component of the job analysis answers the question concerning the overall purpose or the sum total of the task and is the reason for doing the job. The worker also should understand the relationship of his task to other tasks that make up the total job.

Generally, the rehabilitation counselor should attempt to place clients on jobs which they can "handle" and which do not require modification. In some cases, however, minor modifications can be made with little or no reengineering effort. The counselor will have to be careful in suggesting reengineering of a job, since this can be a costly undertaking in many instances. The major objective should be that of helping handicapped workers integrate effectively into the total work force without major modification or change in the work situation.

The following outline can be used in evaluating a job which is to be performed by a handicapped worker:

A. Name Used for Position Surveyed
   1. D.O.T. title
   2. Alternate titles
   3. D.O.T. definitions
   4. Items worked on in plant surveyed
B. Usual Operator
   1. Sex
   2. General characteristics
C. Physical and Psychological Demands
   1. Activities
   2. Working conditions
   3. Skill required
   4. Intelligence

       5. Temperament
       6. Other
   D. Description of Physical Activities
   E. Description of Working Conditions
   F. Description of Hazards
   G. Steps Required to Accomplish the Goal of the Work
   H. Equipment Found in the Particular Plant Surveyed
       1. Identification
       2. Set-up and maintenance
       3. Modification (if required for the handicapped)
   I. Equipment Variations Which May Be Found in Other Plants
   J. Pre-employment Training Required
   K. Training Procedure
   L. Production
       1. Full production definition
       2. Time to reach normal efficiency
   M. Interrelation with Preceding and Succeeding Jobs

RELATING PSYCHOLOGICAL DATA TO JOB ANALYSIS INFORMATION IN VOCATIONAL PLACEMENT

As a first step in getting to know clients well, the counselor should make arrangements to secure appropriate psychological information about them. He should either complete job analyses or use available job evaluation data to make decisions about types of information which will be of value to his clients in the job selection and placement procedure. In many instances, however, the counselor fails to synthesize information obtained from two of his most important sources: the psychological evaluation and the job analysis.

The counselor should take five basic steps, as described by Hardy,[6] in developing a successful procedure for interrelating and using important information. He should:

1. Study the needs of the client and the types of satisfaction meaningful to him.

2. Make certain that valid psychological and job analysis data have been gathered.

3. Review the requirements of the job and evaluate the individual traits needed to meet job requirements.

4. Consider the environmental pressures with which the individual must interact.

5. Discuss the job analysis and psychological evaluation with the client so that he will understand what the work will require of him and what it will offer.

Both client and counselor need to have an understanding of job requirements in order to make realistic decisions. One important move should be structuring a set of goals—a guide to help the client avoid useless foundering that gets him nowhere. What satisfactions is he seeking? What is important to him in the long run and what types of work or work settings will provide these satisfactions? These are questions which the counselor must help the client answer.

Maslow[12] has suggested a hierarchy of the individual needs which the counselor must understand in order to evaluate a client's psychological status—his satisfactions and frustrations. In the usual order of prepotency these needs are for (a) physiological satisfaction; (b) safety; (c) belongingness and love; (d) importance, respect, self-esteem and independence; (e) information; (f) understanding; (g) beauty; and (h) self-actualization.

In our society, there is no single situation which is potentially more capable of giving satisfaction at all levels of these needs as a person's work, and it is the responsibility of the counselor to help his client plan for future happiness through adjustment on the job.

The worker needs to help his client become fully aware of the social pressures of the job because these are as important to the individual as the actual job pressures. A client's ability to adapt to the social interactions of the work environment will directly affect his job performance.

The counselor always must ask himself what the requirements of the job are. This question can be answered superficially or in considerable detail. A lay job analysis can give superficial requirements, but the responsibility for an in-depth job description belongs to the expert—the counselor who will often have to give direct advice to the client.

Effective placement requires effective planning. Planning cannot be really useful unless appropriate information has been obtained, interrelated and skillfully utilized so that the client and the counselor have a clear understanding of possible problems and possible solutions.

FOLLOW-UP AFTER PLACEMENT

A rehabilitation counselor often is tempted to consider his job completed when the client is placed on a job which appears suitable for him; however, the phase of rehabilitation which begins immediately after the person has been placed in employment is one of the most complex. Follow-up involves the counselor's ability to work as a middleman between employer and client in order to help the client solve problems related to his handicap which may arise after being hired. The counselor must be diplomatic and resourceful in maintaining the employer's confidence in his client's ability to do the job. At the same time, he must let the client know that he has full faith in him. The counselor, however, must somehow evaluate how his client is performing on the job and make certain that he is available to help if problems arise which the client cannot solve.

In addition to the worker's service to the client during follow-up, this period can offer real public relations opportunities for the counselor, especially when the employer notes the interest with which the counselor "follows" his client. The frequency of follow-up varies according to the counselor's judgment of the client's job ability and adjustment.

Agency regulations usually require that a final follow-up be done after thirty days in order to make certain that placement is successful before a "case" can be closed as rehabilitated. Counselors should also consider follow-up periods of sixty to eighty days after placement. Again, this helps reassure the client of the interest of the agency and the counselor in his success and can be of value to the counselor in further developing employment opportunities for handicapped persons.

In follow-up after professional placement, however, the counselor must forget the sixty- to ninety-day period which is usually adequate in the placement of clients in nonprofessional jobs. A longer period will be necessary and this period will vary with job complications and severity of the client's handicap. Bauman and Yoder[2] have recommended six months to a year for follow-up for most cases of blind persons placed in professional work.

Counselors will probably wish to schedule specific days for follow-up in the field. Generally, the period of follow-up is a time when the counselor sees the efforts of the entire rehabilitation process coming to fruition. If the job has been well analyzed and the client well evaluated and placed, follow-up will be pleasurable experience for the counselor.

SUMMARY

The counselor's responsibility in vocational placement must not be underrated. The decisions made at this stage in the rehabilitation process not only affect the client's immediate feelings of satisfaction and achievement but also, of course, his long-term physical and mental health. The counselor has a real responsibility to "ready" the client for employment by giving him the type of information that he needs about the job and about holding employment once it is achieved. Placement should be "client-centered" with strong emphasis given to the client's opinions about work and how it will affect him and his family. Counselors must be ready to answer the questions that employers will ask about hiring handicapped persons and about the rehabilitation program. Vocational placement is high level public relations work.

The counselor must be knowledgeable about job analysis and must interrelate all medical, psychological and social data with job analysis information in order to be successful in client-centered placement. Once placement has been achieved, the counselor must "follow-up" the client in order to make certain that he is doing well on the job. The client should have an opportunity to evaluate his job and also the efforts of his counselor in helping him decide on and obtain the job. Effective placement requires effective planning, and counselors must constantly evaluate their knowledge of the world of work and their ability to interrelate information in order to assure real placement success.

REFERENCES

1. American Mutual Insurance Alliance: *Workers Worth Their Hire*, Chicago, Illinois.
2. Bauman, M.K., and Yoder, N.M.: *Placing the Blind and Visually Handicapped in Professional Occupations*. Washington, D. C., Office of Vocational Rehabilitation, Department of Health, Education and Welfare, 1962.
3. Bridges, C. C.: *Job Placement of the Physically Handicapped*. New York, McGraw-Hill, 1946.
4. Department of Veterans' Benefits, Veterans' Administration: *They Return to Work*. Washington, D. C., U. S. Government Printing Office, 1963.
5. Hardy, R. E.: Counseling physically handicapped college students. *The New Outlook for the Blind, 59, (No. 5)*:182-183, 1965.
6. Hardy, R. E.: Relating psychological data to job analysis information in vocational counseling. *The New Outlook for the Blind, 63 (No. 7)*: 202-204, 1969.
7. International Society for the Welfare of Cripples: *Selective Placement of the Handicapped*. New York, 1955.
8. Jeffrey, David L.: *Pertinent Points on Placement*. Clearing House, Oklahoma State University, November 1969.
9. Lofquist, L.H., and Davis, R.V.: *Adjustment to Work—A Psychological View of Man's Problems in Work-Oriented Society*. New York, Appleton-Century-Crofts, 1969.
10. McGowan, J.F., and Porter, T.L.: *An Introduction to the Vocational Rehabilitation Process*. Rehabilitation Services Administration, July 1967.
11. McNamee, H.T., and Jeffrey, R.P.: *Service to the Handicapped 1960*. Phoenix (Ariz.), Arizona State Employment Service, 1960.
12. Maslow, A. H.: A theory of human motivation. *Psychol Rev, 50*:370-396, 1954.
13. Office of Vocational Rehabilitation: *Training Personnel for the State Vocational Rehabilitation Programs—A Guide for Administrators*. Washington, D.C., U.S. Government Printing Office, 1957.
14. Sinick, D.: *Placement Training Handbook*, Washington, D.C., Office of Vocational Rehabilitation, 1962.
15. Stalnaker, W.O., Wright, K.C., and Johnston, L.T.: *Small Business Enterprises in Vocational Rehabilitation*. Washington, D.C., U.S. De-

partment of Health, Education and Welfare, Vocational Rehabilitation Administration, Rehabilitation Services Series No. 63-47, 1963.
16. Thomason, B., and Barrett, A.: *The Placement Process in Vocational Rehabilitation Counseling*. Washington, D.C., U.S. Department of Health, Education and Welfare, Office of Vocational Rehabilitation, GTP Bull. No. 2, Rehabilitation Service Series No. 545, 1960.
17. U.S. Employment Service: *Dictionary of Occupational Titles*. Washington, D.C., U.S. Government Printing Office, 1965.
18. U.S. Employment Service: *Selected Placement for the Handicapped* (Rev. ed.). Washington, D.C.; U.S. Government Printing Office, 1945.
19. Weiss, D.J., Davis, R.V., Lofquist, L.H. and England, G.W.: *Minnesota Studies in Vocational Rehabilitation*. University of Minnesota, Industrial Relations Center.

PART FOUR

THE REHABILITATION PRACTITIONER IN A WORK SETTING

Orientation of the Counselor in the General Rehabilitation Program

Cooperative Programming

Administrative Concerns in Cooperative Programs

The Vocational Rehabilitation-Public Education Cooperative Program

The School Unit Counselor

The Correctional Institution and Vocational Rehabilitation

Rehabilitative Counseling in Correctional Settings

The Mental Health Rehabilitation Counselor

Providing Counseling Services to Blind and Severely Visually Impaired Persons

12

Orientation of the Counselor in the General Rehabilitation Program

Parnell McLaughlin

The Graduate Rehabilitation Counselor
The Counselor Trained in a Related Field
Summary
References

THE REHABILITATION counselor position is the basic position in the provision of services to clients in the state-federal program of rehabilitation. The program over the past fifty years has been successful because the counselor provided services to clients on a person-to-person basis. The other positions in the program provided supportive services for the position of the counselor. The same situation holds true today. The disabled person receives the attention of the counselor and is treated as a person worthy of the time and effort of the counselor. In this chapter we are concerned with the orientation the counselor needs to understand the position he is accepting. Orientation training will vary according to the type of training the individual has received before being accepted for employment with the state agency.

The counselor carries a general case load in a district or regional setting or he may be assigned special duties in reference to a disability group. The needs of each counselor from the standpoint of an orientation program are to enable him to handle his duties and will be much the same regardless of the assignment. The training will be such that he should have the required knowledge to provide the services of a rehabilitation program to those individuals eligible for the services. In order to understand the duties of a counselor, I would like to review what may be expected of the person who accepts such a position in the state rehabilitation agency.

First, the person must like to work with people and must realize that each person should be treated with courtesy and respect. A person is not coming to the rehabilitation office to be judged or to receive charity but to secure help from a person trained and knowledgeable about the techniques, services and procedures to provide the help in accordance with the needs of the individual. It is presumed that the counselor who is hired will be able to meet people. He may or may not have some background in the rehabilitation process. Such knowledge is helpful, however.

Second, the person choosing to become a counselor should have an interest in people and in their problems. The counseling role is a demanding one and it is expected that a person will have good health and be stable emotionally. In order to provide quality services a person should be mature in judgment. The counselor has to work closely with the individuals in his case load and must be practical in working through the rehabilitation program with each one. In considering the role of the counselor, it is important for the individual to relate to his clients; his manner and appearance, therefore, become of major importance. If the behavior, dress or grooming is too bizarre or unusual, the client coming to the program may wonder about the individual counselor and may wonder what his problems are, and as a net result the counselor may be of little help to those coming to the agency.

Third, the counselor must be able to evaluate on an individual basis and to analyze each case to provide the necessary services for each person. People may come to the agency and say they have one disability, and as we go through the process of providing services, we find that the individual may need help with disabilities other than the one he says he has. The counseling which is required in a case may be vocational; it may deal with family problems; and often a major counseling problem may be finances. The individual seeking to become a counselor must be willing to spend extra time on the job because of the community involvement which will be necessary if he is to become a valuable asset to the agency and the handicapped people he is serving.

Training programs for rehabilitation counselors are fairly new. Prior to 1954 there were no such programs.[1] Counselors had training in related programs, such as guidance and counseling, education, psychology, social work and sociology. Many persons serving as rehabilitation counselors in the early program had little special training before accepting the position as a counselor. Their knowledge and training was acquired by experience on the job, by short-term training conferences and institutes, and by communication with other persons working on the job in another district or state.

In the legislation of 1954, provision was made for the funding of rehabilitation counselor training programs at the college and university level. This was placed on the graduate level and usually required two years of work. The state agencies who hired the graduates of these programs realized that although the knowledge and theory of the rehabilitation process and many of the various techniques of working with the handicapped had been mastered by the new counselors, the agency still had to provide an in-service orientation training program. This orientation program included a discussion of the agency philosophy, the agency structure and organization, the channels of communication in the agency, and specific rules and regulations that governed the operation. The day-to-day operation and many other aspects of the rehabilitation program varied greatly from state to state, and still does.

THE GRADUATE REHABILITATION COUNSELOR

The person who has a background in rehabilitation counseling will be able to complete the orientation training in a very short time in comparison to the person being hired with no knowledge of the rehabilitation process and program. The agency hiring the trained rehabilitation counselor will need to develop a training program that will cover the following specifics so that the counselor will have the knowledge to enable him to fulfill the duties of the position. This training program should cover the following items in detail:

A. Philosophy of the Agency
   1. Scope of the population to be served (Definition of the disabled)
   2. Limitations (May be defined by federal or state requirements)
   3. Emphasis (Special disabilities may be emphasized, such as the deaf, the mentally retarded and the mentally ill).
   4. Priorities (May be assigned, such as those on welfare or those with greatest financial need)
B. Rules and Regulations
   1. Published rules of the agency, such as those governing employees (annual leave, sick leave, travel policy, et cetera)
   2. Ethical conduct (The counselor must be aware of his actions because of the counseling position)
   3. Responsibilities of position (The position is such that the counselor must remember he is the representative of the agency and he has a responsibility for the clients in the case load)
C. Forms—State and Federal
   1. *Why*—to enable the counselor to perform and provide services in an organized procedure.
   2. *When*—in accordance with procedures of the agency.
   3. *How*—use the forms when they are needed to provide a service or to make a report or record an important item.
D. Organization
   1. Federal-state relationships
   2. State organization
   3. Channels of communication
   4. Procedures to be followed
E. Supervision in Program
   1. State
   2. District or regional
   3. Office

F. Case Supervision
   1. Case flow
   2. Reporting procedures
   3. Documentation requirements
G. Duties
   1. Particular assignment
   2. Part in the program
   3. Counselor responsibility
H. Procedures of Operation
   1. Interviewing
   2. Coordinating services for client
   3. Case flow
I. Referrals
   1. How are they started in the process?
   2. Evaluation and diagnosis—what does this mean in this particular agency?
   3. Acceptance
   4. Plan development
   5. Implementation of plan—scope of services needed to complete the plan
   6. Client responsibility
   7. Case movement in the program
   8. Training—suitable in terms of interest, disability, aptitude, job possibility
   9. Placement—suitable in line with training
   10. Follow-up—length of time may vary
   11. Closure—meaning of closure. How does the agency deal with quotas? Is this a necessary measurement? Is it a valid measurement criterion? Should it be eliminated or should it be one of many factors used to determine the value of a particular program?

THE COUNSELOR TRAINED IN A RELATED FIELD

This individual will require a much greater length of time to become a fully-trained, qualified counselor. In addition to the orientation training which the agency will provide, the training must cover the areas in which the graduate rehabilitation counselor received training in his school program. This type of training may be secured through the cooperation of a college or university by providing opportunities for this person to take the training for a rehabilitation counselor. If no such training program is available, then the agency will have to accept the responsibility of providing the necessary knowledge for the individual. This may be provided by an extended in-service training at the district level, by making use of short-term training institutes which may be provided by the regional Rehabilitation Services Administration office or by special institutes or seminars sponsored by various training agencies or by the state agency. Most agencies make use of all these opportunities. This was the way the original counselors in the rehabilitation program gained their knowledge and received training.

In order to make certain required training is received, there are areas which must be covered in some detail.

Interviewing

The interview is an important part of the acceptance of the rehabilitation program as far as the client is concerned. The interview should be handled carefully from the very beginning.

First, the counselor needs to realize that the client may be somewhat anxious because this may be a new situation for him, and the counselor, therefore, will need to take time to put the client at ease. It is during this first period that you can explain the services of the rehabilitation program to the client; how we work; and, in general, create the feeling that this is a service that is available to him should he choose to make use of it.

Second, the counselor should remember that he must take time to "sell" himself in the initial interview as well as to "sell" the program. If you can establish in the mind of the client you have a feeling of confidence in yourself, the counseling you do in the rehabilitation process with the client will be much easier.

After this is done, then you may explain that you need to gather information about the client in order to help him evaluate his total situation and to help him make use of his abilities. This may be followed by filling out the survey sheet and making the necessary arrangements for medical examinations and perhaps the special psychological or vocational information or measurements which you may wish to provide for the client. This first interview may last for a full hour and should always be considered as a very important interview, as the client will think in terms of the program and what it has to offer by the way in which the first interview is handled. The counselor should be aware of the fact that under no conditions do we talk down to the client nor in any way make him feel inferior. We must get across the viewpoint that this is the client's program and we are here to help him help himself.

Counseling

This is a term which must be definitely explained because it is easily misunderstood. In defining the process of counseling, the old definition of "vocational guidance," as developed by the National Vocational Guidance Association[3] as revised in 1937, is very helpful. "Vocational guidance is the process of assisting the individual to choose an occupation, prepare for it, enter upon, and progress in it. It is concerned primarily with helping individuals make decisions and choices involved in planning a future and building a career—decisions and choices necessary in effecting satisfactory vocational adjustment."

Rehabilitation counseling is a process which helps the individual to become aware of and evaluate his assets. He has to consider carefully each factor which may affect his selection of a vocational occupation. The counselor is able to assist the person to interpret the findings in each and every area and to arrive at a satisfactory choice in each case.

Rehabilitation counseling is broader than what is normally thought of as vocational counseling because of the medical information and social history which must be considered. Rehabilitation counseling still leaves the decisions to the individual after he has had an opportunity to evaluate all the information. Rehabilitation counseling is a process that continues during the entire time the individual is in the program. The program has developed the performance evaluation to help in instances when it is impossible to determine the rehabilitation potential in the usual procedure. This development followed the broadening of the rehabilitation program to consider behavior disorders, as well as offering services to the more severely involved, physically disabled, as well as the moderately mentally retarded. This provides a method of evaluating the work potential of an individual which may not be possible to determine by other means.

Acceptance

What does this mean to the program? It means that following diagnosis and evaluation, the individual does meet the criteria for eligibility as required in the vocational rehabilitation regulations if there is the presence of a physical or mental disability with limitations; the limitations, because of the physical or mental disability, constitute a substantial barrier to employment; and there is a reasonable expectation that through provision of rehabilitation services, the individual may be made employable.[3] Acceptance means the individual is eligible for those services which he may need to make him employable. He may need only counseling and placement, or he might need many more services, such as physical restoration, training, supplies, transportation, et cetera.

Physical Restoration Services

Physical restoration sometimes is a very misunderstood service. It is provided only after a total evaluation and only in relationship to the attainment of the vocational objective or, if necessary, to enable the agency to determine the vocational potential of an individual. Many counselors have raised objections to the provision of only a single service, not realizing that counseling is such a service. For example, some have said you could not only provide glasses for a rehabilitation client. Glasses may not be provided without the proper examinations and without determining the need in relationship to the vocational objective. However, if the evaluation is made and the individual needs glasses to proceed with the rehabilitation plan, they may certainly be provided.

Plan Development

The plan is developed after the psychological information, the social history, the medical information, the work history and the various observations that may affect the program have been brought together and interpreted to the client. His interest, aptitudes and abilities are interpreted to him in order that he may choose a suitable vocational objective. Following this choice, it will be necessary to develop the plan which will enable him to follow through and attain the objective he has chosen. The various services needed should be listed, the place where they may be secured, and all the details should be worked out during the plan development period. Following this, steps should be taken to implement the plan.

Training

Training for the client will be that which will enable him to achieve the objective which has been chosen. Training may consist of on-the-job training, short-term specialized skill training, or college or university training leading to a professional career.

Reporting

Reporting becomes necessary to justify the need for services. The provision of services to the handicapped are very important and it is through the reports that are received that additional services may be developed and provided. Many counselors have believed that the reporting is unnecessary and a waste of their valuable time. The agencies agree that it is important to provide clerical assistance to the counselor so that much of his time may be free from the actual work of preparing the reports, but the counselor must accept the responsibility for reporting on his cases. No other person is able to do so accurately.

Documentation

Documentation is a simple, brief record of the contacts made by the rehabilitation counselor with the client. It will provide a record of services rendered, decisions reached and the reason for the decision, the development of the plan and all the services rendered so the plan may be completed. Documentation will provide accountability of a counselor's work and justify the expenditures made in behalf of a client. The record also will help to evaluate the adequacy of the state's program and to account for the time spent on a case by the counselor.

Closures

Closure is a term which means that the individual client has completed his rehabilitation plan, has been placed on a suitable job and has been followed for a period of time to determine that:
1. All needed services have been provided.
2. The job is suitable.
3. The client is satisfied.
4. The employer is satisfied.
5. The client will have some permanency on this job.

In many instances in the past, some have thought undue emphasis was placed on "closures." The philosophy is that the counselor render services necessary to the client without undue delay and that closures will be realized as a result. The problem is encountered, of course, when the case flow is not maintained. Cases then become delayed in the process and as a result an individual counselor may not be appearing to fulfill the objective of provision of services to clients as he should. This may show up in other steps of the process as well as in the lack of closures. Such problems should not develop if a counselor has adequate time for his casework and has adequate help from the supervisory staff.

In-Service Training

The in-service training should be developed in line with the needs of each individual counselor. However, it is difficult to develop orientation plans separately; therefore, the needs of the newly hired counselor should be studied and a program developed in accordance with the training and background of each counselor, perhaps with emphasis on special needs. It is the opinion of the writer that there are certain types of orientation which are necessary soon after the counselor is employed. This is information that would be necessary in order to make the counselor feel more at home in his new setting and would consist of the explanation of the program, the personnel who work in the program, the overall philosophy of the program, the written rules and regulations pertaining to employees, specific duties which the counselor may be assigned and the items which may have to do with pay, retirement, leave, et cetera. This period of early orientation should probably be handled by the training officer and the personnel officer in the department, as well as appearances made by perhaps the regional representative and the state director of the division or department. It is my belief, then, that after the counselor has worked in his setting for a period of time, varying from three to six months, that a follow-up period of orientation training should be provided which might last for another ten days or two weeks period of time. At this time it would be valuable for him to receive instruction in reference to the various forms, how they are used, why they are used and when they are used, as he will have had some experience with them and will now understand why many of the procedures are used in the program. This discussion will be much more meaningful to him at this time than if it is given earlier in his training program. Many new counselors have been overpowered and confused by the number of forms and the amount of knowledge which they are expected to retain, if all of this is given to them early in their employment period. The counselor, by the time he comes in for the second orientation period, should have an acquaintance with the office procedures and also should know many of the other employees in the organization and perhaps will feel more secure in asking questions in reference to aspects of the program which may not be understood. It should be the endeavor of the training officer to see that people are present who can answer all the counselor's questions and who are willing to take the time to explain them to the counselor so that he will feel that he is an integral part of the total program of rehabilitation.

In reference to the orientation training which a new counselor receives, it should also be pointed out that the state staff usually sets the tone and determines the dedication of the people in the program. The goals and objectives of the rehabilitation program should be set forth by the director, deputy director or someone from the state staff in such a way that the new counselor will get the idea that this is not a job but a career field he is entering and that in this field you will find many people dedicated to the goals of helping the handicapped citizens of our state and our nation in order that they may attain a rightful place in society.

The program is an investment program in people and one which every person who works in it should feel is worthy of their support and their best effort. This is not a position where you will be able to work without being completely involved. You must be interested in the people who come to you and in their problems as well as be able to help them to understand their difficulties and how to overcome them.

Counselor training is becoming very important in this endeavor as we accept the responsibility for the more difficult cases, such as those who come to us with character disorders and emotional problems. It takes a great deal of time, effort and understanding on the part of the counselor to work with these more difficult clients and to carefully evaluate them in terms of their total rehabilitation potential. The counselor who is working with the correctional cases, the alcoholic or the drug user certainly is going to have to recognize that he is in a field that is very challenging and one which will require his utmost efforts in helping these individuals to overcome their problems and to again secure a place in society. Although these may be difficult cases and the gains may appear to be small, the rewards are great when a rehabilitation closure is secured with one of these clients. The satisfaction that the counselor has when a difficult case is placed and retains the job over a long period of time, without becoming involved again in the same pattern of behavior, cannot be measured in dollars and cents.

Vocational Evaluation

The counselor must recognize that determining the important factors to consider in the vocational evaluation are his area of responsibility. Help will be received from the medical consultant in reference to the limitations imposed by the particular disability. The counselor must be certain that the knowledge he needs to be secured and analyzed is available. The interpretation of all the information and its importance to the vocational selection must be explained to the rehabilitation client. This information must include the medical, psychological, social, educational and work reports. Many times the information overlooked, omitted or not considered important enough to secure causes the plan to fail. In working with people it is recognized that sometimes the plan fails for no apparent reason, so everything that is found out in reference to the individual and the success of a plan must be taken into consideration. The more carefully the plan is detailed before implementation begins, the less opportunity there is for problems to develop because something was not spelled out and discussed thoroughly with the client.

In the rehabilitation program as it is developing today, the cases that are worked with require more understanding. They are those classified as behavior disorders, severely physically handicapped, who, in turn, have psychological problems and anxieties, those that apparently lack motivation to become self-sufficient and appear to be satisfied to remain as a dependent person with relatives, friends or taxpayers providing for their needs. The counselor who faces these cases on his rolls certainly needs the training to be able to cope with the needs and problems of these individuals on a day-to-day basis. Somehow, training in the psychology of disabilities must be provided for in the in-service program.

Family

An area which becomes important in the total evaluation of a client is the family structure and relationships. Understanding of family pressures and expectations is necessary to the success of a rehabilitation plan. The client who has been the breadwinner and suddenly becomes disabled presents a very different problem than the 18-year-old client who has a family to support him and back him up. Each individual is different and so the counselor must recognize the difference and work out a rehabilitation program with the individual to provide for the different needs.

SUMMARY

The overall objective of all the training, in-service orientation and graduate rehabilitation counselor training is to provide the person representing the agency with the knowledge, the skill and the procedures necessary to render adequate services to help the disabled to help themselves. It is the goal to see the handicapped accepting a place in the community and the community accepting them. It is, and has been true in the past, possible for a fully-qualified counselor in the regular program to become overloaded with referrals, with waiting for help in the necessary processing, with the reporting to such an extent that services to the cases in his case load have to wait, and he may, in turn, become frustrated and unhappy with the agency. This is something that most every agency has had to deal with. The problem is threefold: not enough money in many instances, not enough professional staff and not enough clerical staff.

In order to retain the qualified counselors and to be able to render adequate services to the disabled citizens of the state, many programs are more fully implementing an educational and public relations program. The objective is to educate the general public, the legislative members and other facets of the community in reference to the value of the rehabilitation process to the economy and to society. This is an ongoing process and takes much time and effort. The counselor going into the field has a definite part to play in this endeavor. The work of the counselor and how it is accomplished provides the foundation for a public education and public relations program. If a high percentage of the cases the counselor works with are successful in the rehabilitation process, these may be used to explain and discuss in terms of services needed in order to have an adequate program for the handicapped.

In order to turn the spotlight, so to speak, on the counselor and the rehabilitation program to secure adequate staff and financing, it must be recognized that each and every case we serve must be carefully evaluated and documented. Each plan for an individual must receive careful consideration and must be developed from a practical point of view. This approach with careful follow-up studies will enable the agency to request the necessary financing and staff to enable each counselor in the program to adjust his case load in order to provide adequate rehabilitation services to each person in his case load. The size of the case load may vary from program to program, but there should be a maximum and minimum range. A counselor should not be pressed every moment of the day, but his case load should also be large enough to keep his time fairly occupied. He should be able to follow his case load closely but still have some time to visit establishments where there are employment possibilities.

One area that is important to the rehabilitation counselor is the possibility for future development in the program. Is the counselor position the utmost that he can hope for in this program and must he leave to gain a promotion? It is important in the orientation process to point out the possibilities in the rehabilitation field. If a new counselor realizes that opportunities for advancement do exist within a program, he may be more satisfied to remain with the agency. The agency must also realize that the time, money and effort that is expended on the training of the counselor is considerable. In order for the agency to benefit, the counselor must work for a certain period of time after he has become a fully qualified counselor.

REFERENCES

1. Public Law 565, 83rd Congress, 2d Session. 1954.
2. Public Law 89-333. The Vocational Rehabilitation Amendments of 1965.
3. Report of the Committee of the National Vocational Guidance Association: The principles and practices of educational and vocational guidance. *Occupations (The Vocational Guidance Magazine), 15:*772-778, May 1937.

13

Cooperative Programming

William A. Crunk

Definition and Discussion
Cooperation with Private Agencies
Cooperative Programs Using Third-Party Funds
Conditions Governing the Use of Third-Party Funds in Cooperative
  Programs
A Guide to Planning
Development of Program Plans
Historic Perspective

It remains a matter of deep concern for all citizens that in this land of super abundance there remains a significant segment of our people who do not share in this bounty. This is a matter of special significance for those who are involved in planning and directing the Nation's attack on deprivation, dependence and disadvantagement—the prime elements characterizing the unemployed and underemployed in our society.

A most acute aspect of this problem is represented by the millions of persons made dependent by disability. Significantly, for a large segment of these disabled, the problem confronting them is one of unemployability rather than unemployment. This is frequently characterized by both the lack of capability to work and the motivation to work. This incapacity is not based solely upon physical or mental disability but is frequently aggravated by a strong overlay of cultural, educational and economic deprivation as well.

Thus, the design of contemporary rehabilitation programs

must recognize the need for new approaches and services which can deal with the special characteristics of the disabled such as
- Social and economic immobility
- Inadequate education
- Marginal health
- Loss of hope and expectation
- Meager (or no) job experience background
- Frequent rejection and hostility toward the helping services

While the foregoing is a generalization, it represents factors that illustrate the complexities inherent in comprehensive rehabilitation planning with a disabled individual.

DEFINITION AND DISCUSSION

A relatively new approach to rehabilitation planning for priority or "target" groups of disabled persons has been *cooperative programming*. Simply defined, cooperative programming as used here means concerted program planning and action by the public vocational rehabilitation agency and one or more other public or private agencies in an effort to maximize their effectiveness in restoring disabled individuals (and their families) to economic and social independence.

Early target populations for which cooperative programs were designed included the mentally retarded, the mentally ill and the unemployed disabled. Subsequently, programs have been developed for the public offender, the disabled welfare recipient and, to a lesser degree, for the older adults, the deaf and the blind. The most recent group targeted for cooperative programming is miners disabled by pneumoconiosis and other dust diseases. Thus, agencies most frequently entering into cooperative agreements with the public vocational rehabilitation agency are the public schools; correctional, welfare and mental health agencies; workmen's compensation boards; and nonprofit, private groups such as sponsors of workshops and facilities.

Cooperative program development means more than just the provision of services from the two (or more) agencies to a common clientele group. As conceived by this writer, it involves the formalized commitment (written plan) of the agencies involved to plan, organize, improve and focus in the most effective way their respective services on the needs of the disabled to be served through the joint action program. This means prescribed commitment of resources which might result in new organizational and staffing patterns, new and creative use of staff, development of new programs and facilities and full utilization of community resources. Additionally, the formal commitment must address procedural modification, such as client selection and referrals and changes in administrative policy, institutional or agency rules which might retard program development and operation. Following the development of cooperative program content and procedures, the costs of the program must be determined and budgets established. Financial commitments, it should be noted, are crucial to the success of cooperative program efforts whether or not the mechanism of third-party funding (which will be discussed later) is employed. Finally, joint decisions must be reached and recorded as to responsibility for program evaluation and accountability.

While cooperative program planning and implementation is not an easy task, its effectiveness cannot be disputed. Literally hundreds of cooperative programs are in operation throughout the nation. Scores of such endeavors are underway within single states. Probably the most numerous outside of workshop and facility programs are public school vocational rehabilitation programs. Among the earliest cooperative programs established were those for the mentally ill. Several states now have cooperative programs at each of their mental hospitals and have extended this approach to community mental health centers as well. Most cooperative programs are developed between the vocational rehabilitation agency and one other agency. In Kentucky, an exciting cooperative effort is underway which envisions statewide correctional rehabilitation services for eligible, youthful and adult public offenders. In this effort, five public agencies developed cooperative program plans to coordinate the delivery of services to eligible persons within this target group. Thus, it is self-evident that through appropriate administrative and staff action, joint action programs can be developed which provide the basis for long-term commitments to an effective interagency operating pattern resulting in the optimal rehabilitation and well-being of the disabled persons served.

The California Department of Rehabilitation, in a report to the State Legislature on April 1, 1969, pointed out some general benefits of cooperative programs as follows:

> It has been possible for the Department of Rehabilitation to bring its services to larger groups of mentally and physically handicapped persons. It has been possible to do this while conserving the state general fund, and at the same time, maximizing federal funding participation. It has permitted the cooperating departments to enrich and expand their programs to the benefit of their clients. Lastly, the cooperative programs have provided a guide for the diverse vocational interests represented in the various departments so that maximum gains were achieved for the eligible client population.

While cooperative program planning is frequently difficult by the nature of the task, it can be further complicated by applicable state and federal laws and regulation as well as by the "professional jurisdictions" sometimes "staked out" by one of the partnership agencies. However, there is no mystery surrounding their development as some imagine. Such planning is almost always successful when conducted by persons who have sincere concern for the well-being and betterment of the clientele group to be served, who are creative and not fearful about trying new approaches to rehabilitation and self-support and who are willing to invest in hard work to assure that the cooperative effort will be successful. Since all sections authorizing funding of services under the Vocational Rehabilitation Act, as amended, are on a project basis except for Section 2 (basic support to State Vocational Rehabilitation Programs), cooperative programs as discussed in this chapter relate to programs for which the public vocational rehabilitation agency *elects* to use the latter source of funding (Section 2) for its share of cost in such activities.

COOPERATION WITH PRIVATE AGENCIES

The fact that the private sector has benefited from cooperative programs is attested to by the hundreds of workshops and rehabilitation centers that have been started or expanded since 1954. Hundreds of such facilities have been assisted and many states have statewide networks of such resources which make possible services to thousands of disabled persons who could not otherwise be served. Assistance to workshops and facilities included remodeling, renovation, expansion of the building, equipment and initial staffing. Until 1965, the total cost of such workshop improvements was borne essentially by the state agency.

In 1965, Congressman Melvin Laird initiated an amendment to the Department of Health, Education and Welfare's Appropriation Bill that made possible the earmarking and use of contributed funds by local nonprofit organizations as the state's share for earning the federal share in these projects. The Laird Amendments were continued from around 1965 through 1968. The 1968 Amendments to the Vocational Rehabilitation Act incorporated all authorities allowed under the amendments to the Appropriation Act and added provisions to provide new construction of workshops and facilities. The 1968 Amendments also provided for new construction of such facilities.

A further note on the Laird Amendments: Cooperation among agencies—public and private—is being extolled today as a necessary approach to the resolution of problems confronting our society. It is a "theme song" at all levels of government and a similar chorus is heard from various segments of the private sector. The Laird Amendment was responsive to an early recognition of such need by the enlightened leadership in vocational rehabilitation at the time—federal and state—and by members of both Houses of the Congress. The uniqueness of using an amendment to the Appropriation Act as a vehicle in achieving this specific purpose and the support of such amendments through the years without dissenting votes in either House reflect the degree of approval this pioneer effort received in Congress.

The success of state and local private agencies and organizations was significant in securing passage of the 1968 Amendments to the Vocational Rehabilitation Act which, as now evolved, probably represents the most liberal and enlightened piece of social legislation in existence. Beneficiaries from such legislative authority in the private sector has included many independent community workshops administered by local boards of directors and organizations providing services to disabled persons such as associations for retarded and crippled children, organizations for the blind, Goodwill Industries and others. Of course, the real beneficiaries have been and continue to be the disabled, many of whom receive concurrent services from the private facility and the public vocational rehabilitation agency.

COOPERATIVE PROGRAMS USING THIRD-PARTY FUNDS

As noted previously, the Laird Amendment and subsequent changes in the Vocational Rehabilitation Act permitted the use of private, nonprofit funds as the state's share in attracting Federal Section 2 funds for use in "establishment" and construction of rehabilitation workshops and facilities. Similar provisions apply to the public sector as well. In other words, state funds available to public agencies other than the public vocational rehabilitation agency can be used to attract Federal Section 2 funds.

The use of the "other" agency's funds, both private and public, is conditioned on a number or requirements. The latter (public) presents a more complex set of conditions due to the various federal and state laws applicable to each agency and the resultant and traditional functions of the agencies involved in cooperative programming.

Such funds, when made available from another public agency, are known as "third-party funds" and are defined as follows: Third-party funds are that part of the state's share in the cost of vocational rehabilitation services and their administration which is borne by a state or local public agency under an agreement (and program plan) *and* can be made available in two ways: administrative transfer in cash by the cooperating public agency to the state vocational rehabilitation agency and expenditure of funds (for vocational rehabilitation purposes) by the cooperating agency. Third-party funding, whichever method used, is predicated upon the premise that the cooperative program will result in the reaching and serving of more handicapped persons while improving the quality of rehabilitation services over that which could be provided singly by either of the cooperating agencies.

The evolvement of the cooperative public school-vocational-rehabilitation programs provide a good case illustration for the above premise. During the decade of the fifties, public schools engaged, in a substantive way, the issue of education for the exceptional child. Principal focus was upon the retarded, educable child and, to a lesser extent, upon the physically disabled. In most schools, this response consisted of offering the exceptional child a modified academic curriculum based upon some assessments of ability and achievements and their placement in smaller classes which, hopefully, allowed the teacher more time for individualized instruction, counseling and guidance.

Too frequently, special education classes were compartmentalized within the school program and became relatively isolated from the mainstream of school activities. In the smaller schools, the special education teachers, in addition to their teaching duties, were left to their own devices in developing recreational and other activities that would enhance the personal and social adjustment of the youngsters. Even in the larger, more sophisticated schools where psychological, personal and social counseling and special recreational activities augmented basic classroom work, little attention was given to postschool adjustment needs, including participation in the world of work. As the children initially enrolled in special education classes became older, school authorities recognized that the vocational aspects of their training had not been adequately addressed by the school program. Hence, many schools began making referrals to vocational rehabilitation for assistance in bridging the gap between the school and community.

It soon became apparent to both the school and vocational rehabilitation officials that the referrals to vocational rehabilitation had little readiness for confrontation with the real world of work and frequently could not even cope with the social and personal demands of the community in which they lived.

This problem was rather perplexing to all concerned. Here were two agencies "doing their thing" in a logical, sequential manner. Public schools had the child until it was determined that he could no longer profit from the school program. Logically, wasn't it now time for vocational rehabilitation to pick up and continue the good work initiated by the school? Fortunately for thousands of exceptional children and youth, many local school and vocational rehabilitation administrators were able to overcome this level of mentality. They recognized that while each agency had its responsibility—both legal and moral—there was, undoubtedly, a point in time of a youth's formative years where coordinated, concerted services from both agencies would yield the greatest benefit to his total development. Although oversimplified, the following type of program delineation grew out of this recognition of the problems and needs of the exceptional child:

Phase I
The school had the prime responsibility for the child during the preadolescent years. There should be the heaviest concentration on academic development, activities of daily living, personal and social adjustment training activities and the provision of remedial or health maintenance services. Partnerships at this level in addition to the school would be parents, child health agencies and social-recreational agencies in the community.

Phase II
The program for exceptional youth would be shared beginning about age 14 and continuing until it had been jointly determined that the youth had received maximum benefits from the cooperative school program. At Phase II, a specific vocational character would be introduced to the program. Provisions for continuous vocational assessments of individual students would be incorporated into the school programs. Psychological and vocational testing, prevocational experiences, job tryouts and other modalities would be employed to introduce the concept of work to students and probe for individual strengths that could provide the basis for ultimate successful work adjustment. Vocational counseling and guidance services would be added to ongoing personal and social adjustment activities. Finally, work-study programs would be developed for the older school youth. During this second phase, the school's offerings would become more vocational in content with job information, and related job instruction and academic pursuits would be tailored to meeting the individual needs as determined by vocational assessments, counseling and work experience provided through the cooperative program. The partnerships in Phase I would be continued with vocational rehabilitation

taking more responsibility for vocational counseling, medical services, vocational training and the provision of training supplies, special transportation and other supporting services. Additionally, the employment office and vocational education departments of the school might be brought into the partnership.

Phase III
This phase would see the relinquishing of responsibility by the school and the assumption of full responsibility by vocational rehabilitation for the student-client. Individual rehabilitation plans would be carried out as jointly determined through the cooperative program including any postschool training, job development, placement and follow-up services. As needed, the cooperative program staff would be consulted on modifications in such planning and advised of problems and successes of the postgraduate. Partnerships would be continued until final job placement and case closure.

Before cooperative programming, the service sequence in respect to agency responsibility was from the school to the rehabilitation agency. Cooperative programming with public schools requires at a crucial point in the youth's development a shared responsibility.

Similar approaches can be made in determining needs for services in other categories of disability or with other target populations. It should be made clear here that the vocational rehabilitation services component of cooperative programs with either private or public agencies can be and are frequently planned and implemented without use of local private, nonprofit or other public agency funds to attract Federal Section 2 funds. This is particularly true when state vocational rehabilitation appropriations are sufficient to earn all federal funds. However, this activity is an outreach or service expansion for the state rehabilitation agency which accrues benefits to a clientele group that are the prime responsibility, initially, of the cooperating or host agency. Additionally, many state vocational rehabilitation agencies lacked, until recent years, sufficient state appropriated funds to attach their full allotment of Section 2 funds. Since other funds, under acceptable conditions, could be used as the state's "share," the third-party mechanism became popular with many states and is one very definite reason for the attainment of over a quarter million rehabilitations in FY 1970.

CONDITIONS GOVERNING THE USE OF THIRD-PARTY FUNDS IN COOPERATIVE PROGRAMS

It has already been established that third-party funds may be made available in two ways. Cash transfer to the state vocational rehabilitation agency and/or acceptable expenditures for rehabilitation services (and their administration) by the host agency.

The first method is the easiest way to make funds available. It is a cash transfer and, as such, both the state and federal share of costs for services are expended by the vocational rehabilitation agency. The second method frequently involves host agency staff assignment to the rehabilitation program and other services provided by the host agency such as maintenance, heat and other utilities for cooperative program staff and facilities. In this instance, the cost of staff so assigned and services provided constitutes the host agency's contribution to the program and such costs may be considered the state's share for use in attracting Federal Section 2 funds.

The financial significance of third-party funding to the states is quite clear. Let us assume that the cooperative educational program, briefly touched upon in Phase II of the above public school-vocational rehabilitation program illustration, was priced out at a total cost of $250,000. Further, we assume that the state rehabilitation agency's state appropriation was insufficient to attract all of its Federal Section 2 allocation and that a balance of $300,000 in unearned funds remained in the federal "account" which would be lost to the state.

In this instance, if the school makes available the state's share at the current state-federal ratio of 20/80, it would transfer in cash or "in kind" a total of $50,000. They would attract $200,000 in Section 2 funds in support of the total program budget of $250,000. The school system would have infused into its program a rehabilitation component not previously existing and the state vocational rehabilitation agency, and hence, the state would earn a more equitable share of federal funds available for rehabilitation purposes. In the early days of cooperative programming, as discussed later, guidelines covering program content and funding arrangement were rather meager. Through a vast amount of experiences in mounting such efforts, including the resolution of many audit questions and issues, a sound program and legal base now undergirds this type of program activity.

Where third-party funding is used in financing a cooperative service program, both the third-party share and the federal funds earned must meet certain conditions imposed upon any Section 2 expenditures made by the state vocational rehabilitation agency. These conditions are stipulated in both the vocational rehabilitation regulations governing the vocational rehabilitation program and in Chapter 11 of the *Vocational Rehabilitation Manual*. Additionally, cooperative program activity, if adopted by the state agency, must be covered in the approved state plan covering the vocational rehabilitation program in that particular state. These provide essential references for anyone seriously interested in cooperative program planning and operation. However, it might prove useful to discuss briefly some of the principles and criteria governing cooperative programs as discussed in this chapter.

Source of third-party funds. While either of the methods of making funds available is acceptable as noted it is important to observe here that with few exceptions federal funds cannot be used to attach federal funds. The only exceptions known to this writer are certain Appalachian regional development funds and housing and urban supplemental funds made available to model cities agencies. Otherwise, third-party funds must represent state monies and be subject to verification that they so qualify. Also, the state cannot use the same state monies to attract federal funds from more than one federal source (non-duplicate matching).

Third-party funds must be spent for vocational rehabilitation purposes. This simple statement becomes more complex in its essence when we realize that many agencies provide rehabilitation type services. Since it is not the purpose or intent in cooperative programs to supplant existing and adequate rehabilitation services or finance existing services of the third-party agency for which a handicapped person *would be entitled if he was not an applicant or client* of the vocational rehabilitation agency, we reach this important conclusion. Rehabilitation services for which third-

Cooperative Programming 285

party expenditures are claimed must represent *new* rehabilitation services or *new patterns* of rehabilitation services which are not available through the cooperating agency and such expenditures for new or new patterns of services must be under the *control* of the state vocational rehabilitation agency.

The principle of *control* derives from legislative requirement that the state vocational rehabilitation agency must be the final authority on the quality, kinds, scope and extent of vocational rehabilitation services provided disabled people with the funds, from whatever source, for which it is responsible. Also, the agency is required to determine eligibility, rehabilitation potential and scope of services to be provided a handicapped individual. Control, as used here, is not the harsh requirement as it might seem. We are talking about new services or new patterns of vocational rehabilitation services which are nonexistent without the development of the cooperative program. Also, the cost of these new or changed services is borne principally by the state vocational rehabilitation agency (80% Federal Section 2 funds) which becomes involved in the provision of services *after* careful joint planning and agreement as to program content, priority for services in respect to the clientele group and similar program content has been completed. After these discussions, and only then, does the state vocational rehabilitation agency exercise its responsibilities under state and federal laws requiring such control over the vocational rehabilitation part of the program. The cooperating agency would likewise be expected to administer, according to applicable laws, its part of the program.

Additionally, control of expenditures for either new or new patterns of services may be achieved through direct expenditures by the state vocational rehabilitation agency or the disbursement by the cooperating agency when made in accordance with the cooperative program plan, budget and agreement and by such method that satisfies the vocational rehabilitation agency as to fiscal accountability.

New rehabilitation services are those services which are not and have not recently been a part of the cooperating agency's program. They may be services for which the cooperating agency is *authorized* to provide but for some reason has not elected to do so. However, they *may not be* services for which the cooperating agency is *legally obligated* to provide. The key words here are *authorized* and *obligated*. It goes without saying that it would be unlikely that a cooperating agency could make funds available to the vocational rehabilitation agency if it did not have the authority to provide the services envisioned. However, state enabling legislation is frequently more specific on obligatory services which a state agency must provide. Rehabilitation agencies could establish services in the former or *authorized* area if they were nonexistent but not in the latter category. State attorney generals can help make such distinctions in applicable state laws, policies and regulations.

New patterns of rehabilitation services might include previously existing services of the authorized category provided by the cooperating agency. The cost of such services, to constitute a third-party expenditure, would have to be modified or otherwise changed and reoriented to vocational rehabilitation. If existing staff (employed by the cooperating agency) is assigned, control in terms of program assignment and supervision would become the responsibility of the state vocational rehabilitation agency. Thus, the new pattern must provide discernible contrast favoring vocational rehabilitation activity. Occupational therapy, although previously existent might be either medically or recreationally oriented in a setting such as a psychiatric hospital. This modality might be redirected to provide personal adjustment or vocational evaluation services within the cooperative psychiatric rehabilitation program established at the hospital. Under such circumstances, new patterns of services would be established. However, under ordinary circumstances, the psychiatric care and treatment, room and board, medications and similar services for which the hospital is *obligated, under law, to provide* could not be so modified to constitute acceptable third-party expenditures.

A GUIDE TO PLANNING

In an effort to simplify the *approach* to cooperative program planning, the writer developed an outline, with brief comments under each heading, that might be useful to persons interested in this kind of program development. It is a composite outline drawn from several joint action plans now in operation. It is not intended as a prototype plan guide but as a stimulator since each cooperative program opportunity has its own uniqueness for expression in plan development.

A. Introduction

This can be a statement that presents traditional or historical developments or other content which supports, in a general way, the need for and timeliness of the effort to be made. Planners should keep in mind that the implementors might cover a range of professional, paraprofessional and volunteer staff. For educational purposes alone, an introduction or background statement is frequently desirable.

B. Statement of the Problem

This is simply an assessment of the problem as it now exists in respect to the client group to be served, availability of existing services (or lack thereof) and other information that establishes the nature of the problem and establishes the need for a coordinated, concerted joint program effort.

C. Action Plan Development

1. Goals and objectives

Certain program objectives might be specified here and then the establishment of more specific goals in terms of numbers of persons to be served and rehabilitated.

2. Priorities for services

This is a critical plan provision which is required since joint agency resources are rarely adequate to serve a total population group. In correctional rehabilitation planning, for instance, will the program be directed toward youthful or adult offenders, long-termers or those on probation and parole? It is also important, since it establishes, quite specifically, the target group for participating agencies.

3. Selection criteria

    To assure controlled and effective referrals to the program and to assure referrals of those who can profit most from a concerted program effort, it is usually accepted practice to establish such criteria. They can be modified as the program matures to expand coverage.

    Another reason for selection criteria should be to establish an automatic referral and acceptance procedure. If selection criteria is jointly determined then it follows that the host agency—mental hospital, school or welfare agency—would automatically refer those meeting the selection criteria and vocational rehabilitation would automatically accept them for evaluation to determine eligibility for services.

    It is, of course, hardly necessary to mention that the criteria for extended evaluation under the vocational rehabilitation service program would constitute two of the selection criteria.

4. Services to be provided by vocational rehabilitation
5. Services to be provided by other cooperating agency (ies)

    Under each of these headings a concise description of services to be provided is presented.

6. Case planning and management

    Describe how the counseling and planning required to develop and activate a rehabilitation program for the individual is to be carried out.

    In the mental hospitals, for instance, the cooperative program unit is usually located in space made available on campus by the hospital administrators. The client served through the unit is also a patient in the hospital. This poses questions as to the role of the hospital's social workers who obtain intake data, social histories and the like. Frequently, hospital social workers are assigned to the unit staff. How does her role change? Is the counselor's role modified following such assignment? Considerations should be given to all aspects of case plan-

ning and management including plan development, progress reports, case reviews, case closures and so forth.
7. Plans for housing
   In institutionally based programs the plan should provide for adequate housing of professional and support staff assigned to the cooperative program and for adequate evaluation, adjustment and training areas. Such space is made available by the host institution and is frequently renovated or remodeled by vocational rehabilitation. In cooperative programs with public welfare and similar community-based programs, joint housing of social workers and counselors may be desired.
8. Commitment of resources
   Each agency should indicate the extent of financial and staff commitment. Programs utilizing third-party funds will develop operational budgets and, after the first year, prepare expenditure reports as well.
9. Target coverage area
   Cooperative programs, except those directed toward residents in the big city ghettos and in specified rural areas, such as Appalachia, should ultimately be planned for statewide coverage. Orderly program implementation, tight money conditions or other reasons might require phasing in of the new program in selected geographic areas or selected institutions.
10. Staff development
    Should be jointly planned, funded and carried out.
11. Interagency reporting system
    Should be adequate for purposes of each cooperating agency.
12. Public information system
    Usually describes the method used for making known to potential clients and others the services available under the program plan.
13. Supportive services from other agencies
    Usually indicated here are services from other agencies that will be utilized in the cooperative program such as

- Services under Medicaid
- Crippled Children's Service
- Day-Care Facilities and Services
- Manpower Programs

14. Program evaluation

    Describe here the method and procedures jointly developed for use in measuring the strength and weaknesses of the program operation including results obtained.

DEVELOPMENT OF PROGRAM PLANS

In view of the possibilities for joint cooperation, state administrators should review their existing relationships and methods of operation to determine most effective means for achieving a major expansion of services for target groups. They should jointly set in motion steps that will result in a program plan which would be expressed in a formal cooperative plan of operation.

Specific actions in planning and initiating the cooperative program which might be taken by program administrators include the following:

A. The appointment of an interagency task force to be charged with
   1. The development of the program plan, including the identification of agency resources each agency plans to commit and use in achieving program goals.
   2. Assignment of responsibility for its implementation following administrative acceptance.
B. The establishment of target dates for program implementation, including sequential target dates for statewide coverage (if not initially planned).
C. The preparation of operational manuals and guide material for use in implementing and operating the program.
D. The development of material for use with the information media to interpret and explain the program to the general public.

HISTORIC PERSPECTIVE

Strong advocates for the use of third-party funding to carry out vocational rehabilitation service programs emerged at both the state and federal levels in the early fifties. In fact, some of the more aggressive state directors were experiencing audit problems prior to the 1954 Amendments to the Vocational Rehabilitation Act. These Amendments vindicated such cooperative program practices including funding arrangements by legitimizing such practice in federal laws and "grandfathering in" or covering many of the prior activities of state agencies for which audit exceptions were pending.

The strength of character of those state directors and those at the federal level who supported their cause in forcing changes in vocational rehabilitation legislation and practice in the recognition that a disabled individual was a total being, with sundry and complex problems requiring an array of social, medical, psychological and vocational services beyond the capacity of any one agency to provide is to be admired.

Such persons were ahead of their times as can be recognized with today's hue and cry for coordinated, concerted services. Yet, while their intuitive wisdoms of the emerging needs of many of our citizens, disabled and disadvantaged, was denied by policy makers at the time, they and many who followed gave those of us in the rehabilitation movement today ample legislative authority and program experience to provide aggressive leadership in developing new and innovative cooperative programs for the disabled (and if required, the disadvantaged) during the decade of the seventies and beyond.

14

Administrative Concerns in the Cooperative Program

Joe C. Morrow

Program Initiation
Program Administration
Program Organization
The Administrative Role of the Rehabilitation Counselor in Client
    Evaluation
Summary

IN THE EARLY DAYS, when the idea for cooperative programming in rehabilitation was originally conceptualized, program development normally was initiated by the vocational rehabilitation agency. As rapid development occurred the agency experienced growth pains of an intensity which was unanticipated. This phenomenon, coupled with the encumbrance of the additional federal money being received by the state agency, as provided by P.L. 565, slowed the agency's effort to initiate new programs. Consequently, requests for the development of cooperative programs are presently usually initiated by local educational institutions and facilities. State office personnel, usually in consultation with field administrators and supervisors, negotiate with the school the agreement which enunciates the operation of the cooperative program. This initial agreement specifies the resources which each agency will invest in the program and describes the program's general operational procedures.

There are program development activities, however, for which staff members of an established program must be responsible.

These can best be described as developments which refine the original agreement. Local vocational rehabilitation personnel and the educational staff assigned to the individual program should constantly be in the process of evaluating the needs of their constituents as related to conditions in the immediate community so that appropriate changes in the program can be made as needs are better defined and/or conditions change. An organization, at the unit level, for program evaluation needs to be created in order that continued program development is not left to chance or does not become a reaction to difficulties that arise.

PROGRAM INITIATION

Once an agreement for the establishment of a cooperative program has been reached between the vocational rehabilitation agency and a school unit or system, it becomes a responsibility of an agency staff member responsible for the unit to introduce the program to the school's staff. This may be done by attending regular school staff meetings and explaining vocational rehabilitation to the staff as a whole and discussing with them how a cooperative effort between vocational rehabilitation and the public schools may be beneficial to both agencies and the people which they serve. Cooperation is the key to the successful operation of a joint program; without it there is no justification for the program.

With this fact in mind, one can readily see that this introductory period is of critical importance since the character of many relationships is determined by initial impressions which are formed at the time of introduction. Therefore, the agency representative and the principal or similar school administrator should plan a careful strategy for achieving a favorable first reaction, by affected school staff. The report of the Bridgeport Project (Lane, Soares, Silverstone, 1968) suggests the following:

> When? When is the most appropriate time for introducing the rehabilitation counselor and his program to the high school? Should he be introduced immediately when the new school year begins? This is probably not the most appropriate time because the school itself is adjusting to a new year. The teachers and administrators are concerned with unforeseen interruptions in schedules and procedures, due to many uncontrollable conditions—therefore, the rehabilitation

counselor should not be introduced to the school system until at least one month after the regular school period has begun. This plan has four advantages:

1. It allows the school system to settle down into a regular routine.
2. It enables the principal to set into motion the procedures he feels are necessary to properly introduce the rehabilitation counselor and to effect those procedures which enhance his position.
3. It affords the opportunity for the rehabilitation counselor to be properly introduced.
4. It grants to the rehabilitation counselor the opportunity of becoming known to teachers in a manner which will enhance his reception by them, and for developing a program on a carefully prescribed basis.

PROGRAM ADMINISTRATION

The vocational rehabilitation agency is a state-federal program, and the administration required is sometimes more complicated than that of other service programs. Justification for expenditure of funds must be provided to the state and federal government and, in a cooperative program, justification must also be made to the county, city or other third party to the cooperative arrangement. Therefore, it is extremely important to keep detailed and accurate records, especially, if the program is funded resulting from the cooperative agency providing services "in kind" as its financial contribution to the program. Each client case record should clearly indicate how vocational rehabilitation staff, and school personnel certified as program staff, have worked together toward the achievement of the client's rehabilitation. Counselors, some administrators and school personnel perceive this task as being an administrative burden that is almost impossible to satisfy. Such is not the case. The idea behind cooperative programming was to combine the efforts of two or more agencies. The cooperative program was to offer individualized services in the tradition of rehabilitation services. If a cooperative program is operating as it should, cooperation is occurring and can be described in the case record. Recording these activities is not for administrative purposes only but is also in the interest of

Administrative Concerns in the Cooperative Program

good casework performance. If rehabilitation personnel are having difficulty documenting that school personnel are performing a rehabilitation function, they should evaluate their program to see if they are offering stereotyped client services instead of services based on the needs of each individual client. If documentation of cooperative effort is impossible, rehabilitation staff have no business being located within a school facility because it is evident that they do not have an understanding of the dynamics of cooperation.

If I were working in a school unit, I would want its funding based on the certification of personnel time instead of cash contributed to the agency for matching purposes. The funding mechanism used to finance a cooperative program has a definite effect on the teamwork which exists within the program. Cooperation and teamwork are commodities difficult to fabricate if the continuation of a program is not contingent upon their existence, because the temptation for professionals to go their way and do their own thing is too great to avoid. Without cooperation and teamwork pervading throughout all program efforts, the advantage of vocational rehabilitation being in the school unit is lost, and the result is that you have a traditional rehabilitation program located within a traditional school program that has been modified in ways that have little real meaning except that the school is relieved of responsibility for the student during part of the day when he would ordinarily be receiving some sort of service from the school. To bastardize the concept of a cooperative program in this way is unholy.

Record keeping has been discussed as a casework tool and as a mechanism which can be used to justify program expenditures and the continuation of financial support. Another very obvious administrative use of records which does not receive adequate attention is their value in program modification for improvement or assessing the effective use of current operational procedures and available resources.

Rapid social change is a common topic for discussion and evidence of it can be seen daily. Social scientists philosophize about how these changes create new or different individual needs and the implication these needs have for changed social programs. However, social service programs are modified slowly, and their relevance to recently acquired needs is subject to question.

The nature of change is peculiar. Change seems to occur spontaneously in societies, the universe and in those areas of life that are not being consciously controlled and structured. Once the need for change is identified and provisions are made for it to occur in an orderly sequential flow on a predetermined path which, hopefully, will lead to a chosen destination, the preexisting order of things becomes rigid and inflexible. The physical "law of motion" apparently applies to social programs. Once a direction is established, the inertia generated by movement tends to perpetuate that direction regardless of the observable desirability for change. Resistance to change is a condition for which every professional needs to treat himself constantly.

Societal, psychological and biological alterations are inevitable; thus, the service needs of our clients change resulting in the need to modify the service program, which we operate, if it is to be responsive and serve its true purpose. Why is it difficult to achieve organizational flexibility which will allow or, better still, nurture desirable program modifications? Contrary to popular theory, the answer is not human recalcitrance or reluctance to forego the comfort recognized in conventionality. The real reason for the resistance to change is the new or different service needs are inevitably so subtly expressed by individuals and/or small populations that the need for program modifications is obscure.

The purpose of the preceding discussion is to provide a rationale for the following germaine points:

1. Because of evolving social changes which modify the needs of the individual, any program, regardless of its original degree of effectiveness and efficiency, must perpetually be modified.

2. Need for program changes are often so subtle they are obscure, but the knowledgeable professional knows that such needs are developing.

3. Program personnel need to create a mechanism for monitoring their programs to increase their sensitivity regarding what

is happening in their program so they can quickly see indications for change.

4. All program personnel should be schooled regarding the existence of a monitoring device, its purpose, how they can use it and how they are expected to contribute to it.

5. Case records can be used as one source of information for program evaluation only if standard criteria are established and maintained for recording and data collection.

6. A method for utilizing recorded case and program information must be formulated and a regularly scheduled time and procedure established for its use before it will be used or can be of real value in day-to-day programming. This aspect of administration needs at least monthly attention if it is to have casework value.

7. All personnel in the cooperative program should be involved in the program analysis, not only for the contribution each has to make but also to foster and further define cooperation.

8. Administration should recognize responsibility for two distinct functions: program operation and case service. If it addresses either one properly, the other will be adequately served.

PROGRAM ORGANIZATION

In any type of endeavor it is mandatory to identify goals and to plan how the goal or goals of the endeavor are to be achieved. The general process of reaching an aspired goal is to identify the steps or task which must be completed before the goal is realized. After identifying the various steps involved in accomplishing a purpose, the resources available must be assessed and a sequence established which is believed to have qualities to expedite completion of the job being undertaken. Planning and organization for the accomplishment of a job is of eminent importance. In a program as complex as the school vocational rehabilitation cooperative program, planning and organization is of such importance that they cannot be overemphasized. The importance of the planning function remains relatively constant regardless of the number of people involved in the work to be done. However, organization grows in importance in direct proportion to the number of people upon whom a successfully completed job depends. Since the achievement of a cooperative school program is dependent on the skills and contributions of many people, organization must be given a great deal of attention. Rehabilitation personnel have primary responsibility for devising an organizational structure capable of producing the results desired from the program.

Prior to mentioning some specific operations of the cooperative program for which an organization is needed, brief consideration should be directed to the general subject of organization. There seems to be a common belief in today's society that as the size of a program increases, the organizational structure necessarily must develop greater complexity. Although this is a general trend the end result is a loss of efficiency and effectiveness. To the extent that an organizational structure can be kept simple, program efficiency should be maximized.

A structure for communication must exist and be functional. The purpose of organization is communication and coordination. If the organization serves these two purposes, cooperation among all staff members toward achieving specified behavioral objectives may be expected. An organization cannot be expected to serve other purposes, so complicating it by many layers of supervision and extraneous formality and structure is an exercise in futility. The effectiveness of an organization is contingent upon the interpersonal and interprofessional relationships which exist among the individual members of the organization. It is therefore incumbent on an organizational leader to stress the concept of teamwork as a function of mutual respect, a willingness to give support whenever needed and to share responsibility for achieving a common objective.

Two of the most important tasks of an organization are:

1. To provide each member in the organization with a precise understanding of his own job duties and responsibilities. Modern management techniques indicate that the individual member be allowed the opportunity to participate in defining his role. This practice can be implemented only to the extent that the individual knows and understands the entire organization and its objectives.

2. To provide each member an opportunity to learn the duties and responsibilities of his cohorts in the organization so he has insight regarding his relationships to them and how his own and other organizational members activities are interdependent.

It is of utmost importance for a vocational rehabilitation staff member to assume responsibility for building an organization within each school unit that has a cooperative program (an organization with the potential for performing the operations enunciated above). Organization, as has been discussed thus far, is a structure or framework within which an individual, or more commonly, a group of individuals, strives to accomplish certain objections. Organization in another context may be described as an entity which operates as a body for the purpose of performing a function. In a cooperative school program there is a need for such organizations, which are generally referred to as committees. The principal purpose of these committees is to expedite the achievement of program goals. The creation of committees in the cooperative program and the definition of their purpose is a function of vocational rehabilitation personnel. The following are committees which have demonstrated their value in many existing cooperative programs but which are not formally organized and functional in many others:

1. *A screening committee.* The function of this body is to assist with the identification of students who should be accepted into the cooperative school program. The membership of this committee should probably consist of the principal or his assistant, a guidance counselor, the school psychologist, special education teachers, any other special service personnel on the school staff and the vocational rehabilitation staff. An important consideration for organizing this committee is the establishment of a formalized referral system which will prevent the counselor (vocational rehabilitation) from being overwhelmed by referrals coming to him from all directions and in a confusing variety of forms. A good operational system has the advantage of helping the counselor give more consistent consideration to all potential clients in the total student body.

2. *A staffing committee.* This committee's function is to consider the details of diagnostic evaluations performed on students

referred to the cooperative program and to assist in the formulation of a plan of action which will help the individual achieve a status of rehabilitation. This committee should also periodically review case progress in order to evaluate the appropriateness of the rehabilitation plan and strategy for the provision of services. The makeup of this committee may be identical to the screening committee except that there may be some question regarding the necessity for having a member of the school administrative staff devoting time to case staffing. There may be, however, advantages for having as little overlap in membership as possible since this would afford the cooperative program with the ideas of more professionals and would get more personnel actively involved with the cooperative program.

3. *An advisory committee.* This committee should be comprised of professional persons from the community, interested parents, trainers and local employers. This committee should have the operations and services of the cooperative program detailed for it periodically and be requested to evaluate the program in terms of how well it is addressing student-client needs with regard to the realities of community and vocational adjustment.

The validity for having the above-mentioned committees, and their potential value, is dependent on the leadership provided by the vocational rehabilitation staff member, who has the responsibility for organizing and utilizing the committees. Unless the committees have truly interested members and are actively involved in making real decisions, they will be useless and, in fact, burdensome appendages with which the program must contend rather than groups upon which the program can depend for assistance. Further, to insure real contributions by the committees, definite schedules and procedures must be arranged which are adhered to with diligence.

THE ADMINISTRATIVE ROLE OF THE REHABILITATION COUNSELOR IN CLIENT EVALUATION

The vocational rehabilitation counselor has the legal responsibility for determining an individual's eligibility for vocational rehabilitation services. No public case-service funds from the rehabilitation agency's budget may be expended except for diagnosis until the vocational rehabilitation counselor has certified that the individual meets all criteria for eligibility. The counselor has an ultimate responsibility for the evaluation process. That responsibility involves synthesizing all available diagnostic information into a diagnosis for rehabilitation.

Federal and state regulations have put into motion a mechanism for total client evaluation. This mechanism is the requirement that every client be given a general medical examination and whatever other specialty examinations might be indicated. The acceptance of cases generally served in a cooperative program requires narrative recording to justify the acceptance of the case. This requirement for recording demands the counselor to use information which can only be obtained from school records, the family and other related resources. How the counselor uses this data is of tremendous importance if he is to arrive at a prescriptive diagnosis for rehabilitation. In order for the data-gathering process to have any value, all of the information which he gathers must be interpreted so that he begins to get a picture and understanding of the whole person. This means that each particle of available information has to be related to the total of all information according to weighted values.

A prescriptive evaluation of this type requires the counselor to have a working knowledge of the psychodynamics of human behavior. The rehabilitation counselor must understand and be able to interpret to others in the cooperative program, that behavior is multiply determined by physical, social and psychic needs. All these needs must be examined in the development of a diagnosis for and a plan for rehabilitation.

It may be unfortunate, but the nature of rehabilitation and human beings requires that we make, and settle for, a clinical diagnosis because there are no reliable statistics for evaluating, planning or predicting outcome for rehabilitation. This is so because statistical data is not available for making predictions concerning multitudinous life areas. Therefore, with a great deal of caution (risk) and consultation, the counselor and other personnel in the cooperative program must be willing to proceed in their work on the basis of inferences which can be drawn from diagnostic information. From these inferences, can be drawn tentative conclusions concerning training areas and occupations in which the client can be both satisfied and successful. The validity of the diagnostic conclusions can only be assessed by trial.

Work based on subjective inferences implies that the counselor and other cooperating professionals are required to formulate a theory that is pertinent only to an individual case. The theory from which the cooperative personnel works is based on the data gathered concerning the individual client. This approach to arriving at a rehabilitation diagnosis contrasts sharply with the traditional approach to case planning which tries to fit client data into some general theory for successful life adjustment.

SUMMARY

In this chapter we have discussed how the impetus for initiating cooperative schools has shifted from the vocational rehabilitation agency to local school units and how the responsibility for administration of cooperative programs has become more of a local responsibilty.

Justification for continuing a cooperative program is a primary administrative function of the rehabilitation personnel in local projects. In order to enunciate a rationale for continuing a cooperative endeavor, good administrative and case service records must be maintained. In addition, to this activity's importance for continued program funding, such records have tremendous significance in terms of evaluative research which should result in program changes which are necessary for program services to be viable and vital.

Some difficulties in achieving true cooperation have been discussed and emphasis has been placed on each rehabilitation staff member's being able to describe in some concrete terms the relationships which they have with school and community personnel upon which the success of a cooperative school program depends. Various organizations for cooperation have been discussed which would allow for the establishment of proper program goals and a strategy for reaching those goals.

All vocational rehabilitation personnel in a cooperative school program need to be concerned with the administrative aspects of the program as well as the administration of client services. As personnel become more cognitive of their position in the administrative unit and their responsibility for expediting the development and utilization of a teamwork approach to rehabilitation, the cooperative program will experience increasing effectiveness and efficiency in serving handicapped school age clients.

15

The Vocational Rehabilitation-Public Education Cooperative Program

Joe C. Morrow

Special Education-Vocational Rehabilitation Cooperative Programs
History of the Special Education-Vocational Rehabilitation Cooperative Program
The Purpose of the Special Education-Vocational Rehabilitation Cooperative Program
Essential Components of the Program
The Role of Vocational Rehabilitation Personnel in a Cooperative Program
Program Continuation
Vocational Counseling
References

THESE NEXT TWO CHAPTERS are about educational vocational-rehabilitation programs jointly sponsored by a school system and the Division of Vocational Rehabilitation. The purpose of the program is to identify and serve potentially vocationally handicapped students who are enrolled in the school system. In the early phases of the cooperative effort, the school system itself maintains primary administrative responsibility for services that are rendered to the client. As a student progresses through the program, the vocational rehabilitation agency assumes greater and greater responsibility for program services. Below is a chart indicating the administrative responsibilities for a student's academic and vocational development in a cooperative program.

In this chapter an attempt is made to demonstrate the relevance of the cooperative program to contemporary concerns for

The Vocational Rehabilitation-Public Education Program 305

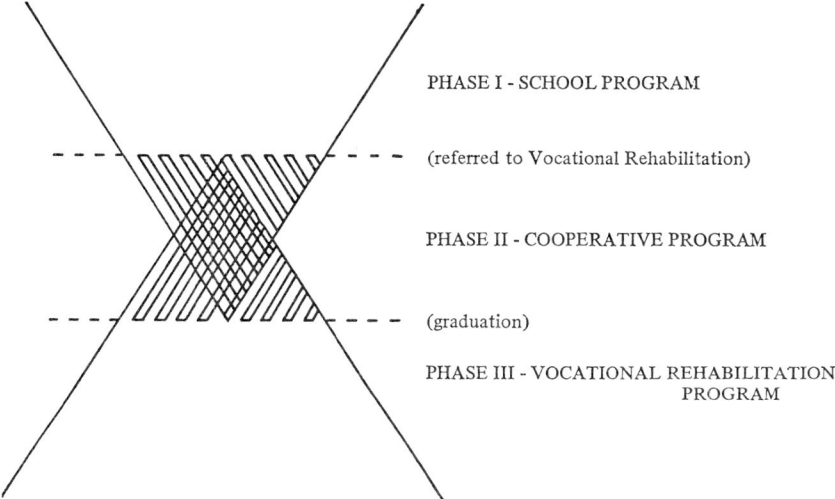

Figure 2. Administrative responsibilities for the student's academic and vocational development.

public education; a brief historical review of education is given; the history of the development of cooperative programs is given attention; and a description of common components of the cooperative program is detailed. Finally, there is a discussion of the role and function of rehabilitation personnel in the operation of the cooperative program and specific attention is given to some very important functions of the rehabilitation counselor.

It is hoped that from this material the reader will gain insights into jobs that should receive daily attention from rehabilitation personnel assigned to a cooperative school program.

The newest concept being echoed across the land, identified as "Accountability,"[7] is seen as being of crucial importance to all social institutions and public and professional services. As applied to public education, this concept implies that the school and its personnel are responsible for learning.

In other words, if a student does not learn—fails to demonstrate facility for acquiring and using new knowledge—it is not the learner's failure but an indication that the teacher has failed to adequately discharge the teaching function. This new concept wreaks havoc with the educators' time-honored explanation for student failure: I can teach, but learning is the student's responsibility.

Accountability is a professionally legitimate concept and the public is entitled to expect professionals and the institutions from which they receive service to accept the responsibility for being accountable. The professional is obligated to insure that services and programs are effective and are related to the attainment of goals that are meaningful to those who are being served. If programs are inefficient and/or ineffective or if they do not have real positive value, the individual practitioner or perhaps the whole profession must reexamine its practices, procedures and/or goals and make whatever adjustments are needed for its activity to produce the desired result. It is illogical and irresponsible to expect the needs for professional services to conform to traditional practices because of procedures arbitrarily established by the profession.

SPECIAL EDUCATION-VOCATIONAL REHABILITATION COOPERATIVE PROGRAMS

Accountability for the result of public education did indeed shift in a proper direction with the advent of special education-vocational rehabilitation cooperative programs. With the coming of the union between this particular school program with this service program for handicapped people, there was for the first time a widespread and consistent educational endeavor in which the involved professional people committed themselves to be responsible for the student's attainment of a specific behavioral objective as determined by the collaborative efforts of institutional personnel, the vocational rehabilitation counselor and the student.

The remaining portion of this chapter will be devoted to describing briefly the elements which should be included in a special education-vocational rehabilitation cooperative school program. More attention will be given to defining the role of the vocational rehabilitation counselor and his functions with the student-client and the system within which he is working. First, however, I would like to call to the reader's attention the reason that the rehabilitation agency has made such an impact on the public school program. There are unthoughtful people who, by looking at the surface success of cooperative programs in relation to the success of traditional special education programs, would say that the vocational rehabilitation agency has added a degree of realism to the school system that was never before there. The same people might be prone to say that the rehabilitation counselor through his knowledge of the world of work and common sense has been able to design a better curriculum for handicapped students. Such an assessment is naive. Vocational rehabilitation personnel cannot compare with educators in their knowledge of child development, the utilization of educational techniques nor the development of teaching materials.

Educational tradition has mitigated against preparing the handicapped individual to make a practical adjustment to community demands; the tradition of vocational rehabilitation has fostered achievement of this goal. Vocational rehabilitation counselors brought with them into the cooperative school unit an individual orientation which the public educator has never had the resources to develop. Because vocational rehabilitation workers have had the opportunity and resources to develop a highly individualized approach to meeting human needs, they possess knowledge and skill in establishing very specific behavioral objectives related to work and adjustment for community living. Some of the obvious weaknesses of public education can be attributed to the fact that education has based its operation on a tradition established long ago in times that were characteristically very different from today's society. The tradition of vocational rehabilitation is of more recent vintage and is, therefore, more keenly in tune with the demands of our modern technological environment.

Although the special education-vocational rehabilitation cooperative program has not been operational long enough for us to adequately evaluate its long-term societal impact, we may speculate, because of the evidence of immediate success, that such programs should be encouraged and their development promoted in all educational systems. Indeed, if longitudinal study confirms their apparent validity, the cooperative program may provide society with the prototype needed for restructuring and strengthening all of public education. If this trend in educational services is ultimately generally adopted, concomitant changes must be made in our manpower development program. Two such changes which I will only mention are training in the meaning and practice of professional cooperation and the real efficacy of working with individuals toward particular goals rather than toward group goals through standardized (stereotyped) procedures.

HISTORY OF THE SPECIAL EDUCATION-VOCATIONAL REHABILITATION COOPERATIVE PROGRAM

Public Law 113, passed in 1943, included the mentally and emotionally disabled in the group of citizens eligible for vocational rehabilitation services. Very little was done by vocational rehabilitation agencies for persons in these disability categories despite the fact that the Congress had given them legislative authority to serve these handicapped people. There are several explanations for this lack of activity in behalf of the mentally and emotionally disabled. Chief among these are the following:

1. Societal attitudes had caused families affected by these disabilities to be reticent about the problem with which they were confronted; consequently, there was little public awareness of the magnitude of these problems.

2. Prognosis for satisfactory treatment or adjustment was poor. An attitude of hopelessness hampered the initiation of attempts to design goal-directed rehabilitation programs.

3. Adequate programming for the physically handicapped (the familiar client population) was overwhelming in view of the limited available resources.

4. Vocational rehabilitation personnel did not have the know-how for programming or providing services to the newly eligible population of handicapped citizens.

5. The legislation was purely permissive; it did not indicate that it was mandating the initiation of programs for the mentally or emotionally disabled, nor did it provide incentives for the ag-

encies—that is, special funding for the development of new types of service programs.

In 1954 Public Law 565 did contain, among other things, a clear mandate for the development of programs for the mentally and emotionally handicapped. It also provided new funding mechanisms which could be used to the advantage of the "traditional vocational rehabilitation program" that fostered the desired new developments. In addition, and a possible rationale for some of the legislative provisions, the Mental Health Association and the National Association for Retarded Children had become quite visible and vocal and had called national attention to the scope of the problems presented by these disabilities. Also, these two organizations had removed enough of the stigma associated with mental and emotional disability that families affected by them were not so hesitant to admit the presence of such a disability or request treatment services. The years between 1943 and 1954 had witnessed the development of tranquilizing drugs by medical research, which had demonstrated the effectiveness of chemotherapy in the management of emotional illness. During the same time period, psychologists and special education teachers had provided the public with a glimpse of the unrecognized productive potential of the mentally retarded.

General pessimism regarding the rehabilitation of the mentally retarded and the emotionally disturbed had by no means been dispelled. When I, as a rehabilitation counselor, was first asked to give up my general case load, with its many bright physically handicapped people who possessed the potential for brilliant careers, to begin work with the mentally retarded I quickly, without hesitation, said "No!". It was inconceivable, to me, that such work could be personally rewarding or very beneficial to society. Once I relented and began working with retarded people, I found that my attitudes could not have been more incorrect. The work was personally rewarding because there was just as much joy in seeing a retarded person become independent and achieve his productive potential as it was to see any other individual achieve this status, even though the retarded person's functioning might be less sophisticated and technical. I soon learned that the beauty of rehabilitation is in beholding achievement which approximates potential rather than in achievement itself.

Vocational rehabilitation programs for the mentally retarded were initiated in an atmosphere of optimism by a few visionaries and skepticism by many traditional vocational rehabilitation personnel and the general public. These new programs, because of funding procedures, were, by and large, cooperative in nature. I doubt that there is anyone who can say with certainty whether the Congress, in its wisdom, structured the enabling legislation as it did in the interest of good programming or because of politically and economically practical considerations.

Regardless of the reasoning, the forces which made cooperative programming mandatory were some of the most positively beneficial the vocational rehabilitation movement and other human service resources have ever experienced.

THE PURPOSE OF THE SPECIAL EDUCATION-VOCATIONAL REHABILITATION COOPERATIVE PROGRAM

The purpose of a school vocational rehabilitation cooperative program is the same as any other public education or vocational rehabilitation program. The objectives for the student-client are the assimilation of all the academic skills which he or she can effectively utilize and the development of appropriate vocational interest, potential and social and personal adjustment necessary for the individual to achieve his highest level of vocational participation. The uniqueness of the cooperative program lies in the fact that a single program has, for once, incorporated all of these highly compatible objectives. Another feature which differentiates the vocational rehabilitation education program from regular educational experiences is that objectives are prescriptive (based on individual evaluations) rather than arbitrarily established objectives formulated for some so-called comparable group.

The school program as an approach to rehabilitation is innovative for vocational rehabilitation agencies also because it represents their original venture into the sphere of prevention. Historically, vocational rehabilitation has been concerned with maladjustment in the world of work resulting from a handicapping disability. The student-client is not vocationally maladjusted since there is no real environmental expected level of vocational performance from an individual until the individual terminates his affiliation with formal educational or training programs. By placing resources into the public schools, the vocational rehabilitation agency is directing attention to the prevention of a developing vocational handicap by early intervention. Although this is a philosophical issue, recognition of this phenomenon by rehabilitation personnel is of vital importance since it has tremendous counseling and guidance implications. The above will be discussed later in the section devoted to the functions of the vocational rehabilitation counselor in a school rehabilitation-cooperative program.

ESSENTIAL COMPONENTS OF THE PROGRAM

The goals of education and vocational rehabilitation are highly comparable although the processes have distinctive characteristics. The following simple breakdown illustrates some of the differences of the two programs.

Rehabilitation	*Education*
1. An individual process	1. A group process (generally)
2. Specific goals	2. General goals
3. Precise objectives	3. Broad objectives
4. A personal and social purpose	4. A social and personal purpose

An oversimplified statement of the differences between vocational rehabilitation and public education is that vocational rehabilitation is oriented toward helping an individual develop the capacity to function within society and that the goal of public education is to develop individuals capable of structuring a productive society.

The combined vocational rehabilitation-school program shares with public education and the general vocational rehabilitation program common concerns; therefore, the cooperative program must have all of the components of both programs participating in the joint relationship.

The necessary components for a cooperative program are described in a series of monographs published by the vocational rehabilitation program operating in the Bridgeport, Connecticut, school system.[4] These publications are probably the most detailed report on the establishment and operation of a cooperative program effort between public education and vocational rehabilitation available today. Program elements described in these monographs which are to be discussed in this section are the following:

1. Systematic case finding procedures
2. Formalized procedures for student-client evaluation
3. A vocational counseling program
4. Opportunities for prevocational training in the program curriculum
5. Exploratory occupational experiences
6. On-campus job training programs
7. Community job training programs
8. Trade or occupational education programs
9. Job placement and follow-up programs
10. Vocational adjustment counseling and guidance (this component pervades the entire system of services available in the total program).

Prior to considering these specific program activities, it is appropriate to direct the reader's attention to a crucial general factor which influences the success of all activities.

Every profession has its own code of ethics which, among other things, establishes professional protocol which must be respected by persons who desire or expect to work effectively with the profession or the establishment within which the profession practices. Anyone with a degree of sophistication regarding relationships with a school unit should be aware that the principal is the pivotal character upon whom the development of a functional relationship with a school unit depends. The principal must be actively involved or, at the very least, informed and actively interested and supportive before a relationship in the school is to be productive. When interfacing with an entire school system, the superintendent commands this position of eminence,

The Vocational Rehabilitation-Public Education Program

but without significantly detracting from the principal's importance in his or her administrative unit. Therefore, negotiations for the development of a cooperative program between vocational rehabilitation and the school must originate with these key personnel. Likewise, any operational changes, additions, expansions or policy changes in an existing program must have prior approval from the school unit and system administrators if they are to be successfully implemented.

Program staff are prone to forget or are unaware of the nature of the administrator's job. For whatever reason, there appears to be little appreciation of the fact that the administrator does not enjoy the staff privilege of concentrating concern on one particular program. This misunderstanding or lack of knowledge often leads to unnecessary conflict between program personnel and administrators, who are accused of "dragging their feet" or of being unconcerned about a certain group of employees and/or certain constituents. If program people are thoughtful enough to analyze the administrator's functions and responsibilities, they will exhibit greater tolerance and patience in seeking administrative sanction for their program activities. This implies that the program personnel should deliberately and carefully develop a clear rationale for activities requiring administrative approval before seeking an audience with the administrator to ask for his endorsement of a proposal. Also, they should attempt to anticipate problems which may arise in other areas of the administrative unit resulting from an opportunity to operationalize their request and seek to develop a strategy that they can suggest to the administrator which would eliminate or at least minimize these anticipated problems. An administrator presented with a well-conceived and well-structured plan, accompanied by a rational approach for dealing with problems that accompany change, is very likely to respond favorably. This approach to selling program ideas is difficult for the practitioner to learn because his familiarity with the program and its needs make the need for recommended changes so obvious that there seems to be little reason for detailed justification for the request. However, if the administrator is viewed as a reasonable person who is probably as interested as anyone else in the development of good service programs and if attention is focused on the reasons for his being sometimes difficult to deal with, rather than condemnation of his actions or inactions, mutual respect and understanding leading to cooperation between administrators and program personnel will usually evolve naturally.

Case Finding

"Before a handicapped person can receive vocational rehabilitation services, he first has to learn about the existence of rehabilitation agencies in his community." (McGowan and Porter, 1967). The above quotation is the introductory sentence in a section on case finding in one of the basic documents about the vocational rehabilitation process. One of the unique features of vocational rehabilitation, as a social agency, is that it actively seeks people who need its services. Generally, service agencies are content to let contituents seek out their services unless they are dealing with contagious problems which have the potential for immediately endangering others in the environment unless the problem is isolated and controlled. Because successful rehabilitation has positive effects for the whole of society, as well as for the individual and his immediate family, case finding is an important concern.

A multitude of research studies has shown that the vocational rehabilitation agency has a very low public visability, and consequently many persons who are most in need of rehabilitation services do not receive them because they are unaware of this existing resource. Community surveys also indicate that there are numerous people who know that there is a vocational rehabilitation service but who do not avail themselves of the service because of misinformation or various apprehensions, for example, fear of corrective surgery. For a local rehabilitation program to maximize its productivity, thought and effort must be directed toward developing and maintaining an effective case finding program.

In the school, with its captive audience which is confined to a highly structured, evaluative regime, case finding would not seem to be a problem, but it can be. Many students have correctable problems which escape the attention of school personnel, particularly if the student is "getting by" in classes and is not being disruptive.[9] Others may be improperly labeled as a result of their "acting out" and poor performance even though their behavior may be unrelated to a disability.

Still another problem which compounds case finding efforts is the identification of a handicapped student whose parents, because of guilt feelings or anxiety, refuse to admit the presence of a problem which needs special attention.

A school unit is actually a buzzing community characterized by fast-paced hustle and bustle. There are always many diverse activities occurring and/or developing concurrently, just as in any other active population center. Also similar to community life is the reality that individuals in the school unit usually know little about what is going on in areas of activity in which they are not participants. It is therefore common for a teacher to recognize that a certain student may have a problem associated with a disability, but being unaware of a helping resource within the school system, she is likely to make a decision to handle the problem as well as she can while looking forward to being relieved of this responsibility when the student is promoted.

A program-oriented case finding problem is that there are usually enough students in the school's special education classes who, by virtue of their educational placement, are prime candidates for vocational rehabilitation services, so there is a real temptation not to seek out additional work in the form of handicapped students who may be in the regular school program.

Recognizing that every handicapped person has the right to be considered for rehabilitation services, the vocational rehabilitation counselor in a school unit is obliged to interpret the services of his agency and the cooperative program to the student body and, in particular, to school administrators, counselors, teachers and parent groups. A primary objective should be to make teachers and guidance staff sensitive to the symptoms of disabilty, the presence of handicapping conditions and the eligibility criteria for vocational rehabilitation services. If this responsibility is adequately discharged, the counselor may expect to be literally bombarded with referrals so that it becomes urgent for him to begin the creation of an organized system for screening referrals as they are received. This organizational responsibility of the vocational rehabilitation staff in a cooperative school program will be discussed more fully later in this chapter in the section devoted to the functions of the rehabilitation personnel.

Evaluation

The name of the game is evaluation. To an extent, the preceding euphemism is true, because for any treatment program to be consistently effective, it must be based on an understanding of the problem or problems *and* the assets of the individual from which the solution to his problem of distability must be fashioned. A rehabilitation program is a treatment program in that it seeks to move a handicapped or potentially handicapped individual to a status of being nonhandicapped by introducing the individual into a series of services and experiences which will enable him to accept himself as a worthwhile individual, capable of enjoying a fulfilling life, with the capacity to be functional and productive in his social situation. The extent of the evaluation is determined by the degree of handicap rather than the severity of the disability. This concept is tremendously important and must be understood by the rehabilitation counselor if he is to secure and have the capacity for utilizing information obtained from an appropriate client evaluation.

A minimum diagnostic evaluation is necessary to establish eligibility for rehabilitation services. The purpose of this information, of course, is to confirm the presence of a disability and a relatively favorable indication that the client can realize some vocational benefit from services. This may be the only evaluation needed to help a well-adjusted person with an appropriate occupational goal design and complete a rehabilitation plan regardless of the disabling condition. However, most student-clients in a school-vocational rehabilitation cooperative program are mentally or emotionally impaired and display symptoms of immaturity, dependency, distractability and unreliability, along with a confusion regarding a vocational objective which they desire or can pursue with a sustained effort. To plan with an individual who has characteristics such as those just mentioned, the counselor will undoubtedly need an in-depth evaluation to identify the personality or social factors which contribute to the maintenance of such destructive traits. The following are commonly recognized areas of evaluation important to rehabilitation success:

1. Medical (general and speciality)
2. Psychological (intelligence, personality, aptitude, interest, academic achievement)
3. Social (family, community, peer-group, work group)
4. Vocational (physical stamina, persistence, interest, dexterity, impulse control (acceptance of instructions and supervision)

As important as evaluation is to the individual rehabilitation process, it has particular significance in the cooperative program. Many school personnel perceive the availability of comprehensive diagnostic evaluation services as the primary advantage for having vocational rehabilitation personnel and services operating within the schools. It is incumbent for vocational rehabilitation to protect its privileged vantage for providing services to handicapped students; therefore, agency personnel must be concerned about meeting the expectations of their hosting partner in the cooperative relationship. This rationale for the implementation of a strong evaluation component in the school is certainly a secondary and yet very important pragmatic concern.

Prevocational Training

Prevocational training is one of the many poorly defined terms commonly used in rehabilitation literature and discussions. All of us in the field of rehabilitation speak glibly about prevocational training as if the subject is well defined. I believe that nothing could be much further from the truth. There are many who seem never to have stopped to consider a specific meaning of the term *prevocational training,* and others who have engaged in such considerations have different orientations regarding the nature of this service. There are many who would define prevocational training as an elementary introduction to "trade and industrial or vocational education."[4] Others speak of prevocational training as a socialization process in which handicapped individuals are given instructions (classroom type, charts, notebooks, lectures, *et cetera*) in grooming, dress, personal hygiene and interpersonal relationships.[9]

Because of the broad continuum of ideas regarding the nature of prevocational training, I must explain the context in which I used the term. The definition provided is not offered as "truth" and a definition which should be commonly adopted but is given so the reader may understand the concept of prevocational training as it is being used in this chapter.*

Prevocational training is a component of the cooperative vocational rehabilitation-school program which should be provided to student-clients upon first entering the program. Ideally, this aspect of the program should be instituted at the ninth or tenth grade level. The program should introduce the student-client to the meaning of work in our society, the characteristics of successful employees, the expected characteristics of an employer, an introduction to occupations and the responsibilities of wage earners —that is, payment into social security program, tax contributions and saving for emergencies.

This program also should help the client develop a perception of himself as a producer by his having an opportunity to successfully engage in productive activities. This implies helping the student select projects with which he may experience success and in which he can learn the use, manipulation, care and safety precautions required in the use of basic tools. Much of what should be accomplished in prevocational training requires the active participation of the student-client and is more dependent upon the relationships between the client and others involved in the program than upon instruction or the use of academic materials.[8] It is my personal opinion that prevocational training should provide the mentally retarded youth, or otherwise developmentally handicapped individual, a developmental experience which will pre-

---

*It is my feeling that continuing to use ill-defined terms which are basic to our profession has drastically deleterious effects and the profession should develop a standardized nomenclature.

pare him to participate in and profit from more structured vocational instruction.

Exploratory Occupational Experiences

This is a program that is of great importance to the young disabled person who never has experienced an exposure to the world of work. Such experiences should be made available to every young person prior to a commitment to develop specific occupational skills. Many so-called normal students have exposure to such experiences in the form of summer and after-school employment. It is quite common in our society for disabled handicapped students to be denied these opportunities because parents and employers alike shelter the disabled young person against the possibly frustrating initial job effort. Disabled students enrolled in the regular school curriculum normally are faced with a limited chance of participating in vocational training programs because of fear they may be injured by shop equipment; also if the individual is pursuing an academic curriculum there is usually little time for him to be involved in trade or skill training programs. If, at the conclusion of his program of education, he comes to the rehabilitation agency without having had the advantage of exploring different occupational fields, he is at a definite disadvantage in selecting an occupational objective. Occasionally, exploratory occupational experiences can be experienced in a sheltered workshop.

Fortunately, in a school cooperative program ample time can be structured for this program and numerous occasions developed for the students to work for at least short periods at various tasks related to a wide variety of occupations. Securing student cooperation should not be difficult in that they should be given some remuneration for the work they have done. Teachers, guidance counselors, administrators and school maintenance personnel should be able to furnish a wide variety of one-time jobs for student-clients. If the school system does not have funds to pay for these jobs which can and should be done by student labor, some satisfactory payment in kind should be given the student-client. It may be that after thinking about the importance of such experiences in shaping vocational interest and tolerance, the vocational rehabilitation agency itself would administratively arrange to pay the student-clients for their efforts. Also, the rehabilitation counselors and teachers may want to make known to the community that participants in the cooperative program are available for short-term jobs. Precautions must be taken to protect the student-client from exploitation by the public, but procedures for this purpose can be developed without great difficulty.

On-Campus Job Training Programs

During the eleventh school year the student-client of the cooperative program should be placed on permanent job assignment within the school so that he or she can begin developing some specific vocational skills. Selection of a placement opportunity should be based on the interest, aptitude and potential indicated in the preliminary evaluation of these traits. Attention also should be given to the student's performance and satisfaction demonstrated during the period allowed earlier for exploratory occupational experiences.

While the client is working on an on-campus job assignment, the counselor should carefully reevaluate the individual to make sure that the developing vocational plan is suitable for the individual. This evaluation can be made through frequent contacts with the job supervisor and the client to determine the progress which is being made and the satisfaction of both with the job that is being performed. In addition to reevaluating the appropriateness of the vocational objective, the counselor should be looking for clues concerning specific problems that may be affecting the individual's adjustment and/or job performance. If problems are noted, the counselor, supervisor and student should try to resolve them. The counselor should also report apparent problem areas to the teacher and, in consultation with the teacher, attempt to arrange classroom assignments which will help expedite the student's development of a solution to job-related problems.

The counselor in this phase of the rehabilitation process must be very supportive of the student, the work supervisor, the teacher and the student-client's family if they can be involved in this on-campus rehabilitation activity.

Community Job Training Program

During the student-client's last school year, arrangements should be made for him to engage in a least half-time work in an off-campus job. It should be noted that the program being described in this chapter illustrates a developmental process. Prevocational training leads naturally into exploratory occupational experiences which in turn leads to on-campus job training with enough consistent activities to provide an opportunity for the development of specific occupational skills. The proximity of the client to the school and cooperative program personnel during the on-campus work activity provides adequate opportunities for closely monitoring and supervising the student-client's work, so that any deficiencies in performance may receive immediate corrective attention. A natural progression from this step in the rehabilitation process is to allow the student to begin work in a community concern. In addition to further developing occupational and work skills the individual can, during this phase of the process, learn much about the competitive world of work as it exists in the community. Since for possibly the first time the person is earning a fixed income, he can begin learning how to manage money. Other important information can also be learned: how to arrange for and meet transportation schedules necessary for getting to and from a job; the reality of observing expected time schedules such as coffee breaks, job reporting and quitting time; how to plan for meals during the work day; how to care for uniforms which may be provided by the employer or for personal clothes acceptable in a public job; and certain amenities expected by fellow employees, the employer and patrons.

This job experience should, if at all possible, be located in a competitive agency, institution, business or industry; but if such arrangements cannot be made, it would be feasible to place the individual in a sheltered workshop if one is available. However, placement in the workshop should be terminated at the first opportunity for placement in a community business. If neither a community job training opportunity is available nor a sheltered workshop opportunity exists, arrangements to work at the school with minimum supervision and maximum expectation for production should be made by the counselor. Such an arrangement should not be continued any longer than is absolutely required unless eventual placement with the school system as an employee is anticipated.

A question which often arises is should vocational rehabilitation pay an on-the-job training fee to employers who are working with school cooperative program clients. Generally, the answer is no. If a client has gone through the kind of cooperative program outlined in this chapter, he should be of some value to the employer, even though he is in a continuing training status. If such is not the case, the counselor should question seriously the validity of earlier program phases, the rehabilitation plan or the validity of the community placement. Of course, there are exceptions to this rule; for example, if the client is being prepared for a highly technical job, it may be legitimate to pay an on-the-job fee. However, the counselor should ask himself the following questions: (a) If this client has the potential for learning and adequately performing this technical work, is on-the-job training the best procedure for his developing the skills involved? (b) Is this client mature enough emotionally to begin training for a specific technical skill? or (c) Should he have another year of general educational and job experience during which time he will develop additional maturity before embarking on such a training program? A consideration that should be kept in mind is that a so-called normal student is believed to need all the maturity he can achieve in a twelve-year program of public education before undertaking highly specific technical or advanced academic training.

Advanced Training

Although it is assumed that the enrollee of a cooperative program is a limited student, the counselor should be aware that there are instances when the client should be provided an opportunity for additional training; on-the-job, trade, technical or commercial. If such is the case, there should be no hesitancy to recommend, encourage or sponsor such additional training. Here again it is important for the counselor to evaluate his client and extend the rehabilitation plan if it appears that by doing so the client can make further vocational and adjustment gains.

Placement and Follow-Up

A major ingredient in the concept of accountability, discussed earlier in this chapter, is the establishment of specific behavioral objectives, which may be the expected outcome of a program effort and can be measured. Behavioral objectives for each phase of the education-rehabilitation process should be clearly defined and related to the unique problems, needs and potential of each person being served in the cooperative program. The global behavioral objective of the total process is for each recipient of service, or more accurately, each active participant in the cooperative program, to have achieved at the conclusion of services and participation a level of adjustment which will permit him to participate in a vocation commensurate with his interests, aptitudes and abilities. This is a quantifiable objective which, to a degree, can be measured. Even though criteria for measurement are not precise, a judgment easily can be reached regarding how closely performance approximates the envisioned goal of the rehabilitation plan. If there is considerable discrepancy between what was projected and the actual case outcome, services may need to be extended; however, if a critical analysis of the case contraindicates further professional effort, failure should be admitted and the case studied in an attempt to correct identifiable service and/or program deficits so that a similar "bust" can be avoided in the future. There may be a tendency for some to say, "You can't rehabilitate everyone who is disabled so why worry about failures, when most of the time failure is the result of the clients' lack of cooperation." Such an attitude denies the concept of accountability. Many people who now survive surgery would have died on the table if surgeons had denied the value of postmortems, and I believe that rehabilitation effectiveness will progress very slowly so long as we hesitate to closely examine our failures.

Placement and vocational adjustment are the behavioral objectives common to all service plans developed in the school-vocational rehabilitation cooperative program. Ideally, the student-client who is not to receive postschool training should be employed at the site of his off-campus job training program. The possibility of eventual placement should be considered when the training site is selected, and if such a placement is not possible, the client should be prepared to utilize the services of the Employment Security Commission for finding a suitable job. The vocational rehabilitation counselor may very well need to help his client establish a satisfactory working relationship with this organization. The counselor working with an individual in this situation should be cognizant of the need to caution his client about utilizing private employment agencies whose service is relatively expensive, which is not to say that such private agencies are not legitimate business concerns, but it is well to remember that the level of jobs available to most cooperative program graduates are listed with the public agency whose service is free. At the same time the counselor and client are working with the employment service to locate a job opportunity, other resources, such as the trainer, friends of the trainee, the guidance counselor and the vocational rehabilitation agency's knowledge of the local labor market should be utilized.

A good vocational rehabilitation agency procedure which is helpful in locating employment opportunities is for each counselor in a particular office or locality to add an entry into a central registry, available to all vocational rehabilitation counselors, concerning employment opportunities he has noted through visiting local business and industry. The contents of his entry should identify the person with whom he has talked, the individual responsible for hiring, the general attitude about employing handicapped workers, the types of jobs, shifts, needed skills and employee turnover in the particular business or industry.

The final phase of the rehabilitation process is follow-up with the newly employed person to determine from him his satisfaction with his job and his employer's satisfaction with the person's performance on the job. This can be and often times is a very mechanical procedure, but it may also be a time when the client critically needs counseling services which, if not provided, will lead to job failure and the development of a client who will be more difficult to place on a subsequent occasion. More will be said about the possible counseling needs of the client during this state of development in the section on the role and function of the rehabilitation counselor in a cooperative school program.

The Vocational Rehabilitation-Public Education Program 325

Vocational Counseling and Guidance

As I began to consider writing this chapter on the public education-vocational rehabilitation cooperative program and the functions and responsibilities of vocational rehabilitation personnel in this program, an initial concern about the structure of this chapter was where to include a discussion concerning vocational counseling and guidance. My thoughts ran as follows: vocational counseling and guidance is the foundation of any complicated rehabilitation procedure or program, therefore, a discussion of this subject should precede all other topics. However, vocational guidance and counseling are so integrally important to all phases of the rehabilitation process that it should be explored in the middle or at the end of all other discussions. I finally decided that since it is a continuous service throughout the process, the alpha and the omega of rehabilitation, I would discuss counseling and guidance after giving consideration to all other components of the immediate subject. I want the reader to relate what is to be said about vocational counseling and guidance to all other aspects of the cooperative program previously discussed.

Since vocational counseling is the subject of another chapter in this book, I will not dwell on it at length. I do feel compelled to discuss it briefly, in general, and at greater length as it applies to some specific problems associated with school-aged handicapped people and the mentally retarded who comprise the bulk of the cooperative program case load.

From my frame of reference, the only difference between vocational rehabilitation counseling and any other form of clinical counseling is that the rehabilitation counselor has a unique work setting. He is providing counseling with a specific adjustment objective in mind, and he utilizes special guidance information when his client is ready to use it effectively. I do not think it can be emphasized too often or too strongly that in order for a vocational counselor or a rehabilitation counselor to work effectively with a handicapped person who needs a counseling service, he must first of all be an effective clinical counselor. Rather than concentrating on giving advice, making recommendations, supplying answers to questions or providing solutions to problems, the vocational rehabilitation counselor should view his specialty as the ability to create a climate in which a disabled person can, without intimidation even from himself, examine and get to know himself and become consciously aware of his strengths, weaknesses, self-worth and his potential for enjoying a productive life. The counselor who refuses, or does not have the time, to practice in this manner can be helpful only to those who are fully capable of self-direction and who, if they never had seen the counselor, would have gotten the information or services needed for their rehabilitation. If an individual is to adequately serve handicapped people who have emotional difficulties (as differentiated from emotional illness) he must be a counselor and not just a representative of an agency which can provide a multitude of special services.

Counseling is of tremendous importance in the school cooperative program. Most of the clients with whom the counselor works have developmental disabilities with which they have had to cope throughout their lives. They have experienced oversolicitation from anxious parents or rejection from parents who more than likely never received the help that they needed for accepting their handicapped child; they have lived in a society which puts a premium on normality and have been pitied, scorned, ignored, laughed at and refused or only given an opportunity with strings on it to participate in peer-group activities. Resulting from these negative experiences, the individual needs and generally must have an opportunity to achieve growth in self-esteem and confidence before he can make a valid effort at selecting a suitable vocational objective or successfully engaged in and benefit from a job training program. Growth is also necessary in order for him to adjust emotionally or even tolerate an independent living and work situation.

THE ROLE OF VOCATIONAL REHABILITATION PERSONNEL IN A COOPERATIVE PROGRAM

Diversity in the staffing patterns of cooperative programs makes it impossible to identify the role of specific program personnel. For example, one of these programs may have any one of the following staffing assignments:

1. One counselor: One school unit
2. One counselor: Two or more school units
3. Two counselors: One school unit or system
4. Several counselors plus a supervisor: One or more school units or an entire system
5. A multidisciplinary rehabilitation staff with an administrator (including aides): One or more school units or an entire system

There are also numerous variations of the patterns enumerated above. Other common differences may be the location of vocational rehabilitation personnel; some are housed in the school facility, others in the administrative office of the school unit and still others may be housed with the local vocational rehabilitation office that serves the community's general population. Roles also may be affected to some extent by the funding arrangements through which the cost of the cooperative program is financed. In programs that are financed with third-party matching funds, vocational rehabilitation personnel may not need to document so carefully the interaction between agency personnel and school employees assigned to the program. For obvious reasons, jobs which the vocational rehabilitation staff should be responsible for will be described without an attempt to specify which staff member should perform the function. In one-counselor units, of course, that individual must assume responsibility for the whole host of duties; also, there are certain service functions which the counselor must execute. These duties will be discussed in the last section of the present chapter.

The counselor also should create opportunities for himself to visit individually with as many school personnel as possible. Doing this informally, possibly over coffee in the teachers' lounge, is desirable. He should not be too hasty about detailing his program. Out of sincere interest he should seek to explore and understand the school's problems as much in depth as possible. He should carefully avoid presenting himself as an "expert" who has solutions to the problems being enunciated to him. He should portray himself as a person keenly interested in the problems of handicapped students and school personnel and who wants to be of assistance to both.

The task just described is not a one-time effort that must be attended to only when the cooperative program is in the infant state. In fact, due to staff turnover, it is a process that has to be performed on a recurring basis.

PROGRAM CONTINUATION

For a program to continue in existence its existence must be justified by results. Assuming that the counselor is accepted into and by the school, his continued acceptance is contingent upon his demonstrating the value of having vocational rehabilitation services incorporated into the school program. He must, therefore, present in some systematic way evidence that he is providing concrete services to the student body. Such evidence should be presented both verbally and through a periodic written report which outlines the counselor's activities and the case services which have been provided or initiated. If a newsletter-type organ is used, the counselor should be sure to recognize specific individuals from the school staff who have been particularly helpful. Such a report should be kept simple to avoid the eventuality of its preparation becoming so time consuming that it appreciably detracts from the time for service duties. The suggested report can have a great deal of meaning in developing and maintaining good morale for those who are devoting time to the cooperative program. It not only reinforces a realization that positive benefits are resulting from their program efforts, but it also calls to the attention of other school personnel that the staff members in the cooperative program are achieving very tangible results.

PROGRAM COORDINATION

For a cooperative program to function properly, the activities of many different people and disciplines must be coordinated. For example, the activities of the counselor and the teachers must be complimentary. When the student-client is placed on work assignment, either during the occupational exploration phase of his program, on-campus job training or off-campus job training, the work of the counselor, teacher, and job supervisor must be coordinated so that all are working toward a common objective.

There are rehabilitation services which must be provided to student-clients outside the school setting. Special diagnostic or treatment services and job training are just a few examples of vital off-campus components of the rehabilitation process in a cooperative program which must be coordinated with the client's school schedule. Vocational rehabilitation responsibilities include providing a link between the educational program of the school, the school's maintenance and support staff, professional services in the community and the local labor market.

A nuisance problem which must be given adequate attention and be coordinated effectively is that of transportation needed by the students if they are to participate in the activities prescribed for them in the cooperative program. This is a problem, the burden of which must ordinarily be assumed by vocational rehabilitation personnel.

A large problem that must be dealt with is securing the help and support of all parents of participants in the cooperative program. The agreement upon a specific behavioral objective for a student and the achievement of that objective is subject to parental consent and cooperation. There are several characteristics of parents which make their appropriate involvement a monumental task. Some parents do not have the emotional strength to cope with the idea that their child is limited, or they may overreact to the disability and therefore refuse to agree to or support a program directed at a behavioral objective which they feel is beneath or beyond the capabilities of their child. Many other parents of student-clients are themselves limited; they live in deprivation and do not have the emotional, physical or intellectual energy or inclination to become involved in the educational program for their child. They therefore do not give the child the support from the home which he needs if he is to fully profit from the activities of the cooperative program. A recognition of the strategic position held by parents is a must if the rehabilitation professional is to be successful in working with students in a cooperative program. A great deal of time must be allocated to working with parents to increase the possibility of getting needed support from them.

A resource which can have much influence on the effectiveness of work with parents and their children is the Department of Social Services. Since many families of individuals enrolled in cooperative school programs receive assistance payments from that department, it must be informed of the work being done in the cooperative program and its cooperation solicited in the development of parental support. A historical problem with which early cooperative programs were confronted was the reduction of welfare money payments going into the homes of students who, as a result of their participation in job-training activities, were earning money. The Welfare Department considered this money as a resource to the family and reduced the public assistance payment by a comparable amount. This problem has generally been resolved but there may still be locations where vestiges of his earlier attitude remain; therefore, rehabilitation personnel, especially in newly established cooperative programs, may need to work closely with the Department of Social Services so there is a thorough understanding by that agency of the goals of the program. With such an understanding, the department can, if necessary, establish policies to discount earnings of students in a job-training program as being a resource for family subsistence.

In this section a discussion of administration, organization, coordination and the relation of the school to the family and community has been offered. As was said, in the beginning of this section, no attempt was made to identify by position the duties and responsibilities of members of the vocational rehabilitation team. This approach was taken because of the variations in the staffing patterns of rehabilitation cooperative school programs. Some of the activities discussed may be performed by supervisors, aides, evaluators, job placement specialists, special-education teachers or vocational rehabilitation counselor, depending on the staffing pattern of a given school unit. In the next section there will be a discussion of functions peculiar to the rehabilitation counselor because these are functions which the counselor cannot legally or ethically relinquish. The topics which will be covered are (a) the establishment of eligibility for vocational rehabilitation services and (b) rehabilitation counseling. The discussion of rehabilitation counseling will be limited to some very specific phases of the counseling process that are most specifically related to individuals served by cooperative school programs.

VOCATIONAL COUNSELING

Because of the youth and lack of vocational experience of clients in the cooperative school program, the rehabilitation counselor must devote considerable time and energy to helping his clients choose a vocational objective. Rather than using the traditional sixty-minute counseling session for this purpose, the cooperative counselor will probably make use of more frequent informal (but purposeful) contacts with his clients in the classroom and as they perform in the various job training and experience opportunities provided by the cooperative program. Two major objectives in vocational counseling are the selection of a vocational objective and the development of ego strength needed to successfully complete vocational preparation and adjust to a job situation, which implies satisfactory community living. These are two very distinct functions which will be discussed separately.

The rehabilitation counselor should give serious consideration to development and utilization of group counseling skills. Numerous research projects have indicated that there is no statistical difference in the outcome of individual versus group counseling in the area of occupational choice.[2] Group counseling has been shown by scientific investigation to have some advantages over individual counseling for helping adolescents develop positive attitudes and socially acceptable behavior.[3] A major factor in deciding to start group work is the demands for counselor time, although it will not save time initially, unless the counselor is training in group dynamics he must devote time to preparing himself for this activity.

Occupational opportunities for the majority of students in a cooperative school program are usually limited. In many cases the selection of a vocational objective will be accomplished during the evaluation process, since the client will probably enjoy and be most interested in the job experience in which he has had the most success. I would like to make the following points; however, in 1960, S. A. Fine, in speaking of vocational choice, said that the process can take two forms: that of discovering or invention.[3] (Dr. Fine defines discovery as a hunt-and-find operation for a place or thing that is known to exist by using various techniques, (maps, measuring instruments, et cetera) guidance.) The technique of invention involves defining relevant parameters hypothesizing alternative solutions, counseling and setting on a final solution by testing the various alternatives (counseling).

The discovery method, which is probably most commonly used, may place the client in a passive, nonparticipating role in the vocational counseling process. He is an object for analysis and study from which patterns and profiles evolve. He is lost in the process unless he can accept and utilize decisions made by others regarding what is best for him. Invention, on the other hand, keeps the client, his unique problem, or problems, in focus and has the client involved during every step of developing the vocational rehabilitation plan. The client is an active participant in the counseling process, which enhances the possibilities that the service will be relevant and can be successfully used by the client.

One other major purpose of vocational counseling, for which the rehabilitation counselor needs to assume greater responsibility, is the development of sufficient ego strength for the client to achieve the personal and social adjustment prerequisite for satisfactory vocational participation.

The counselor needs to realize that supportive counseling is particularly indicated during the initial phase of employment. English and Pearson[1] indicate "One of the first emotional problems to confront an adult is his adaptation to the work by which he earns his living." They go on to enumerate facts which may cause conflicts to arise during work adjustment:

> (1) he (the person) never had friends while growing up and may wish to shrink away from human contacts on the job; (2) he fears exploitation, that is, fears doing too much; (3) he wants many people to recognize him; (4) he wants individual attention; (5) he wants his feelings considered in every situation; (6) he is incapable of putting himself in the other fellow's place; or (7) he fears anger, jealousy, and hostility in others and himself.

In the above discussion, the authors are speaking of common

problems experienced by "normal" people as they enter the world of work. The client from a cooperative school program may very well experience these problems which will be exacerbated by his disability and abnormal social isolation.

For years the Vocational Rehabilitation Agency has recognized the need for and the benefits of providing follow-up services to handicapped people once placed in a job. It has been generally recognized that disabled people entering the labor market, to them an unfamiliar and frightening social structure, may have problems with which they need the help of the counselor. Unfortunately, there has not been enough said about supportive counseling as a technique which should be employed by the counselor at this anxiety provoking period in the case.

A primary difference between the client from a cooperative school program and the general population is that the retarded (the bulk of the cooperative program case load) generally have difficulty in forming close and meaningful relationships. The isolated, lonely and bare existence in which many "rehabilitated" handicapped persons are living is not by choice. In a great majority of cases the disabled person lacks the ability to form the kinds of relationship the nonhandicapped have with their parents, churches, friends, husbands, wives, schools, clubs or work supervisors. Because of this quarantine, often self-imposed but encouraged by the environment and lack of opportunity for sharing the day-to-day problems of life, the disabled person may become bewildered. The pressures of such independent living may become painfully overwhelming. I am sure that the reader will develop empathy if he has ever been in a prolonged situation where communication concerning the complexities of life and one's anxiety about them was not possible. A daily solitary confrontation with life's little problems and questions magnify them so that they become intolerable and immobilizing. It is unthinkable that a person can survive alone, especially if the etiology of the loneliness is a feeling of rejection. The problems just described, as associated with vocational adjustment, present the rehabilitation counselor with a real challenge to develop skills in supportive counseling.

If the client is to establish naturally supportive contacts and if the environment is to realistically accept the client, they both must have the counselor's support. Through this support, the client and his community will be in a position for establishing rapport between themselves. To be effective in supportive counseling, the counselor must offer support to the client and the client's community simultaneously. If the counselor allows himself to become the middleman between the client, the employer and others in the community, his good intentions will impede the development of natural supportive relationships. The only way a handicapped client and his community can establish a healthy relationship is through intimate, direct contact.

In order for the client to establish interpersonal relationships, he must have some positive feelings about himself. If he can like himself, others can like him. For the employer and others in the community to form a relationship with the rehabilitated person, they must be given an opportunity to experience the client as a person. He is not a strange phenomenon; he is not a disability; he is not unapproachable. He is more like others than he is different. The community can develop these insights only insofar as they have an opportunity for dealing directly with the individual. Thus, supportive counseling is not just periodic pep talks or the giving of encouragement, nor is it being available to solve or arbitrate problems. Supportive counseling is a process in which a counselee or other person is given an opportunity to talk about anxieties or problems and is given the opportunity to develop his own solutions. The counselor who is providing support has a positive relationship with the counselee based on previous interactions and can therefore give his client strength by his presence, willingness to listen and his ability to maintain composure. If the counselor attempts to verbally reassure the client, deny the reality of the problem or offers solutions, he is in essence indicating he questions the client's adequacy. This is not support. Supportive counseling must provide the client with the chance to exercise his emotional muscles, so they become conditioned through the process just as physical power is conditioned by calisthentics.

Satisfactory community relationships can be developed by the client if the counselor with whom he has been working has made it possible, through support, for communication to occur between the client and others in the community. Once this is accomplished, the client will develop a reserve of natural resources needed for handling life's problems and rehabilitation is completed.

REFERENCES

1. English, O. S., and Pearson, G. H. J.: *Emotional Problems of Living.* New York, W. W. Norton & Company, Inc., 1945.
2. Fine, S. A.: Comments on Dr. Roe's Paper. A report on the Harvest House Conference, University of Colorado, 1960.
3. Fine, S. A.: Group counseling. *J Res Dev Ed, 1 (No. 2)*:Winter, 1968.
4. Lane, Paul A., Soares, L. M., and Silverstone, L. S.: *Objective Vocational Rehabilitation Within Public Education* (Monograph No. 1). Bridgeport (Conn.), SRS Grant No. RD1818G, 1968.
5. Lane, Paul A., Soares, L. M., and Silverstone, L. S.: *Planning Procedures for Vocational Rehabilitation in Public Education* (Monograph No. 3). Bridgeport (Conn.), SRS Grant No. RD1818G; 1969.
6. Lane, Paul A., Soares, L. M., and Silverstone, L. S.: *A Therapeutic Pre-Vocational Training Program.* (Monograph No. 7). Bridgeport (Conn.).
7. Mager, Robert F.: *Preparing Instructional Objectives.* Palo Alto, Fearson Publishers, 1962.
8. Morrow, Joe C. (Ed.): *Final Report of Comprehensive Statewide Planning for Vocational Rehabilitation Services in North Carolina,* North Carolina Division of Vocational Rehabilitation, 1968.
9. *Preparation of Mentally Retarded Youth for Gainful Employment.* Washington, D.C., U. S. Department of Health, Education, and Welfare, Rehabilitation Services No. 507, Bulletin No. 28, 1959.
10. Rogers, Carl R.: *Freedom to Learn,* Columbus (Ohio), Charles E. Merrill Publishing Co., 1969.

16

The School Unit Counselor

Edward F. Rose and Harold F. Shay

The Student
Parents
School Personnel
The Community
Generalized Functions of the School Unit Counselor
The Texas Plan
Varieties of Coordination
References

THE SCHOOL unit counselor concept evolved during the sixties. It is not a new concept; it is based on an already established system which has been honed and refined as a result of experience and knowledge gained. Rehabilitation counselors had for years been assigned to schools on an itinerant basis which often meant that their contacts with handicapped students came late in the students' high school careers. All too frequently the student received little or no realistic preparation for the pursuit of a vocation or continued training and education. The usual practice was to offer no services until the student either graduated from school or dropped out.[2] This arrangement often meant that the rehabilitation counselor was providing services that were too late to be fully effective.

The development of school units, which contain representatives from the several disciplines necessary to fully serve the handicapped student, is directly related to availability of grant funds for the support of cooperative agreements between special education and vocational rehabilitation. This is a natural bond when the school administration has been sold on rehabilitation counseling, evaluation, placement assistance and other services necessary for the handicapped student to make a better transition into an adult world. Unfortunately, a universal acceptance or implementation of such a plan has not occurred and many school systems still must be convinced of the value of such a venture.

The counselor who enters the rehabilitation field as a member of a school unit can be faced with a variety of approaches and program formats. However, each plan will have several things in common—the client, parents, school personnel, community and other rehabilitation personnel.

THE STUDENT

The first thing to remember about a handicapped youth is that he is "more *like* his peers than unlike them." He has the same desires and ambitions and will strive as hard to obtain his identity as a member of his peer group as a nonhandicapped youth. Many factors may vary, such as how well adjusted he is to the world around him and especially how well he accepts his handicap. Very often, his contact with the rehabilitation counselor will be his first contact with someone solely concerned with his future as an adult. The counselor, therefore, carries the awesome responsibility of providing the transition from a semisheltered way of life to one in which the client must make some decisions on his own.

The counselor must be the instrument of change—a change which may shatter the comfortable world of the youth and his family that has developed over a period of ten to twelve years. The counselor who knows that he must effect the change will be well on the way to recognizing the conflicts that have to be resolved by the school unit. This is especially true where the retarded are concerned. It must be kept in mind that the retarded are functioning at mental ages below those of their normal peers, but they are being forced to enter an adult world ahead of what is expected of normal youth of the same chronological age.

Regardless of the type of handicap the student may have, the counselor has the responsibility of making sure that the student understands the occupational limitations and attributes inherent in his handicap. In many cases this will not be an easy task. Many handicapped youths have been encouraged to seek unrealistic occupational objectives as a means of motivating them to do their best or exceeding their limitations. This is well and good until they are confronted with the real world of advanced education or work. The counselor faces the challenge of getting the handicapped student to accept a realistic evaluation of his potential and still maintain his motivation to achieve. How to do this requires an awareness of the many influences the handicapped youth must cope with and gives the counselor the opportunity to carry out his function as "coordinator" mentioned in much of the literature.[3] The counselor in this role is too often in definite conflict with others who enter the picture—teachers and parents. Frequently, he must convince all parties of the need for personal-social adjustment training of handicapped students during the last years of high school.

- Do get to know the student beyond his test scores and evaluations.
- Don't allow the student to use his handicap as an excuse to get out of difficult situations.
- Do determine the relationship that exists between student and parents.
- Do insist that the student make as many decisions for himself as possible.
- Do explore the aspirations of the student as they relate to his limitations.
- Do evaluate the student's total social, avocational and personal adjustments as they interface with his vocational progress.
- Do attempt to get the student to align his aspirations with the level permitted by his disability.
- Do expect him to make and keep employment interviews on his own.
- Don't make an exception of an exceptional person.

PARENTS

For the parents of handicapped youth, the school unit counselor will be most likely the first contact they have with someone who will insist that their child be oriented toward the world of work. Parents will vary as widely as the youth; for example, from the unconcerned to the overdemanding, from the protective to the permissive or totally rejecting parent, from the passive to the militant. The most common factor shared by parents of the handicapped, and not too well expressed, is their worry and concern for the child's future. When expressed, it comes out, "What's going to happen to my child when I'm not around to look out for him?" The counselor must directly or indirectly alleviate this concern before he can have reasonable success in directing the youth's rehabilitation program.

The parents' concern for the future of their child may manifest itself in such ways as being overly concerned that their youth (a) be placed in employment as soon as possible, (b) be placed at a higher level than his capabilities warrant, (c) be allowed to pursue education or training when evaluations indicate that this approach would not be wise and (d) the opposite of each of the three. The mother will be the dominant parent in most cases and the father may be difficult to draw into conferences. However, it is very important to involve *both* parents in the vocational rehabilitation process. A good rule, where possible, is that no decision-making contacts with the family be made without the presence of both parents. This prevents or at least minimizes the misinterpretation of decisions and very often brings the parents together in their first joint decision for the youth's future.

Two points to keep in mind when dealing with parents of handicapped youths: (a) Frequently a mother's devotion to her child is directly related to the fact that she delivered him and, (b) a father's lack of involvement may be due to his ego which does not accept the fact that he participated in the creation of something less than a perfect child. Showing empathy toward these unexpressed feelings will do much to enhance a more successful dealing with the parents.

A counselor is wise to convey to the parents early in the counseling process his inability to fully appreciate the many problems they face because he has not had the same experience of living a number of years with a handicapped child. He should attempt to reassure the parents that he is serving as an empathetic team member in their decision-making process. The importance of developing that kind of rapport with parents cannot be overemphasized.

- Do make the parents full partners in the rehabilitation process.
- Do help them relate the limitations of their child's handicap to realistic educational and employment goals.
- Don't assume that the parents have accepted the handicap of their child, even as late as high school.
- Do have empathy—being a parent of a handicapped child is not easy.

SCHOOL PERSONNEL

The school unit counselor, who must establish a functional school unit, is faced with a difficult task in developing an understanding among professional disciplines. This is especially true when the unit is being established using federal funds and, as a result, school personnel must take directions from state vocational rehabilitation agency staff personnel. This conflict has been treated lightly in most publications[1] and generally slanted from the writer's professional point of view. Often it is masked in a suggestion that school personnel remain under school supervision and vice versa for rehabilitation personnel. This arrangement might minimize the problem but certainly will not eliminate it. In all honesty, it needs to be admitted that suspicions and conflicts between school and rehabilitation personnel hinder the success of many joint ventures. The school unit counselor holds the key to the situation. He must gain the confidence of the school administration with demonstrated evidence that his integrity is above reproach. He can do this best by keeping everyone concerned informed of contacts with students and parents and decisions which require the school's involvement.

Basic to problems dealing with school personnel is that schools have for years operated with autonomy, with no other professional discipline having the right or privilege of participation in this coveted process. The rehabilitation counselor, if not a direct threat, is an intruder who tends to remind the educator of the shortcomings of many school systems in preparing handicapped youth for the world of work. Rather than all this negativism, the team of school and rehabilitation personnel should devise ways of instituting changes in curricula and programs which could greatly enhance the future of the handicapped.

Many teachers of the handicapped are aware of their lack of understanding of the workaday world and the school unit counselor can provide this necessary understanding, as well as being an active contact with the adult world beyond an educational setting.

- Do maintain a healthy climate of mutual respect between the rehabilitation unit and school educators.
- Don't expect school personnel to be familiar with the rehabilitation process—help them to understand how your objectives relate to the curricula and the school setting.

THE COMMUNITY

Although handicaps have been a part of society throughout the ages, communities as a whole continue to lack understanding of the needs of the handicapped. The business world in particular has in only recent years begun to recognize its social commitment to fully utilize the handicapped as contributing members of society. From a pragmatic and strictly economic viewpoint, the education of the handicapped is a costly effort. The average yearly cost per student equals or exceeds twice the cost of a "normal" student. Communities have been slow to enter into extensive programs for the handicapped for this reason. For instance, less than 40 percent of the retarded people in this country are in public school classes. The physical or orthopedic handicapped percentage is somewhat higher, since many of them can be absorbed in regular classroom situations with a minimum of investment. Nonetheless, education of the handicapped does require the financial commitment of the community.

Communities abound with organizations which promote understanding of the handicapped—that is, Lions, Civitan and others. These groups provide excellent forums for communicating the educational needs to the people who need to know—the taxpayers. For a school effort in rehabilitation, this is a very important fact of life that must be dealt with from the onset. Individuals can be found in a community who are convinced of the merits of educating young people handicapped by different disabilities, but seldom is there a combined effort to educate and train the wide range of disabilities represented in the general population.

Communities must often have their social consciousness awakened to the basic needs of the handicapped—medical, education, training, employment, recreation, housing and transportation. For a rehabilitation effort to be successful in an educational setting, an extensive plan should be devised to muster all forces of the community toward meeting all needs of the handicapped. Members of the community need to be involved in the planning, establishment and ongoing operation of any school rehabilitation effort.

One technique that has been used across the country to facilitate involvement of the community has been the establishment of "work advisory committees" for the school unit. Such a committee should be made up of leading businessmen and women serving in an advisory capacity on the methods used in training, the things necessary to emphasize on-the-job training and possible opportunities for job placements. Through such a committee, the school unit can contact local service clubs and organizations in order to develop a better understanding of the needs of the handicapped in the community.

The school unit counselor serves as liaison between the school and other community members of the rehabilitation team such as doctors, employers, sheltered workshops, and training and postsecondary educational personnel. The most important facet of this liaison is communication—everyone involved must be kept up to date on the needs and progress of the handicapped student. In so doing, the unit counselor assures everyone of his importance as a team member by keeping him involved in the rehabilitation process.

The following should be a cardinal rule for the rehabilitation unit counselor: Keep everyone informed, involved and busy upholding commitments to the handicapped student.

- Do expect the community to function as members of the rehabilitation team.
- Do ask assistance from members of the community where their expertise can aid specific handicapped people.
- Do identify successful placements in community businesses and give due recognition to the employer who made it possible.
- Do use every communication media possible to bring attention to efforts being made—tax increases to support the needs of the program will be more readily accepted if the taxpayer knows what is being accomplished!
- Don't hesitate to have members of community advisory committees do actual follow-up of placements—they talk the language of other businessmen and often obtain better evaluations than a counselor.

GENERALIZED FUNCTIONS OF THE SCHOOL UNIT COUNSELOR

There are many lists of functions of the vocational rehabilitation counselor in a school unit. The following are paraphrased from several state plans for cooperative programs of special education and vocational rehabilitation:

- Serve as a liaison person between the agency and school; supply information and provide consultative service to the school personnel upon the request of the school administrator.
- Visit special classes for handicapped students so he is well acquainted with the educational offerings in the school and with individual handicapped students prior to their becoming clients of the agency.

- Review the records of handicapped students who may soon need the services of the vocational rehabilitation agency and assist the school personnel in determining vocational needs or work experience needed by the student.
- Identify, recommend and plan with the handicapped youth for services needed to rehabilitate him, either on a long-term or short-term basis.
- Counsel with the individual student prior to any evaluation or work experience in the community.
- Conduct, whenever possible, follow-up evaluation of handicapped youth, following school termination, until a satisfactory adjustment has been made.

Until the sixties, few special education programs were operating at the secondary school level, and many students who were enrolled in them simply dropped out of school when they reached the legal age. Where these programs were operating, the schools were faced with evidence that they were not adequately meeting the needs of the students, since so very few were actually prepared for adult independent living. By the same token, the vocational rehabilitation agencies were aware that many young people referred to them had been exposed to so many years of frustration and failure that their poor work habits and ignorance of the demands of the world of work made them very unlikely candidates for successful rehabilitation.

A new mechanism[2] for rehabilitating disabled students developed in Texas with a plan for a closely articulated special-education-vocational rehabilitation program. The two agencies involved recognized that they shared the goal of providing the mentally retarded young people in special classes in the public schools with appropriate preparation for the kinds of adulthood they might reasonably expect. They tried to design a program with a strong vocational orientation but with a full recognition of the social, psychological and cultural needs of the retarded youngsters they were serving. In their efforts at the Dallas Vocational School, they achieved a dramatic success.

THE TEXAS PLAN

In extending the cooperative approach statewide, both agencies knew that some changes were necessary. The schools, for example, immediately saw that the curricula materials in use throughout the state were too academically oriented, and the classroom procedures were too rigid. Vocational orientation materials were introduced into the classroom and seven flexible levels of development were substituted for the traditional twelve public school grades.

In this approach, the elementary school years are concerned with readiness and instruction in the basic communicative arts and arithmetic skills. In junior high school, the students are introduced to occupational education and vocational exploration. Work stations, established in the school plant, are designed to give the student a chance to explore possible vocations, gain work experience and be provided with an opportunity for vocational evaluation.

In the senior high school, the emphasis is on job training and employment, and the program is equipped to provide appropriate and necessary vocational rehabilitation services to all eligible handicapped young people enrolled in the school district. During the student's high school training period, the teacher may become a vocational adjustment coordinator helping the student adjust to the world of work, learn a particular job, develop vocational and social skills, and improve academic skills related directly to specific jobs. The training stations are maintained within the student's curricula plan and are eventually extended to include training opportunities available within the community. The vocational rehabilitation agency, through an assigned counselor, provides such rehabilitation services as vocational evaluation and planning, job training, and job placement and supervision.

Within the high school curricula, there is a focus on competing in the open labor market, securing and retaining a job, and demonstrating acceptable adult behavior. The vocational rehabilitation counselor and the school staff work cooperatively with individual students and families until job and personal adjustment stability is assured. When it appears that this has been achieved and suitable job placement is a reality, the student is eligible for school graduation. After graduation the vocational rehabilitation counselor maintains contact with the student for as long as this follow-up is needed before officially closing the case.

The major innovation in this approach is disarmingly simple. It is no more than the acceptance of the fact that although certain services to handicapped youth may be the overlapping responsibility of both special education and vocational rehabilitation, it is far better to define which agency will actually carry them out than to leave the job undone or inadequately done. Those activities which are traditionally and legally the functions of special education remain the responsibility of the special education agency and the cooperating school district. Similarly, those activities, traditionally and legally the functions of vocational rehabilitation, remain the responsibility of the state division of vocational rehabilitation. Although the agencies' responsibilities remain the same, their complementary relationship emerges in the unified program as something quite different and quite remarkable in its effects on special education during the sixties.

Since its development, the cooperative approach has spread quickly throughout the country and has been modified to make it more responsive to local special class needs and school capabilities. Today, cooperative school programming is found in virtually every state, but there are many variations in the focus and the structure.

- Generally, mentally retarded students have been emphasized in the cooperative program, but physically handicapped, emotionally disturbed, minimally brain injured and other disabled young people are also being served.
- In the beginning the programs seem to have been located primarily in schools in smaller cities, but recently they have been developing in large urban high schools serving young people from disadvantaged neighborhoods.
- Occasionally, vocational education resources have been utilized to complement the special education and voca-

tional rehabilitation services, but usually the cooperative effort is limited to vocational rehabilitation and special education.
- Often, the vocational rehabilitation counselor maintains an office in the school and works with disabled students referred from regular classes in the school, as well as those enrolled in special classes. Usually, however, counselors visit a number of schools on a regular basis to supervise the rehabilitation dimensions of the student program and work primarily with the students in special classes.
- At times, substantial physical alterations have been made within the schoolroom to improve equipment and organization, in order to provide vocational programming and to modify it into a rehabilitation facility.
- In some programs, work laboratories are utilized to provide an evaluation of the students and sometimes even vocational training.
- Still other types of cooperative programs depend on community sheltered workshops to complement the program of both the school and the rehabilitation agency. Students are released from classes to receive extensive vocational evaluation and training services in a workshop.

A full list of ways in which cooperative programs vary would be endless. Part of the reason for the great variation lies in the fact that special education has developed to different degrees in different communities and operates under different types of legislation. The vocational rehabilitation program, on the other hand, has the same potentials in each state. It, therefore, has a flexible capacity to complement existing special education services in a school district in such a way as to produce a program providing essentially the same level of service in each school.

As the cooperative programs have grown, they have contributed to the acceleration of some of the trends currently characterizing special education. School curricula are developing stronger vocational orientations, and more educational and vocational materials are available for use in special classes. There is an overall change in the attitude of the school and the community, with special classes for older handicapped youth being expanded throughout the country and special community support being extended to the cooperative school program.

There has also been a strong influence on the effectiveness of vocational rehabilitation. The programs have enabled increased placement of handicapped young people into full-time gainful employment. There are more job opportunities for cooperative program graduates and they have been placed into employment at higher incomes than have those who have been enrolled in other teacher education programs.

Follow-up studies have shown that handicapped youngsters involved in these programs tend to remain in school longer. Dropout rate has been reduced. There has been a significant increase in job placement by vocational rehabilitation agencies.

Cooperative school programs have done much to show that terminal education programs are a bridge rather than a finishing point. Some people think the purpose of in-school rehabilitation programs is to get youngsters with special problems out of school as quickly as possible. It does not make sense to expect the handicapped adolescent to be ready for community responsibilities at a younger age than his nonhandicapped peers. In-school rehabilitation has been an effective means of keeping disabled young people in school until they really are able to make an adequate and successful transition to the world of work and to hope for a successful future.

With the enactment of the Vocational Education Amendments of 1968, rehabilitation in the schools is beginning a dramatic new phase. Vocational education programming has previously shown little interest in persons with special needs, such as the handicapped, and vocational education and vocational rehabilitation have seldom combined resources in any program. The Vocational Education Amendments of 1968 not only earmark 10 percent of the funds for programs serving the handicapped but also call attention to the experience of the public rehabilitation program in helping handicapped people. Vocational educators have been directed by Congress to work cooperatively with special education and vocational rehabilitation programs to serve handicapped young people more effectively.

Vocational education—semantically, at least—links special education and vocational rehabilitation. Vocational education and special education share the focus on "education"—the orientation toward a program of studies, the idea of an educational experience available to everyone. On the other hand, vocational education and vocational rehabilitation share the focus on *vocational*— a specific goal—oriented kind of preparation made available to those who need it most.

Somehow, in practice, special education and vocational rehabilitation have skipped over the vocational education linkage. The new vocational education legislation assures that the cooperative approach to in-school rehabilitation will be a three-way arrangement in the future.

VARIETIES OF COORDINATION

Throughout the country similar coordinated programs are being developed to meet the particular needs of the community in which they are being established. The scope of coordination is broad and varied. The most significant dimension of each effort is the willingness of the participating agencies to pool resources to provide desirable and necessary services to retarded young people. Examples of this expression of cooperative willingness are numerous. In some states, many schools in rural areas are made available during after-school hours for personal adjustment training, with the schools providing the instructors. Another example of coordinated effort provides for a residential school for the mentally retarded which gives evaluation, personal adjustment training and occupational training to students in their last year of public school. At another residential school, special education and vocational rehabilitation personnel are extensively involved in providing combined services for the mentally retarded. Still other ways in which retarded youth are aided may be cited. Vocational rehabilitation counselors have been employed to work exclusively with the mentally retarded in areas where strong special education programs are in operation. Another approach calls for the assignment of special education teachers to a vocational rehabilitation unit located in community workshops.

As a final example of cooperative interaction, school districts in one county have combined into a cooperative centralized program to meet the needs of the high school educable retarded students.

Programs of this type have spread to almost every state in the country. In some, the coordinated approach was first undertaken as a Vocational Rehabilitation Administration research and demonstration project. In others, it was started as an extension and improvement project of ongoing state vocational rehabilitation services. In most of the states, however, it has been developed and financed under the vocational rehabilitation basic support program, starting in one or two school districts and spreading rapidly to other districts which have special education programs to which the vocational rehabilitation components can be added.

REFERENCES

1. Hensley, Gene, and Buck, Dorothy P. (Ed.) : *Report of Conference–Cooperative Agreements Between Special Education and Rehabilitation Service in the West.* Western Interstate Commission for Higher Education, June 1968, p. 15.
2. Shay, Harold F.: A decade of development. *Rehab Rec,* March and April 1970, pp. 22-26.
3. Stussman, M. B., Haug, M. R., and Joynes, V. A.: The modern model of rehabilitation counselors roles. *J Appl Rehab Counseling, 1 (No. 3):* 6-13, Fall 1970.
4. Vocational Services Committee: *A Guideline for Cooperative Vocational Services for Handicapped Youth at the High School Level.* Illinois commission on Children, 1965, p. 22.
5. West, James A.: *A Coordinated Program of Rehabilitation and Educational Services Leading to Permanent Job Placement for Disabled High School Students. Final Report.* July 1964, p. 43.
6. Younie, William J. (Ed.) : *Guidelines for Establishing School Work-Study Programs for Educable Mentally Retarded Youth.* Special Education Service, State Department of Education, Vol. *48 (No. 10),* June 1966.

17

The Correctional Institution and Vocational Rehabilitation

Craig R. Colvin

General Overview
History of Vocational Rehabilitation's Involvement with the Public Offender
Counselor's Role in the Correctional Setting
The Rehabilitation Counselor's Relationship with the Public Offender
Complementary Programs and Their Participation in Public Offender Rehabilitation
Summary
References

GENERAL OVERVIEW

VOCATIONAL rehabilitation's collaboration with correctional institutions has become a reality. The rationale for its existance is supported in the recent Federal Offenders Program publication[1] outlining the future of correctional rehabilitation. The writers of this enlightening research project state that in addition to the humanitarian aspects inherent in the rehabilitation movement, the primary impetus for creating a treatment program for the public offender emerged from the complementary needs of vocational rehabilitation and corrections. This research study continues by saying that vocational rehabilitation was eager to develop a new source of clientele and had developed the resourcefulness to serve such a population. If one examines, even superficially, the composition of several correctional facilities, he will see that they have an abundance of clients with insufficient community resources to provide at least minimum treatment services.

Therefore, it becomes obvious that these two agencies, vocational rehabilitation and corrections, should join forces in an attempt to provide meaningful services which will increase the probability of the public offender returning to the community as a respected and trusted citizen.

Even though enthusiastic advances have been made, in the majority of articles pertaining to public offender programs, *rehabilitation* of the inmate within the institution has never quite caught up to the age-old concept of *restraint* and, to some degree, *retribution*. To be effective with this population, it is mandatory that professionals realign philosophies regarding institutionalization. The present-day ideologies existing in our country are undergoing massive and sometimes disruptive changes. This writer is confident that vocational rehabilitation can play a vital role in the assertion of rehabilitation techniques and methodologies enabling the inmate, after a predetermined treatment program, to reenter the community (society) as a productive member.

The mere act of putting grandiose ideas down on paper will not produce programs benefiting the public offender; but it is a noble start. This chapter, hopefully, will be the vehicle by which some vocational rehabilitation counselors will become involved in this new field of correctional rehabilitation. If this chapter does nothing more than create an *awareness* within people that public offenders deserve professional guidance, it has served a purpose.

The inclusion of the following editorial written by a prison inmate serves a dual function of introducing the chapter as well as allowing the counselor to read some of the thoughts going through the mind of one man who is confined behind stark barren walls. After all, to whom will the professional be directing his efforts if it is not the inmate himself? Let's read what rehabilitation means to him.

THE GREAT REHABILITATION HOAX*

REHABILITATE, according to the *Webster's Seventh New Collegiate Dictionary,* means: 1a: to restore to a former capacity; to restore to good repute by vindicating; 2a: to restore to a state of

---

*This editorial appeared in the February 7, 1969 publication of the *Prison Mirror*.

efficiency, good management, or solvency; b: to restore to a condition of health or useful and constructive activity. Unfortunately, as often is the case, either my dictionary is obsolete or Webster has failed to grasp the colloquial connotation of the word.

Perhaps I can offer a more up-to-date, workable definition—REHABILITATE: to transform, by some mysterious, miraculous process, convicted felons into model, contributing members of society. This definition seems a little more apropos, and now that we have arrived at a more current definition, let's examine the perpetrators of "THE GREAT REHABILITATION HOAX."

The primary offenders are all those well-meaning judges, social workers, penologists, and pseudo-penologists, criminologists, writers, newspapermen, etc., who persist in misusing and misapplying the term "rehabilitation." Rehabilitation has become the standard one-word answer to a myriad of questions concerning prisons, correctional programs, and penal philosophy. It is the answer that leaves the questioner with that "Oh, I see" feeling, even though he really doesn't "see" at all. "Rehabilitation" has become idiomatic aspirin, to be dispensed by the sociologist as a cure-all for the headache of crime and punishment in these United States.

The aforementioned group of conspirators are not solely responsible for the hoax. They have tens of thousands of "rap partners" inhabiting the prisons and correctional institutions throughout the land—the wise guys and old cons, the youthful offenders who follow idealistically the example of their "elders" and say, "Okay, so rehabilitate me!" It's no secret the vast majority of convicts are waiting for an invisible Merlin to wave a wand, stamp their backsides "REHABILITATED," and send them off to the free world with the keys to a new Cadillac in their pocket and a $25,000 a year income waiting for them, just as soon as they report to their parole officers. Oh yes, to all of "us"—all the smart guys and would-be big shots—half the rap belongs to us.

The answer to the problem does not lie in the application of sociological terminology, for mere words cannot correct a problem of this magnitude. It has taken most of us a lifetime to acquire the ignominy of the label "convict." Words and good intentions are not enough to cure the illness that afflicts us. You sociologists, you penologists—you cannot rehabilitate us! We must rehabilitate ourselves! OOPS! Pardon me, for I have committed the cardinal sin myself. We must HELP ourselves! I think, though, that you must be aware of this fact already, for some of you aren't trying very hard to rehabilitate us anyway.

There is no magic formula that you can apply, no elixir you can prescribe to cure our malady. At best you can but offer the facility, the vehicle, the tools with which we may help ourselves. The degree to which you offer your cooperation and the quality of the tools available will, in the long run, determine how successful you have been. The rate of recidivism is the only yardstick you can apply to measure the success or failure of your part of the bargain, and in the end, one can hardly blame a poor harvest on the man who sold him the seed.

There is one commodity you can furnish—one that has been sorely lacking in the past—EMPATHY! In simpler terms, a genuine understanding of our problems from our point of view and an unqualified belief in the worth of each one of us as a human being. Try to bear this in mind when we approach you with palms extended, asking for a push to get us started. It has taken the courage of a martyr to bring us to this stage. Don't ask us to defend our motives! Don't make us suspects of devious plots and schemes merely because we want to change! The prime mover for all of us is universal—we want to get out and stay out!

The biggest task is ours alone. You cannot make it easy for us, but you can make it difficult. You cannot insure our success, but you can insure our failure. Give us the tools, give us consideration, and above all, be flexible enough to treat us as individuals, and you will have done your job. What remains then is the classic battle—each of us with ourselves. Not all of us will win that battle, some of us will fail and return. To be sure, some will attempt to deceive you from the very first, but more will succeed than are succeeding now!

So far we have uncovered the perpetrators of the hoax, but who are the victims? You are, all of you on the other side of the concrete curtain—you, the taxpayers, that great uninformed electorate, and the conglomeration we call "society." You have bought the "Brooklyn Bridge" of rehabilitation. You have allowed your all too infrequent queries into crime and punishment to be satisfied with the classic one-word answer. You have swallowed the hook and are proceeding to choke on the bait. You've been fleeced and it's your own fault.

Now I've gotten you mad and you want to know why and how you've been taken. It's really quite simple. Your tax dollars have been spent to foster "rehabilitation programs" carried on in every prison in the land. Dedicated men have worked untold hours with us, the convicts, helping us reshape our lives. Time and effort, ours and theirs, and your money are invested in a process which yields a product, the parolee. When that product is placed on the "market" you proceed to destroy it! You saddle it with the burden of a label—EX-CONVICT, which seems to be synonymous with EX-HUMAN BEING—and you ride it into the ground. You beat it over the head with a billy club labeled "Once a thief. . ." You speak aloud of Christian charity and every man deserving another chance, then whisper behind your hand, "They never change." You stretch a thread-like tightrope across the chasm that separates ignominy from respectability, then ask us to carry an elephant on our shoulders when we attempt to cross. Is it any wonder so many wind up on the rocks below?

Why bother to "rehabilitate" us if you are going to allow an attitude to prevail which prevents us from coming all the way back? Our "debt to society" you always speak of, is a debt we have ostensibly paid when we walk out of the shadow of these walls. But somehow you never get around to marking our account "paid in full." Some of us have paid a terrific price to settle that account, perhaps others have not paid enough. But that is a judgment no mortal man can make for certain! So in the end you are like a hunter caught in his own trap. You are your own victim!

To succeed, to re-enter the civilized world of everyday life, we need a tricycle to ride upon. We need the professional guidance and effective administration of dedicated sociologists, psychologists and criminologists; the acceptance of an understanding, unprejudiced society; and the fortitude, the "guts," to start again ourselves. Take away one of the wheels and the ride gets a little shaky—it's easier to ride a tricycle than a bicycle. Take away two of the wheels and it requires the prodigious effort and skill of a unicyclist! To be sure, some of us will find the tricycle too difficult to ride, but don't condemn the rest to that unicycle ride on that account. Give us all the chance to ride the tricycle and rehabilitation will cease to be a hoax and indeed become a reality.

This is the challenge we must accept if there is hope of returning and keeping the public offender within the guidelines established by society.

HISTORY OF VOCATIONAL REHABILITATION'S INVOLVEMENT WITH THE PUBLIC OFFENDER

When considering vocational rehabilitation's participation in public offender programs, one need not go back too many years. To gain a better perspective of this relatively new area called correctional rehabilitation in relation to the total development of vocational rehabilitation, it is imperative to examine briefly some of the legislative movements affecting its growth.

Without repeating the essence of Chapter 1, which is concerned with an overall history of rehabilitation, it is important to look at several of the laws and amendments to see how rehabilitation became interested in serving the incarcerated. This public service organization, vocational rehabilitation, has grown on the concepts of helping one's fellowman. As stated in the introductory chapter to this book, the initial program began in 1918 with the original mandate of providing services to World War I veterans that had been wounded. The ultimate objective was, of course, to place them back into the labor market. It did not take long to see that this program could be expanded to include the civilian population. Even though this author does not have records indicating the provision of services to the public offender population, he is quite sure that a few were accepted for rehabilitation services during these early years.

In 1939, the agency broadened its delivery of services to include a full spectrum of physical disabilities. Prior to this date, the organization had directed its energy toward those individuals with orthopedic handicaps. Again, it is anticipated that a small number of inmates were being provided services under the auspices of vocational rehabilitation even though no formal programs had been developed.

Probably the greatest impetus given to public offender rehabilitation was with the passage of Public Law 565 in 1954 when mental retardation and emotional illness were added to the traditional services which vocational rehabilitation could provide. Studies have indicated that approximately 15 percent of the inmates in penitentiaries have diagnosable mental illness and that 85 percent have some emotional problems.[2] Additionally, and as importantly, research and demonstration projects were approved to be carried out across the nation in specific areas relative to the rehabilitation of various disability groups. Several of these early demonstration projects dealt with the feasibility of working with the inmate population.

Following the 1954 legislation was the passage of Public Law 333 in 1965. Through the expansion of the definition of disability to include behavior disorders, it was determined the public offender could be considered eligible under this category. Within this piece of legislation, vocational rehabilitation states that the socially handicapped were feasible candidates for services; included in this group was the public offender. Research and demonstration projects from previous years supported the rationale for extending services to this group. The 1969 law redefined the disability category of behavior disorders which definitely made the public offender more accessible to the rehabilitation counselor.

Even though adequate legislation has been written at the federal level, all state rehabilitation agencies have not adopted an open-door policy of accepting the public offender as a client. Some states have only "token" programs in which nothing more than an occasional simple physical restoration case is accepted (and usually the inmate is determined feasible only if he has been awarded parole and a job has been secured for him by someone else).

Other state rehabilitation agencies, on the other hand, have accepted the challenge of working with the public offender. California, Georgia, North and South Carolina, Massachusetts and Texas, as well as others, have enacted comprehensive programs with the objective of providing a multitude of rehabilitation services for the majority of each state's respective inmate population. Cooperative agreements have been written—utilizing the broad federal guidelines—outlining the authority, types of services and future direction of participating agencies.

Future developments in correctional rehabilitation will depend upon increased state agency acceptance of the feasibility of working with inmates and the commitment of people to force continued legislation action.

COUNSELOR'S ROLE IN THE CORRECTIONAL SETTING

There is a multitude of variables which must be considered by the rehabilitation counselor prior to his actual contact with clients in a penal institution: The counselor must evaluate his own inadequacies and how they might interfere with the counselor-client relationship; the counselor has to determine to whom he is responsible (the rehabilitation administration or the correctional administration); and the counselor must define his professional relationship with the correctional administration and other members of the prison staff in terms of a treatment approach to inmate rehabilitation. Each of these variables will be expanded to help the neophyte counselor become aware of and adjust to many of the idiosyncrasies prevalent in the correctional setting.

Understand One's Own Limitations

We all have our "hang-ups," both personal as well as professional. Many of us in corrections and rehabilitation envision idealistic approaches to inmate treatment. Before involving many people in a theoretical or academic exercise, a realistic attitude is necessary. This means that the counselor has to maintain a level of maturity capable of functioning within a professional framework.

The quality of maturity is a necessary component anyone working with public offenders must possess. Without it the naive counselor soon will fall to the manipulative devices of some inmates, will be "snowed" under with inmate requests for counseling sessions, and in a short period will become so overly involved with some inmates that the only recourse is to resign.

If a counselor cannot realistically face those problems confronting him, he surely will have a difficult time in the correctional setting. Everyday will be filled with new "crisis" situations that seem to require the counselor's undivided attention. If he is insecure in his personal life, this will soon become evident in the counselor's professional activities. Decisions must be made with professional authority; yet, if the decision is wrong or inappropriate the counselor must have the strength to admit such a mistake.

If, as a professional, you are anticipating a great deal of "success" in rehabilitating the public offender, your expectations will be rather limited. No matter what degree of preparation one might have prior to engaging in correctional rehabilitation, the criteria utilized to evaluate success must be reevaluated. Most publications concerned with this topic are first to mention the failure syndrome surrounding the inmate: he has been a failure in society; he has been a failure to himself; he has even been a failure in crime; and he has been a failure to those people who have tried to help him. No rehabilitation counselor is going to come along and change things overnight. This is not to say that rehabilitation or any of the other related disciplines should not attempt to bring about change. We must design, realistically, a plan for constructive rehabilitation which is relevant to the inmate's own needs rather than the needs imposed upon him by some counselor representing a "bureaucratic organization."

False values, the inability to make decisions, insecurity, a poor attitude toward one's work and other forms of inappropriate behavior will become magnified many times if one enters the correctional rehabilitation field. After all, these types of behavior and personality problems are manifested within the majority of people the counselor has the responsibility of serving! Therefore, prior to accepting an appointment within a correctional facility, it is advantageous for the counselor to examine critically his own behavior and attitudes toward the job. This soul-searching will go a long way if it is approached with conscientiousness. One's assignment in the penal institution can be either a rewarding professional experience or it can become truly a prison of work.

To Whom Is the Counselor Administratively Responsible?

Upon entering professional work in correctional rehabilitation, a question often asked regarding administrative policy is, To whom am I responsible, the department of correction or vocational rehabilitation? Administrative responsibility is directed toward vocational rehabilitation, even though line supervision may be coming from the correctional unit.

For some newly employed counselors there is a tendency to believe that they are accountable to both corrections and vocational rehabilitation. This is true in some situations and false in others. Administrative responsibility is given usually to the agency which has you on its payroll. Since vocational rehabilitation controls the purse strings, it is they to whom you will be directing specific problems concerned with rehabilitation policies and procedures.

Yet, at the same time, there is a fine line separating administrative policies of these two organizations which must be understood. Even though you report to rehabilitation, you must function under the structure of the correctional administration since you share, in most instances, their facilities. This approach "makes for better neighbors."

Delineation of organizational roles is understood better if the counselor can peruse the formal cooperative agreement established. For those counselors working in situations where no formal agreement has been written, specific agency roles and their respective responsibilities will be more difficult to determine. It is recommended the counselor plan a meeting with his immediate vocational rehabilitation supervisor and also a similar meeting with the appropriate institutional supervisor. A get-together of this nature should provide the new employee adequate feedback regarding his responsibility to rehabilitation, corrections and ultimately, the inmate.

The Counselor's Relationship with the Correctional Administration

There are several predominate factors which must be identified prior to becoming involved in any treatment program for the public offender. The rehabilitation counselor must be aware of and appreciate the dilemma facing the correctional institution's administration. This organization has two primary goals which at times may be antithetical—they are custody and rehabilitation.

While it may be objectionable to the newly employed counselor's professional idealisms, the custodial facet of the institution is of the utmost concern to correction's administration. Actually vocational rehabilitation becomes a disruptive influence in the overall operation of a correctional unit. To a prison administrator a rehabilitation program creates more problems than it solves. In a custodially oriented institution a routine is established to maintain order and, in turn, security. If a rehabilitation program is interjected into this routinized system, many changes are required; exceptions to prison procedure which previously were rare now occur with increasing frequency. But in this dichotomy

The Correctional Institution and Vocational Rehabilitation 361

of administrative philosophy the development and support of rehabilitation programs must evolve.

To further define the rehabilitation counselor's relationship with the correctional administration, the counselor has to realize he must function within this militaristically oriented work environment.

Administrative officials have operated penal institutions for decades under a militarily oriented regimen. Such a design allows a few people (with the aid of high walls and iron bars) to control a large number of other individuals. As a counselor one must be cognizant of the realities of such a dehumanizing but essential operation.

Sometimes the stark, raw attitude of prison officials confuses the counselor's expectations regarding prison rehabilitation. The counselor has been taught that a permissive attitude and a humanitarian approach are mandatory requisites for any professional working with clientele such as the public offender. This is not to say that prison officials do not consider the welfare of the inmate. They do; but with the primary objective of maintaining security for the welfare of the institution and its employees, it is difficult for the administration to relax their defenses, knowing well that if they do some inmate will escape or at least attempt to do so thereby endangering lives and property.

The counselor's understanding and acceptance of the administration's security precautions have priority over everything. His personal and professional endeavors to rehabilitate the public offender cannot violate security policies. With this in mind, it is suggested that any counselor considering employment in this challenging area procure and peruse the administration's policies and procedures manual. If there are questions regarding the various areas of this manual, the counselor should make note and attempt to have them answered by the respective prison officials.

Another factor which must be identified and understood in a prison work setting is that there are prescribed channels of communication through which all facets of institutional information flow. If the counselor is to be considered effective in such an organization, he quickly must assess his role and determine how it will fit into the overall plan of the institution. This counselor is obliged to understand the various channels of command and learn how he might interject appropriate comments and suggestions regarding implementation of rehabilitation techniques without feeling or becoming ostracized.

To summarize briefly this section on counselor involvement with prison administration, one must remember that the correctional organization has developed over the years within a very rigid philosophy. Implementation of rehabilitation concepts will not occur without some degree of resistance.

The Counselor's Relationship with Prison Staff

Enthusiasm toward one's work as a correctional rehabilitation counselor is an important asset which should not be stymied by others who, seemingly, do not share this jubilation. Continuous effort must be made to convince the prison staff that dedicated teamwork may eventually result in restoring a percentage of public offenders to a level of behavior acceptable by society. Yet blatant assertion of one's professional role as a vocational rehabilitation counselor will not get you anywhere, especially among members of the correctional institution's staff. Initial involvement with other staff members should be approached with conscientiousness and tactfulness, recalling that to most of the staff adherence to a correctional regimen has become a way of life.

Previous discussion has pointed out the rigid military-like and dehumanizing attitude possessed by some correctional authorities. Many staff members' functioning under this system soon begin unconsciously to imitate and carry out this philosophy in their own work assignments. In relation to the provision of services, the effectiveness of the classification committee members, social workers, psychologists, correctional officers and even chaplains and physicians should be evaluated.

Idealistically, all of these professional groups should be active in every penal institution where inmates reside; but realistically this is not the case. The involvement of these disciplines range from a mere token effort to provide a few basic services to a sophisticated and integrated team approach utilizing every available resource.

Theoretically, the classification committee in most correctional facilities has three fundamental responsibilities: (a) diagnosis, categorization and orientation of the newly arrived inmate; (b) the development of his treatment program; and (c) the establishment of guidelines regarding inmate custody. Under these directives the committee attempts to formulate an individualized rehabilitation program for each inmate.* To facilitate their decision-making processes, a team of professionals is utilized and its contributions are defined briefly in the following paragraphs.

After the public offender's arrival at the institution, he enters the first phase of the classification process. Here he is given a preliminary medical and psychological examination in an attempt to detect physical or mental abnormalities which may need immediate attention. If problems or other deficiencies are noted the inmate usually will receive a more detailed and comprehensive examination.

During his first few days of institutionalization, the inmate is subjected, at the request of the classification committee, to a barrage of aptitude, interest and achievement tests. In part these test results serve as a factor in determining what responsibilities the inmate may have within the unit such as janitorial duties, cooking detail, a maintenance department job or assignment to an educational program. If a gross deficiency pattern is noted from these tests or the psychologicals, further psychiatric services may be warranted.

The reception unit, staffed by social workers, has the responsibility of developing an inmate's social history record. This staff concentrates on the individual's background, pertinent family data, special interests he may have and what role the inmate expects to fulfill within the institution. Due to the ever-increasing admission rates and the pressure to interview a greater number of inmates, the worthiness of such material derived is questioned since the social workers usually have enough time only to record

---

*Realistically, the custodial facet takes precedence over everything. With this in mind it is difficult to envision any program which could be considered effective.

information which is rather objective in nature. An in-depth analysis of an inmate's past cannot be justified when an interviewer has three or four people waiting outside his office.

Also, it should be pointed out that these staff members soon begin to become calloused in their thinking, often forgetting that they are serving someone who most likely has never encountered anyone willing to listen to his problems. This is a rut the professional within an institution easily can get himself into; he soon sees all inmates as the same person, with the same problems, with the same social, educational and environmental history. If we call ourselves professionals we must make a concerted effort to see each inmate as an individual who needs our undivided attention.

There are others who usually see the inmate during this orientation phase; the chaplain, the orientation committee, physicians and dentists. The chaplain tries to get around to each man individually to explain the availability of religious programs within the institution. The unit chaplain attempts to relate with this inmate on an individual basis, letting him know he always has someone to whom he can confide without fear of reprimand.

Most units have at least an informal orientation committee whose primary responsibility is to explain the prison regulations and procedures to the new arrival. The inmate is briefed regarding what is expected of him during his imprisonment and he is told at the outset what consequences will evolve if he violates prison policy.

Medical services are provided similar to those found in the community; a general physical examination along with a blood and urine test, chest x-ray and other diagnostic work-ups are administered. Usually routine dental exams are given each inmate at the beginning of his incarceration.

After all of the above services have been provided, the respective staff reports are typed and sent to the classification committee so that they may use them to carry out their other responsibilities (development of a treatment program and custody assignment).

Classification committees vary in size from three to seven or more members, with one of them acting as chairman. Each member surveys all diagnostic and related material prior to the committee meeting. Following a discussion of the particular inmate being evaluated, specific recommendations are made regarding his rehabilitation program and his custody assignment. As stated in the introduction to this chapter, here we see again the dilemma confronting correctional authorities: rehabilitation versus custody.

Thus far there has been no indication of vocational rehabilitation's involvement in any of the classification committee's activities. Probably the simplest explanation is that in the majority of correctional institutions vocational rehabilitation has not been given the opportunity to help develop constructive inmate rehabilitation programs. Too many facilities feel that vocational rehabilitation is trying to infringe upon their territory. It is imperative archaic attitudes associated with prisons be eliminated and be replaced by professional attitudes which effect positive change.

Active participation on the classification committee should become a personal as well as professional goal of all counselors functioning within the correctional setting. One's involvement at this stage of the inmate's contact with the institution will, more than likely, increase the probability of success once an integrated rehabilitation program can be devised for him. In those few penal facilities where vocational rehabilitation has a clearly defined role, the attitude of correctional staff members responsible for modifying inmate behavior has been positive. Rehabilitation counselors have acted as a catalyst in causing a renewed awareness—on the part of the prison staff—of the public offender's intended life style after release rather than relying only on his life style during imprisonment. The rationale for this is quite obvious: Rehabilitation traditionally has been a community-based program, whereas corrections has divorced itself from the community to become an isolate. Therefore, by joining forces with vocational rehabilitation, the classification committee is in a better position to plan a logical and constructive program facilitating inmate development.

The same holds true regarding the counselor's involvement with the physicians. As in the past, vocational rehabilitation counselors have relied heavily on the medical profession in the free community. This should not change to any significant degree within the institution. Where most of the other professional services found in the community are lacking behind prison walls, the provision of medical services is the least affected.

Counselors should avail themselves to this material and, at the same time, undertake a public relations program promoting vocational rehabilitation. Unfortunately all too often the physicians working solely within the prison setting have removed themselves from the current mainstream of continued professional development. They also are not particularly interested in learning about or becoming associated with the other helping disciplines. Again, the reasons for this should be obvious: Since most institutions do not have adequate legislative and community support, salaries are relatively low in comparison to those same positions outside the walls. This, in turn, creates a vacuum or void which regretfully is filled by the retiring or misplaced physician. Also as it has been stated several times in this chapter, prison staff including the physician, soon depict all public offenders as "con" men attempting to "get something for nothing." As an example one should visit a physician's office inside a prison during sick call. Here one will find most of the waiting chairs occupied by inmates who solemnly attest to the fact that they are in acute pain and are, therefore, in need of drugs. It is true that after a short length of time the physician or any other person for that matter would tire of such actions.

Yet a hardened and negative attitude is not a solution to the problem. Returning to what was said earlier, rehabilitation can become the agent of attitude change. By becoming interested in the physician's role in the institution, the counselor automatically has the chance to increase the doctor's preceptions of vocational rehabilitation and this agency's objective of helping the inmate adapt to the demands of society. Additionally, the counselor can provide the physician appropriate feedback regarding medical information required by vocational rehabilitation to aid in the determination of eligibility. This approach should initiate the doctor's subscribing to rehabilitation-oriented concepts rather

The Correctional Institution and Vocational Rehabilitation

than the antiquated regimen of medical practice solely for maintainance of the inmate while he is institutionalized.

Social workers too can become valuable allies with vocational rehabilitation. Through the coordination of services the duplication of similar programs can be eliminated. Again, as with other disciplines, the combined effort undoubtedly will be greater than the services any one agency could hope to provide the inmate.

There is more to inmate rehabilitation than helping him while he is behind bars; total rehabilitation must extend out into the community once the man has served his time. What better opportunity would the releasee have through the concentrated efforts of these two (and why not other) organizations who have had successful programs in the community for quite some time? If success with the inmate is what we are looking for, we must discard and bury whatever hostilities, jealousies or negative attitudes that have been fostered through the years. A marriage of all disciplines must come about; yet the dissolvance of each organization's professional identity is not necessary nor would it be advisable. Let each agency keep its separate identity; but let each cooperate with one another for the benefit of those people the organizations have said they would serve.

Downtrodden and often neglected, the correctional officer rarely receives the attention he so rightfully deserves. He is probably the most underrated prison staff member though he is the one in the best position to help inmates with their immediate problems. The correctional officer (he has been designated in the past as guard or "turn keys") has responsibility to watch over the inmate twenty-four hours a day, seven days a week, fifty-two weeks a year or until such time release is granted. No one else within the institutional setting has a better chance to influence inmate behavior change. But as evidenced in 99 percent of all prisons, the officer has been relegated an assignment of "watchdog." If an inmate "breaks" or violates any of the outmoded prison rules, he is reported by the officer to a higher level authority who, in turn, continues the transmittal of violation(s) until they have exhausted the chain of command. The point here is that the correctional officer has not been given the responsibility to act on behalf of the inmate as an agent of change; he is there only to carry out the function of surveillance.

This writer feels that if these men were accorded a specific role in the total design of an inmate's rehabilitation program, we would experience a dramatic decrease in recidivism (a public offender's return to prison). Realizing that custody is the primary concern of prison officials there must be an attempt to realign responsibilities so that a delicate balance could be achieved between rehabilitation and custody. Combining both of these facets and having staff control this balance will not be easy, but it is mandatory. If such an effort is to occur it is necessary to involve the correctional officer on the firing line.

THE REHABILITATION COUNSELOR'S RELATIONSHIP WITH THE PUBLIC OFFENDER

Following the counselor's development of an affiliation with those people held responsibile for effecting inmate behavior change within the institution, we finally examine the counselor's own involvement with the public offender. This section will be directed toward several factors that influence the counselor-inmate relationship and how the counselor can improve or strengthen his competency in working with this population.

Utilization of Diagnostic Information

In respect to the history of incarceration, correctional personnel only recently have begun accumulating adequate diagnostic material on each inmate's entering the system. These diagnostic reports or work-ups usually include a comprehensive medical examination with appropriate laboratory tests; a rather elaborate psychological test battery composed of Wechsler Adult Intelligence Scale, Minnesota Multiphasic Personality Inventory, Kuder Preference Record, Bender-*Gestalt* Test, Purdue Pegboard and a host of other personality and achievement tests. With some inmates, a psychiatric examination is necessary. As stated previously a detailed social history is gathered containing educational, religious and economic information.

A thorough and objective analysis of this existing material

should be made prior to the counselor's first interview with the potential client. After a counselor has perused such diagnostic material, he should determine whether or not additional information is required. If such material is deemed necessary, the counselor in conjunction with the correctional unit can activate a program to secure such without breaching security or established prison routines.

Counseling Aspects

Various counseling techniques and approaches *per se* are described in the next chapter and in Chapter 10; even so there are several points which require additional consideration.

Generally, counseling as practiced by vocational rehabilitation counselors does not vary to any significant degree from one rehabilitation setting to another. This is supported in the succeeding chapter by Mr. West regarding the counseling process within correctional institutions. Nevertheless, there is a definite facade existing between a correctional unit counselor and his inmate client which normally does not exist between a field counselor and his client in the community. An "on-guard" or defensive attitude prevails between counselor and inmate which does not lend itself to the establishment of a favorable counseling relationship. The counselor feels compelled to remain "uptight" so as not to become a pawn of the inmate's manipulative devices.

Continuing along this thought and reiterating a point brought out several times in the preceding sections, it is mandatory that the vocational rehabilitation counselor concern himself with security precautions although his ultimate objective is for the rehabilitation of an individual who will be reentering the free world. Without this awareness the counselor may jeopardize his relationship not only with the institution's administration but also with the inmate as well.

For the correctional rehabilitation counselor to be effective in performing his responsibilities, he must discuss his role with the inmate during their initial interview. The counselor must set somewhat rigid limits on the relationship he establishes with this man, yet convince him that he is there to help him rehabilitate himself. As one readily can imagine, such an arrangement is no simple matter that can be sloughed over nonchalantly; to achieve this precarious balance requires a great deal of insight and perceptiveness on the counselor's part.

Inmate Motivation versus Manipulation

Motivation as defined by Webster means a "stimulus to action or something that causes a person to act." If there is one recurring characteristic or quality found within the prison population, it is motivation; but we must ask ourselves, "Motivation for what?" There is both an unconscious as well as conscious desire operating within the inmate that can be defined as motivation. One might even call it a driving impulse which suggests a power arising from personal temperament and desire. It sounds as if the vocational rehabilitation counselor has found the "perfect" client! Again, we have to ask ourselves what the inmate is motivated for or towards. Freedom!

Probably freedom occupies his mind more than any other single facet connected with his institutionalization; his main objective is to get out of prison as soon as humanly possible. Even so, each inmate responds differently to the ever-present desires for freedom: There is the inmate who will resort to escape to reach his freedom; another will quietly sit back and wait out his time in idleness; a third type will try to con his way out; and then there is the individual who will work conscientiously toward earning his freedom by productive work and obeying the institution's regulations.

Vocational rehabilitation will find the greatest degree of success with this last man, and yet it will be difficult for the counselor to separate one from another during the initial interviews. As an example, the motivation of one inmate may be directed toward manipulation of the professional staff. From our side of the fence, we often see this inmate's external behavior as being conducive for positive rehabilitation efforts. Because of the public offender's isolation, he will strive to manipulate or convince some professionals that he is "motivated" toward whatever objective they are wanting him to achieve.

Upon release from the institution, this man usually rejects the likely benefits of rehabilitation programs. As an illustration, in this writer's experience in working with the public offender he has seen individuals really look forward to their training in such areas as bakery, welding, printing and offset. As their counselor, it was felt that adjustment and progression in these training areas was more than satisfactory and that upon release, there would be no difficulty in placing them in the labor market. Prior to their departure from the institution, this counselor made the usual arrangements regarding work and a place to stay for these men. After one or two weeks on the job, the majority of these people came to me to see if they could be trained in some other area. This counselor asked them why and their answer invariably was that the training they received did come from "behind the wall" and it reminded them of an experience they would rather forget; the best way of doing so was to be retrained in another area and go their own way.

Additional Considerations

When the public offender makes a mistake, we have a tendency to ridicule or punish him unduly; if this same mistake were made by one of your clients in the community, it is anticipated that he would not be reprimanded as severely. After all, mistakes are a vital part of the learning process, and we have to examine and, if necessary, reexamine continually the reasons underlying their failure. These "things" called inmates, contrary to much popular opinion, are human—living, breathing, bleeding people with basic desires and behavior characteristics similar to those masses of people called society. We must concentrate and channel our professional efforts toward effecting a realistic treatment program.

By realistic, we mean giving the inmate more responsibility for his actions. As is found in most correctional institutions today the inmate is told when to get up, when to wash and shave, when to eat, when to go to the bathroom, when to go to work, when to participate in recreation, and on and on. What happens to this individual when it comes time for him to reenter the community and face the everyday grind? Self-control has been inhibited or even squelched during his institutionalization and after release we expect him, if by magic, to regain all those intricate components which are identifiable as "normal" behavior patterns exhibited by the majority.

Treatment, rehabilitation, habilitation or any word which expresses a return to normalcy must include responsibility for one's own behavior. This behavioral change process has no predetermined solution which can be applied to all inmates; individual approaches to individual problems are required if we expect to see positive results. Such an approach necessitates greater coordination and teamwork of all disciplines that have dedicated themselves to helping the imprisoned.

COMPLEMENTARY PROGRAMS AND THEIR PARTICIPATION IN PUBLIC OFFENDER REHABILITATION

Thus far we have concerned ourselves primarily with various personnel in the correctional system and the counselor's involvement in public offender rehabilitation. A quick glance at several programs designed specifically to help the individual who has been committed for violating societal laws should provide the reader additional insight into inmate problems and how they might be resolved.

Probation and Parole

A discussion of correctional rehabilitation is meaningless without briefly mentioning two other important agencies and their contributions toward the rehabilitation of the public offender—the probation and parole systems.

Probation as it is known today has changed very little since its inception in the mid-1800's. Those chosen as potential candidates have been screened thoroughly by the probation agency prior to the judge's final sentencing. The probation department's basic responsibility then is to select an individual who has been convicted of a crime and, under a threat of being put into prison, provide him with necessary guidance and supervision in the community. The rationale supporting probation is that if the individual is capable of handling his personal activities, he should be given the opportunity of doing so by remaining in society as a productive member.

Due to vocational rehabilitation's traditional role as a community-based program, it is logical that a cooperative effort should be established whereby both agencies would share in the supervision of the individual on probation. If services are indicated to insure the probationer's remaining on a job, the counselor and the probation officer should collaborate so that complementary services are provided rather than the duplication of services.

The parole system becomes a factor after an individual has been incarcerated for a length of time. The parole department selects certain inmates who have proven to the establishment that they can function readily in the community. Actual work must be available and awaiting the inmate upon release before he is considered eligible for parole. In fact, the philosophy of work is the crux of both the department of probation and the department of parole; without the availability of work in the form of a specific job, an inmate will not be placed on probation or be paroled from the prison. Immediately one can visualize the implications for vocational rehabilitation involvement in both of these organizations as well as with the department of correction. Through a unified team approach a host of interrelated services can be provided with the ultimate objective of placing the inmate back into the community to function on a socially accepted level.

Work Release

The prison work release program has gained wide recognition, especially in the last decade. This program originally began in Wisconsin in 1913 with the passage of the Huber Act. This Act, along with further legislative refinements over the years, capitalizes on or uses as a basis a concept which is one of the most perplexing problems confronting the public offender—unemployment.

Prior to commitment this individual has gotten into trouble usually because he has been out of work. After conviction, the inmate is placed in an isolated environment where idle time or at best limited educational or vocational instruction is provided. Many of the training areas existing within correctional facilities either have become obsolete or are not taught by adequately trained staff. In our highly complex society, job obsolescence becomes a major factor; this means that upon release, the inmate will be entering the labor market unprepared to hold a specific job.

Work release programs, as they are known today, are based on the premise that an inmate must show he can cooperate with and function under authority before he be considered a candidate for the program. Usually it is necessary for him to serve a predetermined prison sentence in order to decide if he can behave accordingly as set forth in the guidelines established by correctional administration.

Through the recommendations of the classification committee, a candidate for work release is transferred to another section of the prison or sometimes outside the unit into a "halfway house" situation. During the day he works on a job *within the community* at this carefully chosen vocation. After work the inmate returns to the work release complex where he spends his nights and weekends. His earnings not only provide him some measure of his ability to reintegrate into the free society, especially the world of work, but this money helps pay for his room and board while at this facility. A part of his earnings are used to help support his family; the remainder of these funds is deposited into a savings account to which he will have access after his release from the institution.

The implications supporting total inmate rehabilitation rather than fragmented rehabilitation are evidenced in the success rates or statistics gathered on the unfortunately small number of work release programs across the country. Of those inmates selected to participate in work release, fewer than 15 percent have failed to complete their sentence without accumulating additional offenses. Most of these infractions were minor in that the work releasee stopped off for a beer on the way back to the unit or the inmate "extended" his allotted time in the community. A smaller percentage forfeited their right to continue on work release after they committed further crimes for which they were reincarcerated.

Some people feel that before work release can be considered a success, it must completely eliminate failure—that is, the inmate will not commit any more crime. This writer feels that such a feat would be next to impossible and that the program is serving its intended purposes beyond the expectations of those who are responsible for its administration. The prediction of inmate success in a work release program is difficult, but as professionals we can eliminate inmate failure by utilizing every available resource at our disposal. Effective screening devices are necessary to select the inmate showing the most potential to reenter the community as a productive member of its work force.

Community Participation in Inmate Rehabilitation

In discussing the challenging field of correctional rehabilitation, it is extremely important to be aware of as many different facets as possible so that one may have a better understanding of the total program. The possibility of inmate manipulation and the rigidity of the correctional unit itself has been discussed along with a brief glimpse of several of the helping agencies working for the inmate's rehabilitation; but we have failed to mention the inadequacies existing within our own community relative to inmate needs. Here is the main problem confronting the newly released individual.

From the very outset of the inmate's institutionalization, the correctional process must be directed back toward the community. It is within the community that either further crimes will be committed or a useful life lived. As a society we have formulated laws which he has violated and, in turn, placed him behind bars; and we have determined the sentence which should be imposed upon him. After he has fulfilled his obligation in relation to the law and the amount of time he should remain segregated from society, he is released. Where does he go? He goes right back out into the community. Instead of accepting him for what he is, we still see him as a "bad guy" or "ex-con" and every other negative connotation that can be depicted. There must be a breakdown in this structure if we ever expect a correctional rehabilitation program to be successful.

Vocational rehabilitation's own field program can alleviate or at least reduce some of the anxiety found within the community. By referring the ex-inmate to a counselor in the field with a complete case history developed by the rehabilitation team within the prison unit, there is a strong likelihood this counselor can become an influencial link in the resocialization of the releasee.

To summarize vocational rehabilitation's overall commitment to the total correctional process and, in turn, the reintegration of the public offender back into the community, Table 1* has been provided.

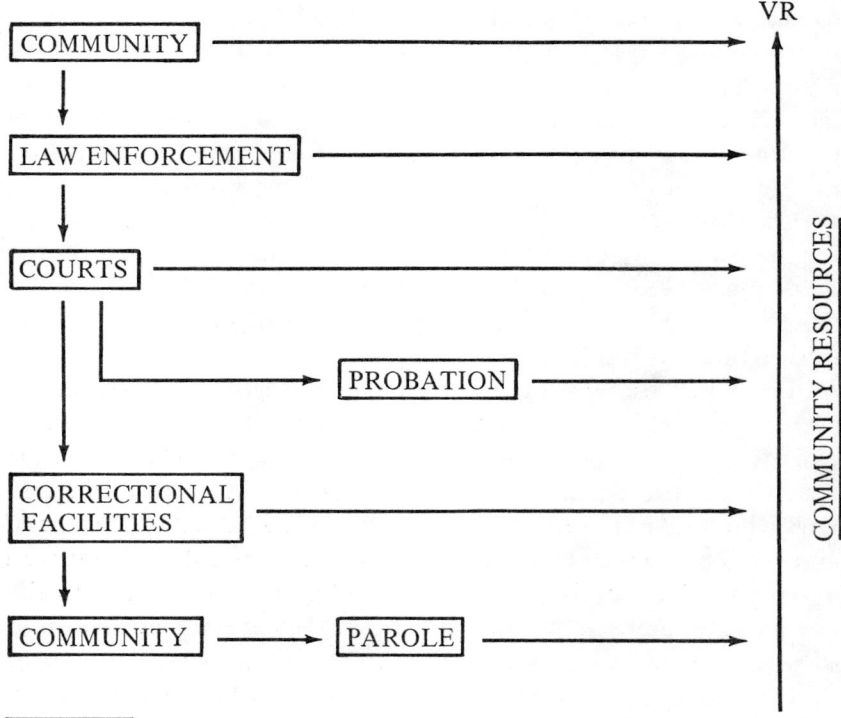

*This table adopted from a seminar presented by Mr. Bob Philbeck, State Coordinator for Correctional Rehabilitation, North Carolina Division of Vocational Rehabilitation. It is reprinted with permission of Mr. Philbeck.

As evidenced in Table 1, vocational rehabilitation can play a dynamic role in each step of the convicted individual's progress through the correctional process. Most often with the inmate human dignity is lost. As professionals we must make every effort to restore or build this dignity into the person. A purpose in life must be found and then appropriate action taken so that he might achieve his goal. Rehabilitation efforts can provide the impetus for the public offender to help himself.

SUMMARY

The extension and provision of limited vocational rehabilitation services to the public offender has been made possible through legislative developments and the determination of a few dedicated people. But before inmate rehabilitation can be considered successful, the counselor must understand his role in relation to the correctional institution and its personnel, his relationship with the public offender himself, and complementary programs outside the institution that provide auxiliary services.

The realization of our rehabilitation efforts can be summarized in the following article by George Fraleigh.*

THE LAST NIGHT

It wasn't so bad while the lights were on. He could pace up and down, making his legs tired, hoping he'd be able to sleep, but knowing he was only kidding himself. He could walk his legs off up to his knees and there would be no sleep for him on his last night.

The lights went out the way they always do in prison, with something akin to a mild shock to him. One minute there was light, then there was darkness, no click of light switch as a warning, just the sudden transition from light to dark and it still was able to shake him up, even after the nights that had gone by.

He stopped his restless pacing and sat on the edge of the bed. Even in stocking feet he might get a rumble from the guy in the cell below. Prisoners are sensitive to even the faint vibration from barefoot pacing on the floor above them and he didn't want to set the

---

*This article appeared in the May-June 1969 issue of the *ISLAND LANTERN*, published by the men of the U.S. Penintentiary, McNeil Island, Washington. Acknowledgement is extended to the author and the editor of the *ISLAND LANTERN*.

joint off into a bedlam of angry shouting and cursing. Not on his last night in this world. Might as well go out with a few good words behind him instead of shouted invective.

He remained on the bed until the steel edge cutting into the underside of his legs stopped the blood and his feet began to feel numb, then prickled with a thousand needle points as he stood up and silently jiggled first one foot, then the other in the air, shaking off the numbness the way he was trying to shake off the terror which was hovering silently over his head waiting for the morning to pounce.

He walked to the barred front of the cell and leaned his hot forehead against the cold steel. Funny how it was always cold, winter and summer the bars were always cold. The cement walls, too, they never warmed up. His hands came up and grasped the bars above his head as high as he could reach while his eyes sought to pierce the darkness over the water that surrounded the island prison.

A tug with red and white running lights fore and aft hove into view, the sound of its diesels a faint chug-chug in the distance, and a few minutes later low lying lights followed, seeming to be riding on top of the water. He knew they were the riding lights on a huge log raft which the tug was towing to the mill. He'd looked out the same window in the daylight and watched the tugs as they strained against the current with their log rafts fighting, inch by inch it seemed, to master the powerful pull of the tide sweeping relentlessly in from the ocean.

The tug and its raft disappeared and he turned wearily away and sought the refuge of his bed, covering his burning eyes with his arms, trying to shut out even the blackness of his cell, trying to escape the spectre which haunted the darkness. Tomorrow it would be all over. They'd come for him early, he knew, they always came early so they could get it over with and go on with their daily routine. They'd walk him down the long corridor, one on each side of him, through the door at the end and there it would be, waiting. He wondered if he could go quietly and expressionlessly the way most of the others went. He hoped so. It wouldn't do any good to make a fuss. Tomorrow morning was his last day and he had to go and all the fighting and screaming and dragging his feet wouldn't change a thing.

He wondered how severe the shock would be. Pretty bad, the way he heard it told, but it only lasted an instant, they said. Maybe the pain came later. He'd never talked to anyone about that though, he'd never seen anyone who'd come back. He was starting to sweat now, could feel the runnels of sticky perspiration coursing down his face, trickling off his chest, sliding down his legs. He leaped off the bed in sudden panic, stood on the cold floor, felt the icy cement through the soles of his stockings, fought the trembling that wracked his body like an attack of ague. Then reason took over, he sank back onto the bed and stared wide-eyed at the ceiling. He wanted a cigarette but he knew it would taste like, hot and acrid in his feverish mouth, so he fought down the craving while he tried to recall events which had led up to this last night. Everything was a confused jumble in his mind and he couldn't sort out the pieces. It had all started too long ago and too many things had happened between then and now, and anyway, all that mattered was that in a few hours he'd be walking down that long, long corridor and through that door. They'd take his prison clothes off him and give him new ones, fresh and clean, and then they'd walk with him through the last door and down the road, put him on the boat, then, turn around and walk away, and he'd be all alone in the free world, all alone .

Will he be alone or will there be someone to help him find his way? This is the challenge of rehabilitation.

REFERENCES

1. Fulton, W.S. (Ed.): *A Future for Correctional Rehabilitation.* Final Report, Federal Offenders Rehabilitation Program, November, 1969, State of Washington, Division of Vocational Rehabilitation, Research and Demonstration Grants, Social and Rehabilitation Services, Department of Health, Education and Welfare.
2. Tessler, B.: In Margolin, R.J., Larson, K., and Vernile, R.T. Jr., (Eds.): *Effective Approaches to the Rehabilitation of the Disabled Public Offender.* May, 1966, Northeastern University, Contract No. VRA 66-35, Vocational Rehabilitation Administration, Department of Health, Education and Welfare.

18

Rehabilitative Counseling in Correctional Settings

James A. West

Difference Between the Traditional Setting and the Correctional Setting
The Counseling Relationship

REHABILITATION counseling in a correctional institution does not differ drastically from counseling in any other setting. Traditionally, a counseling situation presupposes a face-to-face communication by two or more individuals with some goal in mind. The goal of the professional counselor is somewhat different from the goal of the person with whom he is counseling. An element found in any helping profession involves the offer of "expert" experience and training in the service of an individual who is in need of assistance in making positive choices which may lead to a more compatible self-image. The client should experience this relationship in an atmosphere in which he is accepted for the person he is and supported in his search for new goals.

Whether the counselor wishes to utilize direct or indirect techniques in counseling is a matter of choice. As in any other counseling situation, a certain amount of necessary and relevant information is required in order to meet correctional regulations for good bookkeeping. In most cases, the majority of such information can be obtained indirectly during the initial counseling session. Once the information has been obtained, the relationship between counselor and client may develop into a cooperative effort to seek realistic solutions.

Note: This chapter is taken from Mr. West's paper in the report of the Fifth Institute of Rehabilitation Services (1967).

DIFFERENCE BETWEEN THE TRADITIONAL SETTING AND THE CORRECTIONAL SETTING

Undoubtedly, one of the main differences between traditional vocational rehabilitation counseling in the usual setting and that in a correctional setting is the degree of insight a client has into his own limitations. In noncorrectional settings, a majority of clients come to the initial session well aware of their handicaps, physical or emotional. The amputee, the arthritic, the heart patient, and others, have become well aware of their physical handicaps and are usually able to speak about them in a semisophisticated manner. This situation is most often *not* true for the individual in a correctional institution. His first contact with a vocational rehabilitation counselor betrays needs which are somewhat ambiguous and often neither reasonable nor realistic. The inmate may be motivated to seek rehabilitation services for selfish and temporary reasons alone, such as gaining an early parole, personal favors, legal counseling or other nonvocational objectives. On the other hand, he may be realistically concerned about his future and be seeking help in attempting to rehabilitate himself in order to reduce the chances of his return to prison. The salient point is that inmates are, for the most part, unaware or unwilling to admit that they have an accumulation of emotional problems which may have led to their incarceration.

The counselor in a correctional setting must make an initial effort to confront the client with the realistic consequences not only of his past but of his present behavior. Yet, the client should perceive the counselor as something more than just another "square John." If the counselor is identified as an authority figure, effective counseling becomes almost impossible. The client must be made aware that he is accepted as he is and that the counseling confrontation, however painful, is necessary for any growth process. This confrontation must be objective, nonmoralistic and without punitive motivation on the part of the counselor, as a means of helping the client understand himself.

THE COUNSELING RELATIONSHIP

The character makeup of the psychopath or the individual with a character disorder is usually based upon a quasineurotic foundation of defenses in which these individuals must completely fill their conscious lives with rationalizations involving denial of guilt or inadequacy in their own personal lives. Basically, they feel the need to be accepted by others. At an unconscious level, however, they are frightened by warm and close relationships with people. In counseling with these individuals, the relationship must be one in which the client perceives the counselor as a person who is willing to accept him in spite of his deviant, antisocial behavior. If such a relationship is developed, the counselor can more easily confront the client with the reality of his problems in an atmosphere of acceptance and can join with him in an experience of developing new and realistic goals.

The choice of a vocational goal or objective should always be made by the client. The professional responsibility of the counselor is to utilize his academic background and experience to point out to the client any unrealistic or irrational goals which might result in another failure. This responsibility is especially needed in a correctional setting where the average inmate has already experienced far too many failures. Vocational goals should be the result of a broad overview of the individual's life style, taking into account both successes and failures. Most often the task encompasses both vocational and personal counseling.

One of the most important aspects of counseling (as distinct from psychotherapy, for example) is a "reality-oriented" philosophy. Often time is not available for a more analytic counseling approach, and often it is not needed. While the client's past history is of importance, the reality of his present problems should be uppermost in planning for the future. The basic role of the counselor is to focus on present problems and future goals. In the counseling relationship it is not so important for the client to be able to understand in detail the emotional impact of a broken home as it is for him to understand that in spite of a broken home, he must remain a responsible individual in society. In many cases, the very fact that he is incarcerated presents enough evidence that the correctional client has not been responsible in the past. The correctional counselor should explore with the client techniques, changes in perception or other positive means to lead the client toward becoming a more responsible individual both personally and in the society to which he will return. However, the counselor must never assume responsibility for forcing these choices upon the client, for in so doing, he may only reinforce undesirable behavior on the part of the client. The freedom to make choices, good or bad, must remain the prerogative of the client, for without his personal involvement and commitment, little can be accomplished.

QUALITIES OF THE COUNSELING SITUATION

Having covered some of the peculiarities of the correctional setting and of the correctional client, what are some of the qualities of the counseling situation itself? Most authorities are agreed that counseling differs from guidance on the one hand and psychotherapy on the other. Counseling is less problem-oriented and less authority-bound than guidance while being somewhat more personal in orientation. The counseling relationship is usually of longer duration than guidance; a deeper, more meaningful interpersonal relationship than psychotherapy is attempted. Counseling tends to be less analytical, less historical in its perspective and more "adjustment" oriented. Without attempting to delineate where one process begins and another leaves off, one may safely say that any guidance person, counselor or psychotherapist must be aware of the parameters of his techniques and the limitations inherent in his approach whether by dint of his training or of his treatment goals. One does counseling with patients who need counseling and psychotherapy with patients who need psychotherapy. This distinction requires diagnostic and prognostic skills. Many practitioners capable of doing both often elect to do one or the other based upon the requirements of the patients or of the situation.

Ordinarily with the correctional situation a team setting is provided which the counselor represents one professional speciality. Where this is true, the counselor must use caution lest he disturb his client's relationship with other members of the team and create role confusions. Where the team does not exist the counselor must be cautious lest he exceed his limitations or neglect his primary role. Counseling is often the treatment of choice and psychotherapy is often an undesirable alternative.

In general, a majority of correctional clients are not prepared to receive counseling because they reject the frame of reference of the counselor. This is one of the characteristics of the public offender. Without it he would probably not have offended. Therefore, a period of psychotherapeutic intervention should logically precede a vocational counseling approach and once counseling is undertaken the counselor and the psychotherapist should cooperate in dealing with the client jointly for some period of time. If this cooperation is to be developed the roles of the therapist and the counselor must be clearly delineated and each must accept and work within the limitations of orientation, technique and goals of his speciality.

With specific reference to the vocational rehabilitation counselor, this cooperative approach with therapists means that his work with clients should focus primarily on the area of vocational preparation, evaluation, training and placement. As suggested above, the counselor should attempt to remain reality-oriented rather than to deal with the analysis of fantasy. Certainly the counselor should attempt to stimulate insight, but his applications should be present- and future-oriented rather than historical. The basic relationship between counselor and client should remain supportive, permitting ventilation and catharsis, rather than interpretive, utilizing free association or *anamesis*. Counseling is a function of rapport rather than an analysis of transference.

This is not to say that the counselor is limited or restricted in his role. On the contrary, the demands of social reality are so great that a sufficiency of professionally trained professionals is essential. Hence, every counselor should be enabled and encouraged to continually and progressively develop all of his professional skills, preferably in a university-related environment, since all of the personnel involved are college-trained people. In-service training in the absence of formal academic opportunities is inadequate for the development of truly professionalized practitioners. Thus, when in-service training, formal education and adequate supervision are combined, the only appropriate environment for growth is created.

An example of a potentially effective educational and training program would include joint in-service training for classification officers, institutional social workers and counselors combining available academic opportunities with an institutionally coordinated program providing for common communication as well as joint practice and internship possibilities. Such a program would also assist in the integration of new professionals into the institutional program. Another exemplary procedure might include the concept of a horizontal communication structure within the institutional organization itself. This pattern would provide not only for the vertical communication necessary for decision-making and information but also would provide for participation of dormitory officers, work assignment officers and other custodial persons as well as line counselors and other professional personnel. This pattern would accomplish both a necessary communication function, horizontal as well as vertical, and a training function for nonprofessional personnel.

19

The Mental Health Rehabilitation Counselor

Leon Meenach

The Establishment of a Cooperative Partnership
The New Counselor and the Patient-Client
Essential Qualifications
Services for the Mentally Ill
Release from the Hospital
Professional Preparation of the Counselor
Summary

THE ESTABLISHMENT OF A COOPERATIVE PARTNERSHIP

THE COUNSELOR who plans to work with the mentally ill client can benefit from some brief background history concerning the growth of the state-federal program of psychiatric rehabilitation. Although the vocational rehabilitation program was launched in 1920, it wasn't until 1943 that the state rehabilitation agency could provide service to the mentally ill. The 1943 Rehabilitation Legislation was the most significant breakthrough for the mentally ill. Even though the law allowed the state agency to serve the mentally ill, state agencies were slow to provide services to this disability group. During the early years of this legislation the counselor felt more comfortable working with physical restoration cases. It was not until after World War II that any real progress occurred in providing vocational rehabilitation services to the mentally ill.

The program of rehabilitation services for mentally ill in the fifties was usually initiated with the assignment of an experienced general counselor to a mental hospital on a regular visiting basis.

A typical example would be for a counselor to continue to carry his general case load and stop by the hospital on Thursdays to consider any referrals that the hospital staff might want to make. There was usually a patient referred that the hospital staff felt the counselor could not harm. The typical client might be a mentally retarded patient or a chronically ill patient with a long history of institutionalization.

The rehabilitation counselor in most cases was poorly prepared to work with the mentally ill. The disciplines in the hospital such as social service, psychiatry, psychology, physical therapy and occupational therapy, more often than not questioned the competency of the rehabilitation counselor to work with the mentally ill. Such counselors received very little encouragement from his fellow general counselors.

The rehabilitation counselor did bring to the hospital resources and skills that were effective in working with the patient. The counselor brought the community into the hospital and in a small way he was the link that bridged the gap for the patient to the community. The counselor also had the funds to purchase various services available to the clients in the community such as on-the-job training, training, room and board, job placement and follow-up. The most valuable service was the guidance and counseling provided by the counselor. The counselor and the hospital staff become more comfortable and confident with each other as the programs grew. The programs expanded to the point where full-time counselors were needed and requested. Rehabilitation counselors were assigned to the hospitals on a full-time basis and became functioning members of the hospital team. During the fifties, the counselor training orientation was, basically, do-it-yourself and this still holds true in many settings. In the mid-fifties, institutes, seminars and short-term training were developed by the state-federal programs for counselors working with the mentally ill in hospitals. During the fifties, rehabilitation graduate schools began to produce rehabilitation counselors with master's degrees in rehabilitation. Some of these counselors were challenged by this new field of rehabilitation counseling and became hospital counselors.

The 1954 legislation reinforced the 1943 amendments and really opened the door for the patient in terms of rehabilitation services for the mentally ill. The 1954 amendments provided for the establishment of workshops and facilities and research and demonstration projects.

The research and demonstration projects provided the opportunity for rehabilitation agencies and state mental hospitals to join together in demonstrating how they could cooperatively provide rehabilitation services to large numbers of hospitalized patients.

By the early sixties, rehabilitation personnel became a vital part of the in-hospital treatment team. The lone counselor was joined by other counselors, evaluators, instructors, personal adjustment counselors, et cetera, all assigned by the state rehabilitation agency. These rehabilitation workers were joined by professionals in the hospital in serving the treatment and rehabilitation needs from the time the patient was admitted through discharge to the community.

The rehabilitation team worked together with the patient in the development of a vocational diagnosis and a rehabilitation plan of services that would follow the client into the community. During the fifties and sixties, the rehabilitation of the mentally ill involved problems of the type of services to be provided—communication, funds and staff roles. The hospital rehabilitation team had difficulty in working together and there was a struggle for team leadership. Job placement was difficult in the community and the rehabilitation team was often met with rejection by the employers and the community.

There was the ever-present problem of transferring clients to field counselors who already had large case loads and little faith in the new program. There was need to establish after-care facilities such as halfway houses and rehabilitation social centers. These facilities could help the mental patient bridge the gap from the hospital to the community. It was not easy to establish such after-care centers because the neighborhood was fearful of mental patients, their effect on the life of the community and the anticipated devaluation of property.

The decade of the sixties opened the door for the hospitalized mental ill patient. A substantial number of patients received rehabilitation services and moved to gainful community employment and satisfactory social adjustment. By the end of that decade, mental health and rehabilitation agencies in most states had formed solid partnerships.

THE NEW COUNSELOR AND THE PATIENT-CLIENT

Today the new counselor assigned to a mental hospital rehabilitation program or a program serving the mentally ill in the community may come to the job from a variety of backgrounds. He may be a graduate of a rehabilitation counseling program, a school counselor, a schoolteacher, a minister or a general counselor interested in specializing in work with the mentally ill client. Regardless of the route to the job, there are some work experiences that the new counselor needs to be exposed to in order to effectively serve the psychiatric client.

It is essential that the new counselor become familiar with the ground rules in the hospital or community center where he is to serve patient-clients. One of the best ways for a new counselor to become acquainted with the job is to be assigned to work on the job with an experienced and respected psychiatric rehabilitation counselor. The experienced counselor can provide the opportunity for the new counselor to learn techniques, methods and policies of working effectively with the patient-client and the hospital staff. It is the responsibility of the supervisory staff to make effective in-service training available to the new counselor during at least the first six-months of his employment.

The rehabilitation counselor entering the psychiatric rehabilitation field will be serving clients in a number of treatment and rehabilitation settings. The greatest demand for counselor service in the past, and at present, is in a large mental hospital where a rehabilitation program is a cooperative venture between the mental hospital and the rehabilitation agency. The rehabilitation team is made up of assigned hospital staff and rehabilitation agency staff. The team is usually composed of psychiatrists, social workers, psychologists, rehabilitation counselors, vocational evaluators, industrial therapists, nurses, instructors and workshop personnel. The rehabilitation unit will more than likely be classified as a facility and be directed by state rehabilitation agency supervisors or directed jointly with the hospital administration.

The patient in most hospitals will be automatically referred at admission and interviewed within a few days by the rehabilitation team to determine the client's potential for eventual gainful employment in the community. The team approach is generally practiced and the team begins vocational rehabilitation services as soon as the patient can be engaged in the process. After the patient has received maximum benefit from the hospital rehabilitation program and is ready to return to the community, there may be a number of after-care facilities to which the counselor can refer his client. At this point, the hospital counselor will have had the opportunity to work with the patient from the time of referral to the point when he is ready to leave the hospital.

The hospital counselor may actually carry the former patient on his caseload if the client is within a radius of twenty-five to fifty miles of the hospital. Often he will transfer the client to a field counselor or a community facility counselor who works with a team which will provide continuous services after discharge.

The beginning counselor may not start his counseling in the hospital setting, but he may serve in a community-based program where clients are transferred to him from the hospital. He may also handle the processing of new referrals from psychiatrists or community mental health centers.

After the new counselor becomes familiar with his surroundings, the organizational structure, the hospital and rehabilitation personnel, the agency and hospital regulations, the referral procedures, the services available to his client, and so forth, he needs to prepare himself to work directly with the client and with the hospital team in developing a rehabilitation plan for the patient-client.

ESSENTIAL QUALIFICATIONS

If one is to be effective as a psychiatric rehabilitation counselor, there are some essential qualifications: (a) there must be a genuine concern about what happens to the patient and (b) the counselor must sincerely want to do something constructive about the factors that are barriers to the patient's engaging in gainful employment in the community.

One problem in working with the mentally ill client is the simple fact that they often are difficult to like. The new counselor will be working with many people who demonstrate very abnormal behavior. The counselor may develop attitudes of hostility, rejection, frustration, et cetera, that prevent him from working effectively with the patient-client. The counselor must understand his own reactions toward the mentally ill patient-client and remember that the client has been admitted to the hospital or center because the community could no longer tolerate the client's behavior or help him. The case load of the counselor will be made up of clients with a variety of psychiatric diagnoses. Many of these persons will be difficult to deal with in the rehabilitation process. The diagnosis will not be as important as the potential of the patient-client to engage in gainful employment and satisfactory social adjustment.

In many cases the rehabilitation counselor will be able to provide services with very little effort after the patient has responded to treatment. There will be other patient-clients who will need a long period of treatment and rehabilitation services before return to the community is advisable. Often the client's return to the community may be a painful experience and every effort should be made on the part of the hospital counselor and the field counselor to make this experience as comfortable as possible especially during his first few weeks in the community or after-care facility. Chances are that the client will need support services long after he has returned to the community and to a job.

SERVICES FOR THE MENTALLY ILL

Rehabilitation of the mentally ill requires a broad spectrum of services. Today in treatment facilities we find that vocational rehabilitation has an important role in the total treatment process of the patient-client. Frequently the rehabilitation process centers around the return of the patient to work. The rehabilitation counselor becomes an important member of the treatment team providing services that will enable the patient-client to achieve a level of adjustment favorable enough to allow him to engage in a meaningful work experience. Early work experience may take place in the hospital, center, community workshop or actual job placement.

Depending on the hospital or center where the counselor is assigned, he will find a number of services available for his patient-client. The single most important service might be the guidance and counseling that the rehabilitation counselor provides. For the counselor to work effectively with the patient-client, there needs to be cooperation and communication between other members of the rehabilitation team. The team or individual discipline will provide important input that will assist the counselor in developing a realistic vocational rehabilitation plan for the patient-client. Effective communication between counselor and client will be the key to the development of a plan of action for the patient-client. This means the counselor must learn to listen and empathize with the patient-client and be a helping person. When a satisfactory relationship is developed between the client and the counselor, a joint objective can be developed that will facilitate the development of a plan of action. There will be evaluative service, training, group counseling and job training for the client to experience, if needed. Many hospitals operate training programs on the hospital grounds which provide prevocational and vocational training through work assignments in the hospital, in vocational training areas and in the workshop. The in-hospital work experience will be valuable in developing self-confidence, work tolerance, positive work habits and motivation and in establishing realistic work goals. The new counselor must become completely familiar with comprehensive in-hospital services and utilize them for the maximum benefit of his clients.

The counselor also must familiarize himself with available community services and those that will carry over from the hospital into the community. This will prepare the hospital counselor to assist the patient-client in planning for the activities in the community that will be of the greatest help to the client.

RELEASE FROM THE HOSPITAL

When the beginning counselor starts developing his case load and moving the patient-client through the rehabilitation process in the hospital and into the community, he should familiarize himself with the rules, policies, laws, et cetera, that pertain to the rehabilitation agency, the Department of Mental Health and community agencies that are cooperating in the rehabilitation process. In some states, patients may be discharged with full legal rights or the patient may have to have his civil rights restored before he can engage in gainful employment or live in a halfway house or foster home setting. Some states or hospitals may require an attendant with the patient if he is to take part in rehabilitation activities in the community during the day. The counselor should make it a point to thoroughly familiarize himself on the behalf of the client to avoid the delay or disruption of services to the client because of legal problems.

The trend is to the development of community-based programs for the treatment and rehabilitation of the mentally ill. The rehabilitation services in large mental hospitals will continue, but the pattern is for a comprehensive in-hospital program with continuation of services in the community. This continuation of services will be provided in community mental health centers, halfway houses, outpatient clinics, day hospitals and community workshops. Some states are decentralizing their hospitals and building small regional hospitals for short-term treatment and hospitalization. We find treatment and rehabilitation services for the drug addict and the alcoholic in increased numbers in the regional units and community centers. Several states have added rehabilitation as an essential service when planning the services of the community mental health centers.

The psychiatric rehabilitation counselor must become completely familiar with both the in-hospital services and the community after-care services and bring all of these to bear for the benefit of the client. The community-based centers will offer preventive services to help avoid rehospitalization. It may be necessary for the rehabilitation counselor to assume leadership in the promotion and development of programs of services in both the community and the hospital if these are not available to the client.

PROFESSIONAL PREPARATION OF THE COUNSELOR

The counselor working with the mentally ill obviously should be trained in the basic work of the rehabilitation agency function which may vary from state to state. The specialty counselor working with the mentally ill could benefit from having the experience of serving as a general counselor. This is not to say that a counselor with a graduate degree and no work experience will be ineffective as a psychiatric counselor. It will take time, however, for the beginning counselor to develop expertise in working with the mentally ill. A good exposure to psychiatric material and the help of colleagues will be invaluable in acquiring skills and techniques in working with the psychiatric patient.

The state agency usually provides the counselor with opportunities to participate in organized in-service training programs on a continuing basis. Such training involves basic rehabilitation counseling as well as training opportunities developed for the specialty counselor working with the mentally ill. Field trips to other facilities in the state or nearby states provide an excellent opportunity for the exchange of ideas. There are also training opportunities for the counselor working with the mentally ill on both the national and regional levels. A psychiatric rehabilitation internship program is located at the Massachusetts Mental Health Center, Harvard Medical School. It is a six-month program. Candidates are selected from state agencies, are provided a stipend and their state salary is usually continued while in training. There are short-term training programs organized on a regional basis. These are usually located in a medical school or are based in a rehabilitation facility. One of these is located at the University of Virginia and is a six-week training program for the counselors in Region III. This six-week program is spaced over a period of several months and is designed to provide training to the counselor working with a psychiatric case load. There is a trend to expand this type of training to other regions to enable the counselor to receive training for short periods of time while carrying a case load. A number of the schools of rehabilitation counseling provide their graduates with considerable experience in work with the mentally ill. In some graduate programs, the student can serve a field internship in a rehabilitation program for the mentally ill. Although the formalized experiences for training in psychiatric rehabilitation counseling are limited at this time, the future looks bright for extended on-the-job training, formalized training and short-term training on a continuing basis.

SUMMARY

There is an increasing demand for psychiatric counselors. State agencies are moving from the medical model of rehabilitation services to the psychosocial model. In a short time, more than half of all rehabilitation clients will come from recently emphasized groups such as the mentally ill, the public offender, the drug addict, the alcoholic, behavior disorders and the disabled disadvantaged.

Since the state agencies started serving the mentally ill in the early fifties, tremendous progress has been made. Departments of mental health and other community services have joined hands with state rehabilitation agencies to provide rehabilitation services to the mentally ill. Thousands of counselors have joined the staffs of hospitals and community rehabilitation programs designed to serve the rehabilitation needs of the mentally ill. Large numbers of general counselors have performed outstanding jobs of receiving patient-clients from hospitals and providing them with the type of services that result in gainful employment. The surface has just been scratched, but we are learning how to deal with the problem of rehabilitating the mentally ill. New counselors will bring innovations and fresh approaches to our present delivery systems, and this will result in rehabilitation services to thousands of our mentally ill citizens. We are just beginning to meet the exciting challenge of the rehabilitation of the mentally ill.

20

Providing Counseling Services to Blind and Severely Visually Impaired Persons

Richard E. Hardy

What Is Counseling?
Rehabilitation Counseling
Rehabilitation Counseling with the Blind and Severely Visually Impaired
Summary
References

WHAT IS COUNSELING?

COUNSELING has been defined in various terms and by many experts. Gustad[3] has written that "counseling is a learning oriented process, carried on in a simple, one-to-one social environment in which a counselor, professionally competent in relative psychological skills and knowledge, seeks to assist the client to learn more about himself, to know how to put understanding into effect in relation to clearly perceived, realistically defined goals to the end that the client may become a happier and more productive member of his society."

While definitions vary according to the orientation of the counselor, certain truisms have resulted from the enormous amount of research concerning the effectiveness of counseling. These will be explained in the following paragraphs.

No matter what particular school or theory of counseling is accepted by the practitioner, the most important factor determining the outcome of counseling effectiveness is the "personality" of the counselor himself. In other words, whether he counts himself as Rogerian as Ellisonian or eclectic, the personality of the counselor will come through in counseling sessions and affect the outcome to a degree which will determine whether or not the counseling session is effective. Just as teachers can bring about enormous growth and changes in students by modifying their attitudes toward various subject matter, the counselor can bring about substantial changes in his client for better or worse.

Effective counseling requires certain basic ingredients. As the strength or weakness of these ingredients vary so does the ability of the counselor to help the client. There are three basic prerequisites to effective counseling. First, the counselor must accept the client without imposing conditions for this acceptance. He must be willing to work with the client and become actively involved with him as an individual, no matter what the counselee's race, attitudes or mode of life may be. This is necessary in order for the counselee to gain the knowledge that the counselor as a person wishes to help him with his problems and is not prejudging.

The counselor must be "genuine" in that he must function in a way which indicates to the client that he is being true to his own feelings and to himself. To be otherwise is to present a facade to the client—a false image which will act as a deterrent to a successful relationship. Counselors must avoid artificiality in their relationships. If the counselor hides behind a professional mystique, he may find that the counselee is better at "fooling" him than he is at deceiving the client. The professional worker cannot expect his client to be open, sincere and genuine if he himself does not represent these characteristics well.

In addition, the counselor must have an empathetic understanding and feeling *vis-à-vis* the client. He must make a sincere effort to see the client's problem through the *client's* eyes, and he must be able to communicate the depth of his understanding.

Counseling can be considered a relationship between two persons which is conducive to good mental health. Inherent in an effective counseling relationship is the absence of threat. The counselor must remove threat if the client is to grow and be able to solve his problems in an uninhibited manner. Counseling as a relationship is also typified by the types of feelings that many of us have for our closest friends. True close friendships are characterized by honest caring, genuine interest and a high level of concern about helping in a time of need. Real friendships often require one person to put aside his own selfish needs in order to listen long enough and with enough empathy so that a friend's problem may begin to work itself out in a natural and constructive manner.

There are a number of adjectives which apply to various types of counseling (religious, marital, rehabilitation, educational, personal, vocational and others). Counseling services vary according to the needs of the client—not the counselor. A counselee who comes to the counselor for help will often at first outline a concern which is not the real problem. The counselor must have considerable flexibility and insight to know what is required in each individual situation.

REHABILITATION COUNSELING

Rehabilitation counselors are concerned with individuals who have vocational handicaps. These handicaps may result from physical disability, emotional or mental illness, social or cultural deprivation. In each individual case, the counselor must be able to decide what remedy is required in order to move the counselee toward successful personal adjustment in his family, community and on the job.

Rehabilitation counseling requires the ingredients mentioned earlier for effective counselor-client relationships; however, much of rehabilitation counseling consists of advice-giving and coordination of services to the client. In a sense, "rehabilitation counseling" can be considered a misnomer when the term is applied across the board. A substantial number of clients need considerable advice and information which the counselor has to offer concerning social and rehabilitation services from which they can profit. When the counselee needs advice and information, the rehabilitation counselor must be able to recognize this need and provide what is required. There also will be many instances in which the client and counselor must enter into a number of counseling sessions in depth. The counselor must make the judgment concerning what type of help is needed for the client to solve his particular problems. Rehabilitation counselors need appropriate training that will enable them to decide whether or not they are qualified to do the kind of counseling which is necessary.

Many counselors fall into the trap of wanting to play the role of "junior therapist" and involve high percentages of their clients in in-depth counseling sessions. This is particularly true of the graduates of many rehabilitation counselor training programs. Some workers hide behind "counseling" (as synonymous with quality) in terms of their justifying low numbers of rehabilitated clients. There is much talk of quality services and in-depth counseling which require considerable time. The rehabilitation counselor who is an effective manager of his case load can "rehabilitate" the number of persons required by his agency administrator and while doing so can provide counseling services as needed to his clients.

Rehabilitation work requires a broad definition of counseling which includes the offering of some and coordination of other professional services to clients. Generally, agency administrators—especially those trained in counseling—do not accept the explanation of "the time required and quality services" for a low client rehabilitation rate. Any agency administrator or supervisor knows that some cases require much involved counseling and these cases, in many instances, are the most difficult ones. They are time-consuming and can test the fiber of the rehabilitation counselor. Untrained counselors generally cannot handle such cases without help from someone who has had some advanced orientation in counseling. Counselors, however, who play the role of "junior therapist" in trying to become deeply involved with all of their clients—whether or not this type of service is called for—will be ineffective and probably will not remain long in rehabilitation work.

The rehabilitation counselor will find his coordinating and facilitating role highly rewarding when it is done well and gets needed services to the client. One of the greatest satisfactions that the counselor can have is the assurance that he knows when certain types of services are required and whether these should be more therapeutically oriented or oriented more toward advice, information and coordination of community resources and professional services.

Rehabilitation counselors should not rank-order their clients in a psychological need hierarchy which places the individual with severe psychological problems at the top of the counselor's list for services. Certainly, these persons should be served immediately upon the counselor's realization that severe psychological problems exist. They should either be referred to the appropriate psychologist or psychiatrist if problems are so severe that the counselor cannot handle them alone or they should be served by rehabilitation counselors who are competent in the type of service required. The point to be made here is that the rehabilitation process is a complicated procedure; the client who may be adjusting normally to a loss and who does not need substantial in-depth therapeutic involvement is as good a case for services as one requiring more therapeutic work. Coordination of services of supportive personnel and professional personnel is a substantial part of the work of the rehabilitation counselor. In many cases, he will have to bring this team together in order that the client can continue to receive effective and necessary rehabilitation services.

The rehabilitation counselor must actively involve himself within the community in order to be fully aware of the many resources which exist that can be of substantial benefit to his clients. Generally, counselors have indicated that so much of their time is taken with counseling and coordination of services that they are unable to put forward enough effort to learn all that the community has to offer. Counselors who utilize community resources effectively are very familiar with the offerings of various agencies and through coordination and cooperation find that their work load is lessened by the support of other social service programs.

The counselor will wish to offer his services to various types of community agencies. For instance, most counselors can give a great deal of useful advice to such programs as the community action and model cities efforts sponsored by the Federal Government. Agencies and organizations such as family service programs and welfare agencies can be of considerable help in getting needed services for the rehabilitation client. The counselor should take a major responsibility in coordinating efforts of agencies and programs that can help in the rehabilitation of clients, and he should volunteer his time and energies to help strengthen other social service programs.

The rehabilitation counselor must keep in mind that he should be moving the client toward end objectives of independence and successful adjustment on the job. Rehabilitation differs from some other social service professions in the regard that a substantial test of the counselor's work is made at the end of the rehabilitation process. That test consists of the appropriateness of the client's behavior in a work situation.[4]

REHABILITATION COUNSELING WITH THE BLIND AND SEVERELY VISUALLY IMPAIRED

No special counseling theory need be constructed in order for the rehabilitation counselor to serve blind persons. There is, however, a substantial body of knowledge with which the counselor should be thoroughly familiar. Topics include the etiology of diseases related to blindness, problems in adjustment to visual loss including mobility, social adjustment, occupational advice and job placement. The counselor serving blind persons has a real responsibility to undertake considerable study in order to acquaint himself with what Father Carroll[2] has called in the title of his book, *Blindness: What It Is, What It Does, and How To Live With It.*

The rehabilitation counselor serving blind persons has as much or more a coordinating function as does the counselor in a general agency setting. A counselor concerned with the blind will work closely with the educational services specialist, the social worker, the ophthalmologist, the placement specialist, the rehabilitation teacher and the mobility instructor who help in the team effort of moving the blind individual toward adjustment to his visual problem and later adjustment on the job.

Rehabilitation counselors serving the blind, just as counselors working with any other rehabilitation clients, must be certain that their clients are without need of further medical or psychological treatment. In this regard, the counselor helping the partially sighted should make certain that no visual aid or professional service can offer additional help to the client. He should be fully aware of the various problems which go hand in hand with a loss of sight. Persons who are experiencing a severe physical inadequacy lose some ability to be independent. They feel socially inadequate and in some cases may have additional problems which at first might not be apparent to the counselor. Advanced age or other physical incapabilities may add to the blind person's adjustment problems.

The client will be very much interested in the prognosis for his future, and the rehabilitation counselor should make sure that valid information is provided. An effective counselor must be ready to help the blind person understand what his opportunities are for education, employment and social activities. He should also talk with those persons who give information to the blind client, especially those professional individuals such as ophthalmologists, to make certain that they have valid and useful information concerning blindness and the services of the state rehabilitation agency.

Bauman and Yoder[1] have suggested that the rehabilitation counselor must offer

> . . . a combination of several qualities: (1) his own emotional acceptance of blindness (he must be the first person to whom the client has spoken who did not immediately show great pity and anxiety—a helping new experience for the client); (2) formal or informal instruction in procedures which make it easier to live as a blind person (the home teacher and also some adjustment on pre-vocational training can help here); (3) realistic planning for the future, including vocational planning if the age and general health of the client make this appropriate. It is true that all of these may be rejected for a time, in which case the counselor must offer (4) understanding, patience, and a gentle persistence which keeps him available until the client and his family are able to reorient themselves to the future instead of clinging to the past.

In counseling with blind persons, the rehabilitation counselor must remember that he is working with individuals who cannot see or whose sight is impaired. The client will differ from fellow blind persons as much as he will differ from sighted persons.

Some blind persons are very healthy; others are sickly. Some are well adjusted psychologically; others are poorly adjusted. In many cases, blindness will have caused severe psychological stress which has not been overcome, just as an accident or some other type of traumatic experience may have caused either a sighted or a blind person severe psychological difficulty.

Often, reaction to partial vision causes as much or more frustration and anxiety than reaction to total blindness. One reason for this seems to be that partially sighted persons are unable to function normally and do not want to accept their loss of sight as a reality. They live in a no-man's-world between blindness and sight.

The rehabilitation counselor serving blind and severely visually impaired persons must be even more planful and thoughtful than the counselor who is concerned with individuals who are sighted. Often it will be necessary to anticipate problems which may arise for the blind client. For instance, simply getting to and from the counselor's office may become a very troublesome and embarrassing task. The blind client may be traveling over unfamiliar terrain with or without the help of relatives or friends. The counselor, in many cases, may want to initially visit in the home and later during the relationship invite the client to the rehabilitation agency.

The counselor must be very much aware that this blind client is "tuned into" audiology clues ("yes's and "un-hum's" may be helpful), since the usual eye contact and other nonverbal communications are not effective with blind persons. For instance, silence over a considerable period of time often takes place in counseling sessions; but when the counselor is working with a blind client, silence may be interpreted as disinterest or rejection.

It is respectful and appropriate for the counselor to look directly into the face and eyes of the client just as if the counselee were fully sighted. Blind persons are often aware that sighted persons are not looking at them and they get the impression, which may be true, that the counselor is not listening.

Counselors should be particularly careful about shuffling papers, tapping a pencil on the desk or making other sounds that are distracting. They should also be aware that many blind persons, especially the congenitally blind, give the counselor little to go by in terms of facial expression. The counselor who is used to reading emotionality in various facial responses may be at a considerable loss with some persons who have been blind for a number of years and who are not nearly as responsive in this respect as sighted people.[5]

A rehabilitation counselor providing professional services to blind persons must avoid fostering unnecessary dependence. Often counselors, unknowingly as well as knowingly, build their own self-esteem by continually allowing clients to rely on them for personal advice and other services. On the other hand, many rehabilitation counselors are afraid to show sufficient interest in the problems of the client because they are concerned about being forced to give a great deal of time and attention to the client. Neither of these extremes will allow the counselor to be effective.

SUMMARY

It has been said that the most important variable for helping people which the counselor brings to the counseling relationship is "himself." The rehabilitation counselor, whether he is working with blind or sighted clients, must make a substantial effort to maintain genuineness, openness, sincerity, honesty and respect for the client. While techniques and procedures are important in accomplishing goals in counseling sessions, the real key to successful counseling is whether the counselor genuinely cares for the individual. A rehabilitation counselor provides substantial professional and coordinated services from which the client benefits enormously. Most rehabilitation counselors will have certain quotas to meet and the effective counselor through proper case load management will be able to provide quality and quantity services. He will also realize that his coordinative and facilitative function is as important as his counseling function. He must serve clients according to *their needs* and not his own, and when this is done counselees will not claim that his work lacks quality because he will have been much more concerned with them as individuals than with whether or not his services were "professional" in nature.

REFERENCES

1. Bauman, Mary K., and Yoder, Norman M.: *Adjustment to Blindness— Re-Viewed.* Springfield, Charles C Thomas, 1966.
2. Carroll, Thomas J.: *Blindness: What It Is, What It Does, And How To Live With It.* Boston, Little, Brown Co., 1961.
3. Gustad, J. W.: The definition of counseling. In Berdie, R. F.: *Roles and Relationship in Counseling.* Minneapolis: University of Minnesota Press, 1953.
4. Hardy, Richard E.: Vocational placement. In Cull, John G., and Hardy, Richard E.: *Vocational Rehabilitation: Professional and Process.* Springfield, Charles C Thomas, 1971.
5. Jordan, John E.: Counseling the blind. *Personnel and Guidance Journal. 39 (No. 3):*10-214, November 1962.
6. Morgan, Clayton A.: Personality of counseling. *Blindness.* AAWB Annual, American Association of Workers for the Blind, Inc., Washington, D.C.
7. Truax, Charles B., and Carkkuff, Robert R.: *Toward Effective Counseling and Psychotherapy: Training and Practice.* Chicago, Aldine Publishing Co., 1967.

PART FIVE

THE CLIENTS IN THE REHABILITATION PROCESS

I, The Client
Adjustment to Disability
The Rehabilitation Needs of the Older Adult

21

I, The Client

Clayton A. Morgan

THIS CHAPTER has been written in the first person singular. Free use is made of the personal pronoun "I." This approach has been employed in the hope that the reader will be made more sensitive to the world of the client.

Obviously it is impossible to speak for the client in an "Everyman" sense. Each individual comes alive as a personality in his own right.

It is not implied or intended that a universal set of working principles has been identified. On the definitive side, an attempt has been made to stimulate thinking, to highlight some of the considerations and responsibilities implicit when one human being attempts to help another.

* * * * * * * * * * * * *

> Anyone who wants to make a living folding parachutes ought to be required to jump frequently. —GEORGE A. MICHAEL

I wonder if a counselor or helping person remembers what it is like to ask for help...with nothing more than his own personhood as the reason for anyone's lifting even a little finger in his behalf.

Think about that!

Could it be that in order to be able to give help one should first learn how to receive help?

What's it like to go to a rehabilitation agency for help? You sit in the waiting room and a weird mix of questions and thoughts fly through your mind: How will I be treated? Will they be able to do anything for me? And if they can, will they explain to me what they do here and what I can expect? How long will it take? What kind of personal questions will they ask me? Will I like the counselor?

It's almost like having the agency on one side and me on the other. There's little question about who has the visible power and authority in this situation. The symbols are easily seen: the agency name on the door, secretaries, degrees on the wall and desks—small desks in the waiting room, larger desks in the offices. There are certain rituals I must go through before I can see anyone of importance.

Why has society devised so many ways to provide distance and protection for the helping person. When you consider how little protection I have, it seems rather one-sided. For almost anyone can see my incompleteness, my humanity. There are few fig leaves to cover my psychological nakedness. As a referral to a strange agency with a new counselor, few of my strengths seem evident. The emphasis can easily focus on my weaknesses. . .my lacks. . .my reasons for coming to the agency. . .my confusion and uncertainty . . . sometimes my hostility and aggressiveness—or passiveness.

Is it any wonder that one of the first things I want is for the helpful professional to come alive as a fellow human being?

This is not easy. Maybe I am asking for too much. Or is it the least I can ask?

For I start with my impressions of him as a person. I end with my impressions of him as a person. True, he might have gone to school twelve years longer than I have—or be able to use language I do not understand—but instinctively I know that if you scratch him deeply enough he will bleed. Just like me. He may be behind a desk but he is as mortal as I am. I read the birth and death notices and I note there is no respector of persons in these kinds of realities. They put us all on the same level. Every man is but one heartbeat from eternity.

How much of this common ground does his behavior indicate he is willing to freely admit sharing with me?

Does he communicate to me in a thousand subtle ways that he knows we are more nearly alike than different?

I am thinking of the things which make us people. . .like

whistling in the dark when we are afraid. . .clinging to those we love. . .of having to settle for less than we want. . .of reaching out to others in a desire to understand and to be understood. . .of searching for the secret of a better tomorrow. . . .

One might say that these things are incidental—that they are personal matters of small consequence. May I counter suggesting that my impressions of the helping person helps free or freeze whatever skills, talents or understandings he has to share with me. Before I am a child, a father, or mother, or a citizen, I am first of all "people." I operate much of the time at the feeling level. Don't most other people?

I like for a helping person to extend his hand across to me— not down to me. In the warmth of his clasp I want to sense his saying, "As one man to another, we are in this fight together, fellow. We are joined in problems that in one form or another continue to pester me, too." When this happens and he has really come alive as a person, then I'll be in a lot better mood to listen to what he has to offer.

Emphasis in the biblical passage which states "it is more blessed to give than to receive" has been traditionally directed at the "giver." What about the receiver? Am I happy to be placed in a position of either asking or receiving?

What do we mean when we speak of the "dignity and worth of a person"? How can this be enhanced unless there is a built-in quality in the helping relationship which makes me feel that I, too, am giving something in return, that there is a mutual sharing and mutual involvement?

To assist in accomplishing this, I want the helping person to be essentially warm and human. I want him to be secure enough not to feel the need to erect artificial distance barriers or try to impress me as being a gracious dispenser of goods from the "have's" to the "have-not's."

I want someone who is trustworthy. . .who keeps as a sacred charge every aspect of my personal life that is either in the case folder or which I have shared with him in conversation or which he has learned from others.

No one can buy my trust.

No one can force me to trust.

I determine whom I trust—and when—and where.

I want someone who does not take away a hope, a dream or an idea without replacing it with something better. Chesterton said, "Don't take down a fence until you know the reason why it was put up."

I want someone who is willing to start with me as I am. . .who gives priority to me and my needs as contrasted with what he would like to give me or limit his recommendations to the services his agency can offer.

Perhaps the real difference in the way I accept help is in the degree to which I sense a person is giving of himself. Is he willing to care enough to run the risk of being hurt? Sometimes I will disappoint him; sometimes I will hurt him either through ignorance or by design.

In the movie, *Monsieur Vincent,* there is a scene in which St. Vincent de Paul gives instructions to a new nun. Maybe part of the secret can be found in this quote: "It is only for your love the poor will forgive you the bread you give to them."

Help is not easy to give.

Help is not easy to receive.

Why can't people care enough to use language I can understand? I need plenty of opportunities for asking questions without my appearing foolish or stupid. Why doesn't a counselor realize that a word can have dozens of different interpretations? I need someone who deeply appreciates the fact that *meaning is in me,* not in words. I want someone to help who is far too wise to say "but I told him." Blessed is the man who understands there can be a great difference between what a person says or writes and what he is trying to communicate.

I want someone who believes it isn't really too important what he says but rather *what I hear*—and one who is truly aware of the difference when he talks with me.

Pray don't use words to cover up or confuse me when things are uncertain. Sometimes it seems that speech is used to keep things muddled, for keeping people at arms length when there is some kind of threat. What if I do threaten? Isn't the counselor strong enough to "roll with the punch"? What was he learning all those years in school? How to protect himself?

When I introduce a subject that is painful or involves deep feeling, I am discouraged if the response indicates the person ignores my signal—if he plainly shows he would rather talk about something else. I need someone mature enough and accepting enough to let me try to express and clarify my feelings and evaluate my behavior.

Time and again I can tell that people are not really listening to me. Maybe I could better state it the other way—seldom do I enjoy the experience of having someone who gives me his undivided attention. There seems to be so many ready prescriptions for my problem before I have even defined the problem—much less gotten across to the other person what the problem is.

Such ready answers often silence me. There are many ways of silencing me. Sometimes I get the strangest feeling that people kid themselves into thinking when I have been shushed that somehow my problems have been cut down to size—or at least that they are not as serious as I first thought.

Should I be made to feel guilty because I still have problems? Should the atmosphere of the agency ever cause me to feel apologetic because of my trying circumstances . . . even lead me to feel I should approach the helping person, hat in hand, and mumble something like, "Sorry to inconvenience you, sir, but. . . ."

I want a helping person who realizes that the professional mettle of a man is tested by the depth and intensity of the problems he is willing to tackle with me. Such a person becomes excited at evidence of growth and discovery in me. He delights in realizing that he is less and less needed. He seems to meet his own deep personal needs when he sees I am able to do that which he is unable to do or understand.

Please refer me to someone who does not feel the need to make up his mind too quickly about me. Spare me from the person who is frightened by failure. Part of the rehabilitation bill of rights should be the right to make mistakes—the right to fail. Isn't this the price to pay for learning and growing?

What tragic games we play when anyone feels he has graduated to the school of perfection. Then he has a vested interest in his mistakes. He sees himself as a pencil without an eraser. To be teamed with such a "helper" could result in being help-less.

> What happens when the theoretical and hypothetical comes alive in flesh and blood? . . . What is our response when there stands before us a handicapped person with a name, a given set of physical characteristics, a social history, likes and dislikes, strengths and weaknesses: a frail human being?
> How well do we wear the mantle of deferred judgment when we are charged with the responsibility both to know and help him?
> We see him functioning in a variety of circumstances . . . when he is hungry, filled, tired, lonely, cheerful, elated. We see him when he is depressed, when he tries, when he gives up.
> When do we typecast him?
> When do we make up our mind about him?
> Do we give him a batting average after only one time up? What if the first time up he strikes out? Or knocks a home run? Do we then decide his fate the second time he is at bat? Or the third? Or the fourth? When . . . if ever?
> Do we project his tomorrows as an endless repetition of his todays? Dare we let repeated disappointments dull our vision of what he might become, or the next person entrusted to our care, or the next, or the next? Dare we care enough to sometimes be made to look like a fool and yet continue to care in the faith that what we are and how we perform may make a difference—if not to this one then perhaps to the next one, or the next? How can we tell when the most routine everyday act is not a princely opportunity in work clothes?[3]

I want a helping person who is mature enough to face up to the realization that *he can never be sure he is being fair to me*. Then he is not mouse-trapped by the deception of "facts" into thinking that he can once and for all time come to a hard and fast conclusion about me and my inner world and how I will outwardly express what is me. He tends to share with Bliss Carmen the thought, "I often wish I could rid the world of the tyranny of facts. What are facts but compromises? A fact merely marks the point where we have agreed to let investigation cease."

> Man is often viewed as a hopeless clod in much thinking now, not because he was made so by the Creator but because custom encourages him to be no more than that. Bad leadership, bad morals and crass stu-

pidity have made man only a shadow of what he can be, what God intended him to be, and what he eventually will be.

Such concepts about inherent potential will be clear to the man of vision. It will be nonsense to the creature of habit. It will be workable to those who will understand. It will be funny to the so-called old time "business as usual man."

The possible progress is too great to believe by those who cannot dream.[2]

It takes a big person to be able to live with ambiguity. It takes a strong person to be flexible. It takes a rare kind of being "grown up" to find added strength when honestly facing up to one's own frailties.

It is not easy to work with me. Time and again I have tried and have failed. In fact many say I have built a stable life style based on failure. Without help they are probably right; however, intelligent, professional, interested assistance can help me identify my difficulties, assist me in developing my abilities and break this life style of failure. But again, it is not easy to work with me.

When I have tried to change, any lasting results usually come about quite gradually—so gradually in fact that others have difficulty in recognizing any difference. It requires a sort of "second-mile" vision to see that a person can continue to be most "like he was" and at the same time slowly change, develop and grow.

Often I have been told to "build yourself a dream" . . . and "you can make dreams come true." Just like that! The idea is too easy—like black magic—a neat formula which a person can follow to the pot of gold at the foot of the rainbow.

I have found no easy solution. The ideas which others have suggested for overnight results just don't work for me.

I want a helping person who understands that his *insights* and understandings have gradually taken shape over many years. Common with my human brothers everywhere, I would like a ready-made answer. But let's face it, there is no way to give me a painless psychic transfusion which instantly makes it possible for me to appreciate the world through his eyes.

It takes time.

People are not by nature patient. They want closure. Even when a person's future is at stake there are temptations to take shortcuts. Some samplings of what I say and do can be blown up as being "the answer" to what I am—how I feel—how I will function in the future.

Let me suggest some things which will make the professional think twice before looking for simple answers to complex problems. May I start by stating that I want to work with someone who considers me bigger than a psychological report, or medical report, a case folder or any other collection of data.

When will people wake up to the fact that what others say about me *may reveal more about them than it does about me?*

> One more word about time and this is based on the client's need and how time helps to meet that need. Since so few clients react spontaneously because of confusion engendered by their problems and because of the added concern created by the experience of asking for help in a new and strange setting of an unknown agency and in relation to an unknown counselor, the client needs time with himself apart from the worker in between interviews. He needs time to dissipate confusion; time to assimiliate what he has acquired during the interview; time to grapple with it as far as he is able and to bring more of his real self into the next interview. Only then can he be expected to affirm more and more of himself and to take ever greater responsibility for his actions and his part in the helping relationship, so that the total process truly becomes a dynamic experience of interaction. There are both growth and therapeutic values inherent in time.[1]

I am not an IQ score; I am not a label. I am not a word, be it "para," "saint" or "welfare client." I belong also to me. I am not someone's "schizophrenic" or someone elses "case." I hope I haven't relinquished my individual identity or self-ownership by virtue of being referred to you. The case history is not me; dime-store diagnoses give but fleeting, incomplete glimpses of what others consider present reality; the prognosis does not predict all that will happen. I, the client, tower above any piece of paper; I burst the bounds of any label; I dwarf all the typed or scrawled symbols however neatly catalogued and filed.

The helping person's responsibility is not to demonstrate the validity of a test profile—his responsibility is to me; his allegiance is not to carry out the crossed "t's" and dotted "i's" of a plan—his loyalty is to work with me in *process,* as one who is *becoming.* This means, when indicated, *that revision and change are welcomed as a normal part of growth and development.* How tragic when we become slaves to a plan. Should not the plan be our slave? A means to an end?

Solemn consultations in strange language behind closed doors by people with impressive titles could make it appear I am their pawn to analyze and manage as another statistic. Is it this simple? Am I at their mercy? How ironical! Their reputation rests in my hands. My survival is critical to their survival; my success is critical to their success. I am the justification for their professional existence.

Does this mean I would detract one iota from the importance of a helping person? No. I need the doctor, the counselor the psychologist, the social worker and all the others. But they merit their titles and status only to the degree they can help set into motion forces which will better help me help myself.

I am not setting the stage for a contest of wills—a case of my winning—or his—or their—winning. Many of the possible difficulties will have been resolved if the helping person recognizes and uses me as the major resource I am. In what better way can I gain an increased feeling of respect for myself and my abilities? I need a person who will look at me and see *me.* In the final analysis, it is my attitudes, my abilities, my physical, moral and spiritual stamina which will determine whether or not any "plan" succeeds.

There are times I would like to avoid or postpone facing up to the responsibility of who I am and what I am capable of becoming. In my weakness I may take advantage of the easy way out if others find shallow excuses for me. When this happens I come away from the experience questioning, wondering if they have conspired with me to sell a part of my birthright of dignity and worth.

Much of what I have been trying to express ties in with how I see myself as others see me.

What conditions my behavior? What conditions their behavior? Why is it that helping people have often tried to shy away from matters of belief and conviction? They speak of being "objective." Some would have you buy the idea that they can separate what they think and feel from what they do when they are "on the job."

Is there any way for the effective helping person to operate outside of a frame of reference which is the essence of what he is?

How does he define man?

Does he believe that man can be quickly and easily analyzed? Does he casually speak of "that type" or "the kind who"? Does he think man is a bundle of reflexes? A conditioned machine? Would he say that arthritis of the mind inevitably develops with age, that "you can't teach an old dog new tricks"? Does he hang convenient words like "welfare client" or "deaf mute" or "a quad" on a person? Does he have that rare quality of dedication which leads him to shun mind-deadening labels and attempt through never-ending observation and study to understand and describe the unique pattern of individual behavior?

Does he with clear conscience ever say, "I know how you feel" or "I am sure this is the best plan for you"?

Does he believe people can change and grow? What does the word "counsel" mean to him? What are his values about my values?

What does he believe about ongoing professional development? Does he subscribe to the thought that those who dare to counsel must never cease to learn?

If it seems I am asking too many questions, let me remind you that my life, time and interests are at stake. The helping person is supposed to be in business for me. I have every reason to be interested in just what he is trying to sell. Whatever this is and how deeply he feels about it will make a difference—in what he says, in what he does, in how large or small he sees me and my world.

Take for example the person who sincerely feels that he should at all costs try to hide his feelings—that it is "unprofessional" to express emotion or say what he is really thinking. How many times have you ever seen a studied neutrality breed enthusiasm and a desire to achieve? How can a person really have an active concern if he succeeds in keeping this concern "under a bushel"? Does strength find life in thin soil of timidity? Can the spark of faith in one's ability be caught from a face that feels compelled to wear a mask coldly calculated to hide belief and feelings?

No!

If you yourself are not an inspiring example of one who is "becoming" how can you expect me to glimpse the beginning of a new day? What better way to get across an idea than for it to come alive in a person? Enthusiasm breeds enthusiasm; courage is contagious; strength spawns and sustains strength.

The mainspring of human effort is bound by belief and guided by a value system which is part and parcel of what we are and do. This is not to imply that I, the client, would want anyone to shove his philosophy down my throat or try to fit square pegs into round holes. But isn't it possible for helping people to lean so far backward to avoid this charge that they fail in a significant part of their mission—being agents and facilitators of change?

There is a dramatic difference between being exposed to values and having someone try to impose his values on me.

Please be frank with me. Be honest with me. You cannot be believable unless you are genuine. There is an old Indian proverb which states, "Do not speak to me from the book. Speak to me from the heart."

* * * * * * * * * * * * * *

There are many additional items which could be discussed under the broad heading of "I, The Client." Perhaps the gist of what has already been said—and glimpses into some additional things which could be said—is summarized in a paraphrased quote from Gilbert Highet's *The Art of Teaching:*

> A helping relationship involves emotions, which have not been systematically appraised and employed, and human values, which seem outside the grasp of science. A "scientifically" brought-up child would be a pitiable monster. A "scientific" marriage would be only a thin and crippled version of a true marriage. A "scientific" friendship would be as cold as a chess problem. . .helping another human being is not like inducing a chemical reaction; it is much more like painting a picture or making a piece of music, or on a lower level

like planting a garden or writing a friendly letter. You must throw your heart into it, you must realize that it cannot all be done by formulas, or you will spoil your work, and your clients, and yourself.

REFERENCES

1. Blicksler, Paul: *The Helping Relationship.* Lebanon (Pa.), Family and Children's Service, 1950, p. 51.
2. Lincoln, James F.: *Incentive Management.* Cleveland (Ohio), The Lincoln Electric Company, 1951.
3. Morgan, Clayton A.: The personality of counseling. *Blindness,* AAWB, 1969.

22

Adjustment to Disability

John G. Cull

Role of Body Image in Adjustment to Disability
Factors Associated with Adjustment
Role of Defense Mechanisms in Adjustment
Implications for Professionals Working with the Disabled
References

IT IS TRUE that our clients are much more like us than unlike us, but they differ in one major respect. They have suffered the psychological impact of disability and have adjusted or are in the process of adjusting to this impact. In this chapter we shall discuss the factors which affect the psychological adjustment to disability and the mechanism by which an individual adjusts to his disability.

During the First and Second World Wars, behavioral scientists noticed an increased incidence in conversion reactions. Conversion reactions are[1] a type of psychoneurotic disorder in which the impulse causing anxiety is "converted" into functional symptoms in parts of the body rather than the anxiety being experienced consciously. Examples of conversion reactions include such functional disabilities as anesthesias (blindness, deafness), paralyses (aphonia, monoplegia, or hemiplegia) and dyskineses (tic, tremor, catalepsy).

The study of these conditions along with other studies led to the development of a discipline known as psychosomatic medicine.

Psychosomatic medicine is concerned with the study of the effects of the personality and emotional stresses upon the body and its function. This psychological interaction with physiology can be observed in any of the body systems.

After the establishment of psychosomatic medicine, behavioral scientists (psychiatrists, psychologists, social workers, et cetera) began observing the converse of this new field. Instead of studying the effects of emotional stress on bodily functioning, they studied the effects of physical stress on emotional functioning. Their concern was directed toward answering the question, What are the emotional and personality changes which result from physical stress or a change in body function or physical configuration?

ROLE OF BODY IMAGE IN ADJUSTMENT TO DISABILITY

This new area of study became known as somatopsychology. The basis for this study is the body image concept. The body image is a complex conceptualization which we use to describe ourselves. It is one of the basic parts of the total personality and as such determines our reaction to our environment. According to Horace and English[2] the body image is the mental representation one has of his own body.

There are two aspects of the body image concept—the individual's ideal (desired) body image and the actual body image. The greater the congruity between these two images, the better the psychological adjustment of the individual; and conversely the greater the discrepancy between these two parts of the self-concept, the poorer an individual's psychological adjustment. This is very understandable. If an individual is quite short and views himself as such but has a strong ideal body image of a tall person, he is less well adjusted than he would be if his desired image were that of a short person. This is a simplistic example, but it portrays the crux of psychological adjustment to disability.

In order to adjust to the psychological impact of a disability, the body image has to change from the image of a nondisabled person to the body image of a disabled person. Early in the adjustment process the actual body image will change from that of a nondisabled person to the actual body image of a disabled person; however, for adequate psychological adjustment to the disability the ideal body image must make the corresponding adaptation. Therefore, in essence the psychological adjustment to a disability is the acceptance of an altered body image which is more in harmony with reality.

FACTORS ASSOCIATED WITH ADJUSTMENT

There are three groups of factors which determine the speed or facility with which an individual will adjust to his disability. They help an individual understand the degree of psychological impact a particular disability is having on a client and the significance of the adjustment he must undergo.

The first of these three groups of factors are those factors directly associated with the disability. Psychological effects of disabilities may arise from direct insult or damage to the central nervous system. These psychological effects are called brain syndromes and may be either acute or chronic. In this instance there are a variety of behavioral patterns which may result directly from the disability. In disabilities involving no damage to brain tissue, the physical limitations imposed by the disability may cause excessive frustration and in turn result in behavioral disorders. For example, an active outdoorsman and nature lover may experience a greater psychological impact upon becoming disabled than an individual who leads a more restricted and physically limited life, since the restrictions imposed by the disability demand a greater change in the basic life style of the outdoorsman. Therefore, factors directly associated with the disability have an important bearing upon an individual's reaction to disability.

The second group consists of those factors arising from the individual's attitude toward his disability. An individual's adjustment to his disability is dependent upon the attitudes he had prior to his disability. If his attitudes toward the disabled were quite negative and strong, he will naturally have a greater adjustment problem than an individual with a neutral or positive attitude toward disability and the disabled. A part of this attitude formation prior to the onset of his disability is dependent upon the experiences the client had with other disabled individuals and the stereotypes he developed.

The amount of fear a client experiences or emotion he expends during the onset and duration of the illness or accident leading up to the disability will determine the psychological impact of the disability. Generally, the greater the amount of emotion expended during onset, the better the psychological adjustment to the disability. If an individual goes to sleep a sighted person and awakens a blind person, his psychological reaction to the disability is much greater than if a great deal of emotion is expended during a process of becoming blinded.

The more information an individual has relating to his disability, the less impact the disability will have. If the newly disabled individual is told about his disability in a simple, straightforward, mechanistic manner, it is much easier to accept and adjust to the disability than if it remains shrouded in a cloak of ignorance and mystery. Any strangeness or unpredictable aspect of our body associated with its function immediately creates anxiety and if not clarified rapidly can result in totally debilitating anxiety. Therefore, it is important for psychological adjustment to a disability that the individual have communicated to him, in terms he can understand, the medical aspects of his disability as soon after onset of disability as possible.

When we are in strange or uncomfortable surroundings our social perceptiveness becomes keener. Social cues which are below threshold or not noticed in comfortable surroundings become highly significant to us in new, strange or uncomfortable surroundings. Upon the onset of disability the client will develop a heightened perceptiveness relative to how he is being treated by family, friends and professionals. If others start treating him in a condescending fashion and relegate him to a position of less importance, his reaction to the psychological impact of the blindness will be poor. Professionals can react to the client from an anatomical orientation (what is missing) or a functional orientation (what is left). The anatomical orientation is efficient for classification purposes but is completely dehumanizing. The functional orientation is completely individualistic and as such enhances a client's adjustment to his disability.

Perhaps a key concept in the adjustment process is the evaluation of the future and the individual's role in the future. In many physical medicine rehabilitation centers a rehabilitation counselor is one of the first professionals to see the patient after the medical crisis has passed. The purpose of this approach is to facilitate the patient's psychological adjustment. If he feels there is a potential for his regaining his independence and security, the psychological impact of the blindness will be lessened. While the counselor cannot engage in specific vocational counseling with the client, he can discuss the depth of the vocational rehabilitation program and through these preliminary counseling sessions the counselor can help the newly disabled person evaluate the roles he might play in the future.

The last factor which determines the adjustment process is based upon the individual's view of the purpose of his body and the relationship this view has with the type and extent of disability. The views individuals have of their bodies may be characterized as falling somewhere on a continuum. At one end of the continuum is the view that the body is a tool to accomplish work; it is a productive machine. At the other end is the view that the body is an esthetic stimulus to be enjoyed and provide pleasure for others. This latter concept is much the same as we have for sculpture and harks back to the philosophy of the ancient Greeks. Everyone falls somewhere on this continuum. To adequately predict the impact of a disability upon an individual, one has to locate the placement of the individual upon this continuum; then evaluate the disability in light of the individual's view of the function of his body.

As an example of the above principle consider the case in which a day laborer and a film actress sustain the same disabling injury—a deep gash across the face. Obviously, when considering the disability in conjunction with the assumed placements of these two upon the functional continuum, the psychological impact will be greater for the actress; since we have assumed the day laborer views his body almost completely as a tool to accomplish work and the disability has not impaired that function, the psychological impact of the disability upon him will be minimal. However, if the disability were changed (they both sustained severe injury to the abdomen resulting in the destruction of the musculature of the abdominal wall), the psychological impact would be reversed. In this case the actress would view her disability as minimal since it did not interfere with the aesthetic value of her body; while the day laborer's disability would be overpowering since it had substantial effects upon the productive capacity of his body.

The most obvious conclusion to be drawn from the above three factors is that the degree of psychological impact is not highly correlated with the degree of disability. This statement is contrary to popular opinion; however, disability and its psychological impact is a highly personalized event. Many counselors fall into the trap of equating degree of disability with degree of psychological impact. If the psychological impact suffered by a client is much greater than that considered "normal," the counselor will oftentimes become impatient with the client. It should be remembered that relatively superficial disabilities may have devastating psychological effects. The psychological impact of quadraplegia is not necessarily greater than the psychological impact of paraplegia or for that matter, more anatomically superficial physical disabilities.

ROLE OF DEFENSE MECHANISMS IN ADJUSTMENT

While the three groups of factors discussed above determine the length of time required for adjustment to disability, the path to adjustment is best described by defense mechanisms. Defense mechanisms are psychological devices used by all to distort reality. Often reality is so harsh it is unacceptable to us. Therefore, we distort the situation to make it more acceptable. Defense mechanisms are used to satisfy motives which cannot be met in reality, to reduce tensions in personal interactions and to resolve conflicts. To be effective they must be unconscious. They are not acquired consciously or deliberately. If they become conscious they become ineffective as defenses and other mechanisms must replace them. For the major part of the remainder of this chapter we will look at the defenses most often employed by the disabled in the general order of their use.

Denial

Denial is an unconscious rejection of an obvious fact which is too disruptive of the personality or too emotionally painful to accept. Therefore, in order to soften reality the obvious fact is denied. Immediately upon onset of disability the individual denies it happened. He denies his disability. Then, as the fact of the disability becomes so overwhelming to him that its existence can no longer be denied, there is a denial of the permanency of the disability. The newly disabled individual, while utilizing the defense of denial, will adamantly maintain that he shall be whole again. There will be a miraculous cure or a new surgical technique will be discovered.

While there are few steadfast rules in human behavior, one is that rehabilitation at best can be only marginally successful at this point. Rehabilitation cannot proceed adequately until the client accepts the permanency of the disability and is ready to cope with the condition. This is what is meant by many professionals when they say a client must "accept" his blindness or his deafness. Most clients will never accept their disability, but they should and will accept the permanence of the disability. Denial is the front line of psychological defense, but it may outlast all other defenses. It is most persistently used by persons with deafness, blindness and the plegias.

Withdrawal

Withdrawal is a mechanism which is used to reduce tension by reducing the requirements for interaction with others within the individual's environment. There are two dynamics which result from withdrawal. In order to keep from being forced to face the acceptance of the newly acquired disability, the individual withdraws. As a result of the client's changed physical condition, his social interaction is quite naturally reduced. His circle of interests as determined by friends, business, social responsibilities, church, civic responsibilities and family is drastically reduced. Thus, the client becomes egocentrically oriented until finally his entire world revolves around himself.

Rather than functioning interdependently with his environment to mutually fulfill needs as our culture demands, he is concerned exclusively with his environment's fulfilling his needs. As his world becomes more narrowed, his thoughts and preoccupations become more somatic. Physiological processes heretofore unconscious now become conscious. At this point he begins using another defense mechanism—regression.

Regression

Regression is the defense mechanism which reduces stress by avoiding it. The individual psychologically returns to an earlier chronological age that was more satisfying to him. He adopts the type of behavior that was effective at that age but now has been outgrown and has been substituted for more mature behavior—behavior which is more effective in coping with stressful situations.

As the newly disabled individual withdraws, becomes egocentric and hypochondriacal, he will regress to an earlier age which was more satisfactory. This regression may be manifested in two manners. First he may, in his regression, adopt the dress, mannerisms, speech, et cetera, of contemporaries at the age level to which he is regressing. Secondly, he may adopt the outmoded dress, mannerisms, speech, et cetera, of the earlier time in his life to which he regressed. This second manifestation of regression is considerably more maladaptive since it holds the individual out to more ridicule which, at this point in his adjustment to his disability, quite possibly will result in more emphasis on the defense mechanism of withdrawal. This would be regressive as far as the adjustment process is concerned.

If reality is harshly pushed on him and his defenses are not working, while utilizing the first three defense mechanisms he may as a last resort become highly negative of those around him and negative in general. This negativism is demonstrated as an active refusal, stubbornness, contradictory attitudes and rebellion against external demands. He may become abusive of those around him and may become destructive in an effort to act out the thwarting he is experiencing. This negativistic behavior is an indication the defense mechanisms he is employing are not distorting reality enough to allow him to adjust to his newly acquired disabled status. If, however, he is able to adjust and the defense mechanisms are effective to this point, he will employ the next defense.

Repression

Repression is selective forgetting. It is contrasted with suppression which is a conscious, voluntary forgetting. Repression is unconscious. Events are repressed because they are psychologically traumatic. As mentioned above, the attitudes the client had relative to disability and the disabled has a major bearing upon his adjustment. If these attitudes are highly negative the client will have to repress them at this point if his adjustment is to progress. Until he represses them he will be unable to accept the required new body image.

Reaction Formation

When an individual has an attitude which creates a great deal of guilt, tension or anxiety and he unconsciously adopts behavior typical of the opposite attitude, he has developed a reaction formation. In order to inhibit a tendency to flee in terror, a boy will express his nonchalance by whistling in the dark. Some timid persons, who feel anxious in relating with others, hide behind a facade of gruffness and assume an attitude of hostility to protect themselves from fear. A third and last example is that of a mother who feels guilty about her rejection of a newborn child and may adopt an attitude of extreme overprotectiveness to reduce the anxiety produced by her feeling of guilt. This example is seen more often in cases of parents with handicapped children.

In this new dependent role the disabled individual will feel a varying degree of hostility and resentment toward those upon whom he is so dependent—wife, children, relatives and so forth. Since these feelings are unacceptable he will develop a reaction formation. The manifest behavior will be marked by concern, love, affection, closeness, et cetera; all to an excessive degree.

Fantasy

Fantasy is daydreaming. It is the imaginary representative of satisfactions that are not attained in real experience. This defense mechanism quite often accompanies withdrawal. As the client starts to adjust to a new body image and a new role in life, he will develop a rich, overactive fantasy life. In this dream world he will place himself into many different situations to see how well he fits.

Rationalization

Rationalization is giving socially acceptable reasons for behavior and decisions. There are four generally accepted types of rationalization. The first is called blaming an incidental cause—the child who stumbles blames the stool by kicking it; the poor or sloppy workman blames his tools. "Sour grapes" rationalization is called into play when an individual is thwarted. A goal to which the individual aspires is blocked to him; therefore, he devalues the goal by saying he did not really want to reach this goal so much anyway. The opposite type of rationalization is called "sweet lemons." When something the individual does not want is forced upon him, he will modify his attitude by saying it was really a very desirable goal and he feels quite positive about the new condition. The fourth and last type of rationalization is called the doctrine of balances. In this type of rationalization we balance positive attributes in others with perceived negative qualities. Conversely, we balance negative attributes with positive qualities. For example, beautiful women are assumed to be dumb; bright young boys are assumed to be weak and asthenic; and the poor are happier than the rich.

The disabled individual will have to rationalize his disability to assist him in accepting the permanence of the disability. One rationalization may be that he had nothing to do with his current condition; something over which he had no control caused the disability. Another dynamic which might be observed is the adherence to the belief on the part of the client that as a result of the disability there will be compensating factors. For example, many newly blinded persons feel they will develop special competencies in other areas such as music, etc.

I once had a paraplegic client whose rationalization for his disability ran something like this: All of the men in his family had been highly active outdoors types. They all had died prematurely with coronaries. The client was a highly active outdoors type; however, now that he was severely disabled he would be considerably restricted in his activities. Therefore, he would not die prematurely. This logic resulted in the conclusion that the disability was positive and he was pleased he had become disabled. Granted, rationalization is seldom carried to this extreme in the adjustment process, but this case is illustrative of a type of thinking which must occur for good adjustment.

Projection

A person who perceives traits or qualities in himself which are unacceptable may deny these traits and project them to others. In doing so he is using the defense mechanism of projection. A person who is quite stingy sees others as being essentially more stingy. A person who is basically dishonest sees others as trying to steal from him. A person who feels inferior rejects this idea and instead projects it to others—that is, he is capable but others will not give him a chance because they doubt his ability. These are examples of projection. With the disabled person many of the feelings he has of himself are unacceptable. Therefore, in order to adjust adequately he projects these feelings to society in general. "They" feel he is inadequate. "They" feel he is not capable. "They" feel he is inferior and is to be devalued. This type of thinking, normally, leads directly into identification and compensation which are in reality the natural exits from this maze in which he has been wandering around.

Identification

The defense mechanism of identification is used to reduce an individual's conflicts through the achievement of another person or group of people. Identification can be with material possessions as well as with people. A person may derive feelings of social and psychological adequacy through his clothes ("The clothes make the man"), his sports car, his hi-fi stereo paraphenalia and so forth. People identify with larger groups in order to take on the power, prestige and respect attributed to that organization ("our team won"). This larger group may be a social club, lodge, garden club, college or professional group.

In adjustment to his disability the client will identify with a larger group. It may be a group of persons with his particular disability, an occupational group, a men's lodge, a veteran's group, et cetera. But at this point in the adjustment process, he will identify with some group in order to offset some of the feelings he has as a result of the projection in which he is engaging. If successful, the identification obviates the need to employ the mechanisms of denial, withdrawal and regression.

Compensation

If an individual's path to a set of goals is blocked and he finds other routes to achieve that set of goals, he is using the defense mechanism of compensation. A teenager is seeking recognition and acceptance from his peers. He decides to gain this recognition through sports. However, when he fails to make the team he decides to become a scholar. This is an example of compensation. Compensation brings success; therefore, it diverts attention from shortcomings and defects, thereby eliminating expressed or implied criticism. This defense mechanism is most often used to reduce self-criticism rather than external criticism. As the individual experiences successes he will become less preoccupied with anxieties relating to his disability and his lack of productivity.

Identification and compensation usually go together in the adjustment process. When the client starts using these two defenses, he is at a point at which he may adequately adjust to the new body image and his new role in life.

IMPLICATIONS FOR PROFESSIONALS WORKING WITH THE DISABLED

Almost everyone in our society views handicapping and disabling conditions from an anatomical point of view rather than functional. It is imperative that the counselor help the newly disabled view their disability functionally rather than anatomically. The client should gain an appreciation for the abilities he has left rather than classifying himself with a group based solely upon an anatomical loss.

The rehabilitation counselor should make sure the information which the client has is factual, concise and clear. He should be sure the client's perception of his disability is correct and the cause is completely understood. This understanding greatly enhances the adjustment of the client to his disability.

The client should be helped in exploring his feelings regarding the manner in which he is currently being treated by family and friends. Help him to understand the natural emotional reactions he will have resulting from his newly acquired disability; and help him to understand that the feelings of family and friends are going to be different for a period of time while they themselves adjust to his disability. You should help him to understand that negative feelings which result from his dependent role now that he has become disabled are quite natural. As such he should not repress them but should try to deal with them and look at them very objectively.

Do not fall into the trap of thinking that the degree of disability is correlated with the degree of psychological impact. Realize that each individual's disability is unique unto that individual and his reaction to his disability will be unique.

If you as a counselor are able to observe that the client is employing the defense mechanisms of denial and withdrawal, be sure to make efforts to keep him in complete touch with his environment. Allow his environment to be present for him to call upon as much as he would like without it becoming stifling and demanding in areas in which he can not meet the demands. As he becomes ego-oriented, bring in outside stimulation from news and the world at large, family, comments about family, friends, et cetera, so that he can be reminded that he should function interdependently with his environment rather than independently of his environment.

If aberrant behavior is observed which will hold him up to

ridicule as a result of regression, the counselor should point out the manner in which he is regressing. Help him to understand what he is doing; help him to understand some of the mechanics that are going on in his adjustment to disability. However, this counseling should be done in such a manner that will preserve the integrity of the defense mechanism.

Assist him in his fantasy world. If you are fortunate enough to be called in and become part of his fantasy life, be aware of the fact that he is trying on new roles to see how well he fits in these new roles and as such; he is asking you to function as a mirror for him to see how he is adjusting to the various new roles in life.

With the defense mechanism of projection, it is very difficult for him to realize that he is projecting even though it may be patently clear and obvious to you or to any other objective person that he is projecting his feelings onto these other people. Perhaps the only real role you can play here is one which is highly supportive of him and his abilities; but at the same time, he should be required to identify the people to whom he is projecting his feelings of inadequacy and inferiority. In other words, encourage the client to identify the "they" to which he refers so negatively so often.

Lastly, in summary, the most important role anyone can play in assisting a client in his adjustment to disability is to be a warm, empathic, accepting individual who is positive in his regard toward the client and one who is pragmatic in counseling and planning efforts with the client.

REFERENCES

1. *American Psychiatric Association: Diagnostic and Statistical Manual of Mental Disorders.* Washington, D. C., American Psychiatric Association, 1965.
2. Horace, H.B., and English, A.C.: *A Comprehensive Dictionary of Psychological and Psychoanalytical Terms.* New York, David McKay Company, Inc., 1966.

23

Rehabilitation Needs of the Older Adult

John G. Cull

Definition of Older Adult
Emotional Aspects of the Aging
Psychological Aspects of Aging
Employment Needs of the Aging
Social Needs of the Aging
Summary
References

DEFINITION OF OLDER ADULT

THE PURPOSE OF THIS CHAPTER is to outline some of the rehabilitation needs of older adults which might be met in the workshop environment. It will cover some of the emotional, psychological, employment and social needs of these individuals. Before looking at these specific areas, it would be appropriate to identify this segment of our population. In rehabilitation we tend to be quite exact in our functional descriptions or definitions of a disability group. For example, in mental illness there are numerous specific diagnostic categories which describe the psychological function of the individual; in cardiac involvement there is the functional heart classification; almost all state rehabilitation agencies use a rather specific range of IQ to define mental retardation, and IQ is a quantified approach to describing intellectual function; however, the term "older Americans" is filled with ambiguity. We use many other terms which are just as inadequate—the aged, the aging, senior citizens, geriatrics, golden-agers and many others. Not only are the names for this segment of our population indefinite and inadequate, the definitions are just as confusing. Almost all the definitions use age rather than *function* as the criterion. As you will recognize this is foreign to professionals involved in vocational rehabilitation since we pride ourselves on taking the humanistic or functional approach with individuals.

As a professional in rehabilitation, I prefer the term *industrial gerontology* or the *industrial geriatic*. According to Norman Sprague,[5] industrial gerontology is the study of the employment and retirement problems of middle-aged and older workers. It is the science of aging and work.

Industrial gerontology begins where age *per se* becomes a handicap to employment. Age discrimination in employment may start as early as age 35 or 40 in some industries and occupations, and it begins to take on major dimensions at age 45. Federal and state legislation imposes age discrimination in employment policies generally around the ages of 40 to 65. However, as in other disability areas of vocational rehabilitation, this condition (age) becomes a factor of concern only when it constitutes a handicap to employment.

Industrial gerontology is concerned with aptitude testing, job counseling, vocational training and placement. It is concerned with job adjustment, job assignment and reassignment, retention on the job, redesign of the work requirements, vocational motivation and mobility.

I believe the similarity between the concerns of industrial geronontology and vocational rehabilitation and the degree of overlapping in these two areas are both impressive and remarkable. So programs in industrial gerontology are highly significant to the individuals charged with responsibilities for program planning and program development in vocational rehabilitation as well as the practitioner in the field. Historically, vocational rehabilitation has been a medically oriented program. We have worked exclusively with medical disabilities which impose vocational handicaps. There are many in vocational rehabilitation who have been advocating a change in the philosophy of our profession. This change would result in our working with individuals who have a vocational handicap regardless of his physical or medical status. Recently (through P.L. 89-333, 1965) there has been a major step forward in this direction—the expansion of the definition of eligibility to include behavior disorders. This is the first nonmedical, social disorder with which we have worked. I am firmly convinced one of the next nonmedical disabilty groups we will expand our definition of eligibility to accept and serve will be the industrial geriatric. This is why I feel we should start gaining program experience through our workshop programs now.

Before discussing the specific needs of this segment of our population as outlined above, I would like to state a basic position which I feel we all accept but often forget. The similarities between any section of our population and the population as a whole are much greater than the dissimilarities. The industrial geriatric or "older American" is more like than unlike the clients on our existing case loads. Programatic changes which are needed to adapt our services to this population will be minor and tend to be changes in emphasis rather than changes in direction. Programs for the aging in workshops are completely compatible with existing service programs.

EMOTIONAL ASPECTS OF THE AGING

A very interesting trend has occurred in our culture which has resulted in creating emotional needs for the "older American"; age is no longer related to conformity behavior.[1] Traditionally we have revered our elders. In our culture we can see this reverence in the admonishments of the Old Testament. In the Indo-Iranian and Hindu cultures we can turn to the Rig Vedas, the Upanashads and the Bhagavad-Gita for the same admonishments. Since the beginning of time, cultures and societies have turned to their elders for judgments, decisions, values and mores. The elders have determined the future of the tribe, culture or society. This has been true universally until the past generation. The current generation of elders have been socially, economically and vocationally emasculated. They have become a lost generation. They grew up expecting, and with every reason to expect, to mature into a role of influence in our culture. This is a very enviable role and one generally anticipated with a degree of eagerness. To become an elder had meaning, purpose, rewards and status.

However, after the revolution in technology we now turn to younger, more aggressive, more highly trained individuals to make decisions. The demands for speed and innovation are the two factors which have robbed older people of what they viewed as a birthright. Everything which smacks of seniority is under fire —even the committee heirarchy in Congress.

The result is this lost generation of elders have become confused, disoriented, relegated to an inferior role with a great amount of condescending expressions of concern. Rather than arriving at a state which would bring status and reverence and one filled with meaning and purpose, they have been pushed to early retirement, then isolated and forgotten. No wonder many are concerned, bitter and resentful.

The most important need this group of individuals has is to feel useful. While much can be said for our new sophisticated decision-making theories, there is a great manpower pool of years of experience going to waste. This pool of manpower should be mobilized by our workshops for the benefit of both parties. While production and income supplementation will solve some of the problems of the aging, the workshop can solve many others. In workshop operations, it has been found[3] that if older workers are placed with younger retardates, the production of both groups increases and the discipline problems with the retarded youngsters are reduced. This arrangement also seems to be an effective motivating factor for the older worker. Life is becoming more meaningful for them—they are more useful. From the workshop's point of view this arrangement is beneficial since it reduces the need for intensive professional supervision and simultaneously increases production.

PSYCHOLOGICAL ASPECTS OF AGING

When we think of the psychological aspects of aging, we almost automatically think of reduced intellectual ability. Almost all research studies between Galton's in 1883 up to Lorges in 1947 have indicated there is a decline in intelligence with age. The decline was supposed to be progressive beginning after a peak at age 18 to 25. However, more recent studies indicate this is not the case. It appears as if there is a plateau established at approximately age 24 to 25. This plateau is stable until about age 70. The objections to decline in intellectual abilities center around (a) the speeded nature of the tests and the decline of the individual's reaction time as opposed to intelligence, (b) the scores being dependent upon acquired and stored knowledge and older subjects being more remote from the time of schooling and having less schooling and (c) the tests being constructed so they are more appropriate to younger subjects than older subjects. There is little if any reliable evidence that the older individual undergoes significant intellectual decline.

Testing deficits may be explained by a lack of motivation, lowered reaction time, lack of familiarity with the testing orientation, as well as the considerations above.

A second factor to consider under psychological aspects of aging is the pathological mental conditions among the aged. This factor is probably the largest precluding factor in vocational rehabilitation's accepting and serving the aging population. There are statistics which support the position that age invariably brings on mental aberrations. During the last third of a century the admission rate of geriatrics in our state hospitals has zoomed.

There are many articles now appearing in the literature which indicate the state hospital geriatric wards are serving more as human warehouses and foster homes than bona fide treatment facilities. The high rate of admissions is partially explained by social and cultural factors rather than emotional factors. Due to the removal of much of the stigma attached to mental illness, many adults have older relatives committed on the slightest of pretexts since this is a convenient solution to a social problem.

I am not trying to explain away the problems of the aging. Some are very serious and need the attention and concern of all of us; however, the problem is not of the magnitude we in vocational rehabilitation suppose. In the past we have felt the problems were insurmountable so we ignored them. The life expectancy for this attitude is indeed very short. It is incumbent on us as professionals to understand the problems of these people and mobilize our efforts to solve them.

In the psychological aspects of aging one explanation of the increased incidence of a type of mental illness lies in the role they are required to accept. The current life style in our culture leads toward older citizens feeling much less secure, unhappy, nonproductive; they generally live in a home situation in which they have at best an ill-defined role; there is a feeling of dependence rather than independence which leads to self-respect. Their future is narrowing, constricting and bleak with a diminishing health status (physical and emotional).

The last factor I will discuss in the psychological aspects of aging which is related to vocational rehabilitation is the psychological set of the older individual. All of us view ourselves as workers. If we become unemployed we still tend to view ourselves as workers and as such are capable of work. The longer we are unemployed the more narrowed and rigid our view of our capabilities of working become. While employed, our psychological set relative to our capabilities for work is highly flexible. We feel we can do our job and many variations of our job in many different locations. The longer we are out of work the more rigid our psychological set of us as workers becomes, until finally we become convinced we are no longer workers. This is very obvious in the coal miners in Appalachia: They can function only as coal miners in their local area. Since there are no jobs, they are unemployable. They no longer view themselves as workers.

This phenomenon is particularly appropriate with the aging. The longer they have been unemployed and the more they felt pushed out of their last job, the less they will characterize themselves as "a worker" or productive individual. Since the older individual has a rather strong need to be considered a useful person, but is unable to do so, his psychological adjustment to aging will be quite difficult.

The older worker can be a highly productive worker; therefore, a workshop administrator should be keenly interested in adapting and extending existing service programs.

Now, what can the workshop do? First, the workshop should modify its work adjustment program for the older client. As with other clients this should be a sequentially or graduated program providing positive, concrete feedback relative to progress and production and should require not only repetitive tasks but should include a program of graduated decision-making responsibility. Most of us in vocational rehabilitation fail to recognize the need for work adjustment training for the older worker of average intelligence with a work history. We feel he can just go back to work. In our approach to the practice of rehabilitation work, adjustment training is for the client with just the opposite qualities —young, mentally retarded and no work history—but the purpose of the work adjustment training is the same in both instances—the establishment of an appropriate psychological set. With the young retardate, we are trying to establish the self-concept of a worker; with the other worker, we are attempting to reestablish this concept.

Next, I feel workshops should extend their service programs to develop satellites in the geriatric wards of state hospitals. There are many indications that the majority of the patients on these wards are not in need of psychotherapy as much as they need redefinition of their role in society. A satellite program of a workshop can be developed which would incorporate a work adjustment training program and a re-motivation program and would provide many avenues to facilitate the psychological adjustment to aging. The establishment of a program such as this will broaden the client experience background and add depth to the clientability factor of the workshop which obviously will broaden the spectrum of subcontract work the workshop can attract. It is a basic principle of workshop administration that the more heterogeneous the clientele of a workshop the more flexible and diversified will be its negotiations for subcontract and prime contract work.

In the satellite program, which I am proposing, there should be a provision for a full array of services within the satellite for those whose maximum capabilities are at the state hospital terminal placement level as well as a built-in opportunity to progress through interim placement in the workshop and when appropriate industrial placement.

EMPLOYMENT NEEDS OF THE AGING

Employment fulfills many functions and needs for all of us. As individuals we are what we do. In our culture we are identified by what we do for a living. Our economic status, self-concept, social status, friends and community activities are to a great extent determined by our jobs. All of these factors which have direct bearing upon personality integration deteriorate in unemployment.

In the face of economic inflation, more and more concern is being expressed relative to retirement programs which provide fixed incomes. The inflationary spiral which we have had in this country for the last decade has seriously jeopardized or destroyed the stability of fixed income retirement plans.

Therefore, the employment needs of the aging are two faceted —first, employment supplies many social and psychological needs which are essential to the individual, and secondly, and more mundanely, employment needs of the aging include the provision for basic subsistence.

As I have outlined above, the older worker can be a highly positive asset to a workshop since the workshop can uniquely meet many of his needs while he is contributing to the economic stability of the workshop. The productive older worker is interested, in many cases, in supplementing his fixed retirement income; therefore, his employment needs are uniquely adapted to workshop production. His interests and vocational and production capabilities can be developed to the point of permitting the workshop to attract a diversity of subcontract work and if properly planned programs are instituted the workshop will be able to attract national industrial contract work on a long-term basis.

The workshop also can institute a program which will meet the social and psychological aspects of employment needs of older workers who have solved the problems of basic subsistence. For most bright, alert, aggressive retired persons, retirement, unless impeccably planned, soon begins to pall. The avocational pursuits which held so much attraction on the "pre" side of retirement soon become stultifying and deadly on the "post" side of retirement. Fishing, bridge, hiking and so forth soon fail to fill the void left by the demands and rewards of employment. Consequently, many retirees are looking for an opportunity to utilize the talents, abilities and proficiencies they have developed and perfected over many years of employment.

I am amazed that workshops have failed to adapt the SCORE concept (Service Corps of Retired Executives) on the local level. I feel these people represent a vast untapped reservoir of manpower in our communities. In some limited situations workshops have solicited volunteers composed of retired teachers to teach remedial subjects, but we have in our communities retired workers who were supervisors, foremen, managers and executives concerned with purchasing, marketing, production, accounting, plant layout and efficiency, and contract procurement—the same concerns we in workshop administration have. I believe a workshop administration can be highly self-serving and still meet some of the employment needs of retired workers by developing a program to utilize these people's talents in the operation, development and administration of the workshop.

They can be used on a continuing volunteer basis in areas such as remedial education, production supervision, quality control or on a consultative basis for marketing, contract procurement, et cetera. I feel this approach will gain the workshop not only improved efficiency in operations and administration but a wider base and greater degree of community support for its programs.

SOCIAL NEEDS OF THE AGING

It is difficult to separate the social needs of the aging from the other needs discussed above. Almost all of the needs outlined above have direct social implications.

The social needs of the aging, as well as other needs, are the same as for all populations. They need satisfying relationships with their peer groups, security in interpersonal relations (they need to know who they are and have a sense of identity), recognition for achievement and acceptance.

Generally the aging process is also an isolating process. As people grow old and retire from work their environment shrinks drastically until, in many instances, the individual withdraws into isolation. In this situation he becomes highly ego-oriented, selfish and preoccupied with himself and his bodily functions to the point of becoming hypochrondriacal. If the social needs of the individual continually fail to be fulfilled, this psychological and physiological deterioration will continue. Once established, this pattern of isolationism is extremely difficult to break since chronic behavior in the aged is relatively easy to establish and the drive for change and new experiences is subdued in them. Individuals in this social isolation system are so obvious or noticeable, regretfully they form the stereotype we have of the older persons. This is an unfair stereotype but as all stereotypes, it is a highly persistent image highly impervious to change.

Most of the suggestions made above regarding the extension of service programs in the workshop to meet the various needs of the aging will also meet the social needs of the aging. Perhaps a specific action the workshop could take would be the development of a service center for the aging. This action would be directed objectively at the social needs.

SUMMARY

In summary, I feel it is particularly good workshop administration to plan for a workshop to become the focal point of services to the aging population within a community. I feel:

1. The workshop should create and develop an administrative policy and an operation climate which will attract older citizens to contribute to the goals of the workshop.

2. Workshops should extend the orientation of their existing service programs to include the aging—this includes all programs from work adjustment training through terminal placement.

3. The workshop should establish satellite programs in areas with a high concentration of older nonworkers—state hospitals, senior centers and homes for the aged, et cetera.

4. The workshop should be flexible in its approach to workers. It should permit and encourage part-time workers—workers

who produce according to their own needs and schedules rather than adhering exclusively to the workshop's schedule.

5. The workshop should mobilize the retired people in the community to contribute their talents to the objectives of the workshop. In this I am advocating a local adaptation of the SCORE (Service Corps of Retired Executives).

There are several other areas in which a workshop can become involved in the needs of the aging, but I feel these are perhaps the prime areas.

REFERENCES

1. Cull, J. G.: Age as a factor in achieving conformity behavior. *Industrial Gerontology*, Spring, 1970.
2. Galton, F.: *Hereditary Genius*. New York, 1891.
3. Johndrow, R. F.: Personal communication, 1970.
4. Lorge, I.: Intellectual changes during maturity and old age. *Rev Educ Res*, Vol. 17, 1947.
5. Sprague, N.: Industrial gerontology: A definition and a statement of purpose. *Industrial Gerontology*, Spring 1970.

PART SIX

WORKING WITH OTHER PROFESSIONALS IN THE REHABILITATION PROCESS

Working with the Physician

The Psychologist and Rehabilitation

Planning For Psychological Services In Vocational Rehabilitation: A Priority Consideration

State Rehabilitation Administrators' Views on Psychological Evaluation

Working with the Rehabilitation Facility

Working with the Community

24

Working with the Physician

Leslie F. McCoy

The Role of the Counselor
Informational Needs: Evaluation and Reporting
Board Certified Versus Board Eligible
Selecting a Physician
Utilization of Existing Medical Information
The Counselor-Physician Relationship
Ethical Considerations
The Physician as a Source of Referrals and as a Referral Source
The Medical Consultant in Rehabilitation

THE PHYSICIAN is a major contributor to the rehabilitation process. He provides information on the presence and extent of physical and psychic impairments, their remediability, their probable course and their functional implications. Medical therapy lessens the level of impairment for many.

The counselor, the principal person in vocational rehabilitation, has responsibility for assuring that the physician's full potential contribution is harnessed for the benefit of each client. If only minimal physician input is utilized in the counselor's decision-making, the result will be a needlessly high incidence of poor rehabilitation results.

To permit greater specificity, this chapter has been written about the counselor-physician relationship as it exists in the state vocational rehabilitation agency setting. An understanding of this material will, however, facilitate the counselor's interacting effectively with physicians in other settings as well. Much of what is written also holds true for the counselor's relationship with dentists.

Much of the character of the counselor-physician relationship stems from the counselor being the generalist in vocational rehabilitation and the physician being the specialist. The counselor is the generalist because of his application of a wide range of subjects to the client's plan development and services. The psychological, social, educational, vocational as well as medical factors must be considered by the generalist counselor whereas the physician looking only at the medical factors is in their relationship a specialist.

THE ROLE OF THE COUNSELOR

The above concept leads us to the following important deduction as to roles: The counselor carries overall responsibility for the client's rehabilitation and therefore is the decision-making authority. The physician as a specialist is a consultant and an advisor. He has a better grasp of the facts and their implications in the medical sphere but a lesser grasp of either the facts or their implications in the nonmedical sphere. Thus, the competent counselor will outperform the physician in the field of vocational rehabilitation and their respective roles must reflect this.

Common sense dictates limitations to the application of this role statement. When various disciplines are represented on a rehabilitation team, all of whose members are knowledgeable about rehabilitation, no subject should remain the exclusive domain of any team member. Likewise, in the nonteam setting, when the medical considerations in a given case so overshadow other factors as to make them comparatively trivial, the sensible counselor will recognize that the generalist is little needed.

A final word of caution in the counselor's exercise of his prerogatives: The counselor should not substitute his own medical judgments for those of the physician. Of course over a period of time, the counselor will encounter poor medical judgments and in time often will be able to identify much of the questionable physician performance. But the wise counselor will recognize his own limitations in this highly technical field and seek additional physician advice on the questionable items rather than resorting to his decision-making prerogatives.

The responsibility which the counselor carries for the overall success of his client's rehabilitation spawns certain component responsibilities. One of these is responsibility for the adequacy of the medical support which he and his client receive. As the manager, he must assure that the amount, quality and timeliness of the physician's contribution are satisfactory. Incidentally as the public's purchasing agent, he is also responsible for value received for the tax dollars spent.

Many counselors are troubled as how to discharge this responsibility in view of their disadvantaged bargaining position relative to the medical community as described later. Many in fact discharge this responsibility poorly.

There is no denying that the counselor does not have things all his own way when holding the medical community accountable. However, a large portion of the performance failures of the medical community in serving vocational rehabilitation has nothing to do with bargaining strengths but result from communication and coordination problems, pure and simple, where all concerned would prefer to do better, once what is needed is clearly perceived. Physician performance failure of this type might more accurately be classified as counselor performance failure. More importantly, it is largely remediable by either.

INFORMATIONAL NEEDS: EVALUATION AND REPORTING

A common and serious shortcoming in physician evaluation reports is the absence of the particular medical information which the counselor needs to make his decisions. The absence of this report content is understandable when one stops to realize that the average physician knows little or nothing about the vocational rehabilitation agency, what it does, what use it will make of the information he gives and what are its informational needs. Because of their own objectives in patient care, many physicians are accustomed to record, after patient evaluation, only the diagnosis. Treatment is recorded usually as it is given. For example, the physician treating the heart attack patient will not usually record in advance in the record when he expects to get the patient out of bed, out of the hospital, back to work and with what anticipated restrictions. Such recording would serve him no useful purpose.

The solution to this physician performance failure begins with the counselor's communicating to the physician his informational needs.

In addition to the diagnosis the counselor needs to have physician guidance on:

1. What is his client's functional level? This needs to be as specific as possible. Can he be on his feet all day, climb stairs, lift; and are there limitations in amount, duration or rate?

2. Are certain work environments inappropriate to the patient's health; for example, dusty surroundings, irregular hours, proximity to heavy moving machinery?

3. What is the probable future course of this impairment; for example, indefinite stability at present level, frequent periods of relapse with good function in between, inexorable deterioration leading to bedfast status or death in three to six years?

4. Can therapy partially or completely remove the impairment or halt its advancement, and, if so, to what degree?

It is acknowledged that the agency's medical form may indicate the informational needs. This is an insufficient communication, however, to many busy physicians who spend most days struggling to keep up with their scheduled work and without time to reflect on where their contribution fits into the scheme of things. A personal note attached to the form or the evaluation authorization by the counselor to the physician highlighting a particular informational need regarding this client will help clarify for the physician what is wanted in this case and, over a period of time, clarify for him what is commonly needed by counselors. Other techniques for getting these points across are suggested later.

One obstacle to quality medical evaluation and reporting is the amount of time the physician has or chooses to expend to render this service. His time demand problems may cause him to adopt the attitude, "I'll do what I can for them in the next fifteen minutes." The counselor can lessen this quality problem somewhat by seeing to it that the time the physician spends with the client is not partially consumed with tasks that the counselor

Working with the Physician

himself could have performed. Reports of previous examinations, recent hospitalizations, laboratory and x-ray work should be obtained by the counselor and attached to the service request.

Obtaining these reports will not only save the physician time but also will improve the quality of his evaluation inasmuch as he seldom will take time to request these reports from their various sources on his own initiative. Additionally, such reports contain evidence he would not have had otherwise which will increase the validity of his conclusions.

In many agencies, procedures call for the counselor to ask certain screening-type health history questions of his client. The physician may then confine his questioning to those subject areas wherein the screening questions elicit possible clues of abnormalities. If this pattern is used by one's agency, the counselor should, in addition to recording the screening history specifically, call the physician's attention by personalized note to client answers which may point to abnormalities to assure that they are not overlooked.

Regardless of the cause, the counselor must seek a solution to the problem posed by inadequate evaluations or reports by physicians, particularly if the physician is one whose services are important to the agency; for example, the only ophthalmologist within twenty miles or a general examiner used by many of the client group.

An initial approach can be to have the agency representative, usually the counselor or the office's medical consultant, call on the physician and briefly explain the rehabilitation program and its importance to society and the handicapped, what use it makes of the medical data provided and, specifically, what additionally is needed that it has not generally gotten from this physician. Every effort is made at this point to assist the physician to bring his evaluation and reporting up to standard including bringing clients back for additional examinations. The objective is to obtain a fully adequate physician participant for the program. Emphasis in the discussion is on meaningful services for the client and what the agency can do to assist the physician in his role rather than on agency rules, bureaucratic procedure and physician shortcomings to date.

When an adequate attempt fails to result in satisfactory performance by a physician, the counselor has an obligation to no longer use public funds to purchase services from him. In reaching such decisions the agency's regular medical consultant should be a major participant.

The decision to discontinue use of a particular physician must not be ducked when his services to the agency are irremediably unsatisfactory, yet it must be taken thoughtfully and carefully. "Governmental action" against a colleague can arouse emotional support for him among his fellow physicians who may be much valued by the agency. The agency must not be, or even seem to be, capricious in such decisions. Mere agency inconvenience resulting from a low level of cooperation by a physician may not be as troublesome as the consequences of never using him provided that the agency is able to get good quality services to its clients by this practitioner.

The decision not to use may also be influenced by the available alternatives. For example, a rather frequent use of second evaluations by an internist for clients with more complicated medical problems may be preferable to discontinuing all use of a practitioner who is the only one available within reasonable distance for a significant portion of a counselor's territory.

Once the decision is made, the agency medical consultant should assist in minimizing the possible resulting hostilities and in dealing with future clients so as to take the agency out of the position of appearing to judge the performance of the physician as a practitioner working with his own patients. For indeed, the latter may be exemplary even though his service to vocational rehabilitation may be too unsatisfactory to continue.

A parallel and less troublesome question is what the role of the counselor should be in steering clients to use a physician whose services to agency and clients are highly satisfactory. I believe the answer to this is, Yes, he should steer selected clients.

There are, however, real advantages in having a client evaluated by his regular physician if he has one. This examiner often is able to evaluate more adequately this client because of his observation of him over a longer period of time and knowledge of past medical events. Particularly for treatment, the client may much prefer his usual physician and indeed decline to be sent elsewhere.

The counselor also seeks to receive and serve referrals from all of the community's physicians. Confining his utilization of physicians to a small percentage deprives the counselor of a closer working relationship and the understanding of his program by other potential physicians.

When the client has no ties to any physician, the counselor ordinarily will make the referral to a physician whom he knows provides the agency with particularly helpful evaluations.

For certain specialized medical problems, the importance of specialty competence for achieving the most effective evaluation or treatment outweighs the importance of use of only the generalist physician, even though the latter may perceive the client more comprehensively, have an existing and productive relationship with him and be conveniently nearby. In these situations, the agency's responsibility is to have the services rendered by the appropriate specialist. Happily, the great majority of physicians fully subscribe to referring work which others can do better on to these others and will decline to undertake it themselves.

BOARD CERTIFIED VERSUS BOARD ELIGIBLE

A helpful clue as to the competence of the physician specialist is his certification by the American Board. Certification by this Board requires a period of generally three to five years of postgraduate training in the specialty followed by a written and a performance examination. The term "Board—eligible" refers to the person who has completed the required training but has not yet taken (or has failed) the examination. Such persons generally are regarded as also well qualified.

Standards specifying qualifications of specialists, established by rehabilitation agencies, hospitals or others, often will group Board-certified and Board-eligible physicians together in one class.

A universal limitation in the prediction of the probable performance of a professional, based upon his qualifications, is the failure of standards to take into account such key matters as the personal qualities of the practitioner classified. Thus, in medicine as in other professions, there are individuals with less formal study or experience who nevertheless have great competency resulting from careful, extensive reading; full learning from the experience they have had; and systematic approach to problems. There, of course, are certified specialists with sloppy work habits, limited study since certification and so forth. The observant counselor will identify in time the most competent physicians in his geographic area through his own experience in using them and through the guidance of his agency's medical consultant.

SELECTING A PHYSICIAN

Many clients are not sophisticated in obtaining medical services. They may have little basis for choice of a physician especially when a specialist is needed. The counselor must provide the needed guidance and assistance. Commonly, he will make the arrangements and set up the appointment.

In joining with his client to choose a specialist he should give considerable weight to the one suggested by the examining physician. Of course, agency standards for qualifications for specialists, adverse agency experience with a given individual or the advice of the agency's medical consultant may bring about a different selection. Departures from the preference expressed by either the client or the client's physician are sufficiently sensitive to dictate the counselor's seeking guidance from his agency's medical consultant.

The preceding remarks pertain to the situation wherein the client is not under current *treatment* by a physician.

When a client is under treatment by a physician and the counselor considers sending him elsewhere for agency-sponsored care, a major question of propriety arises. It is highly inadvisable for a client to be under the simultaneous care of two physicians for the same problems unless they are carefully coordinating their plans of care. Interruption of an active physician-patient relationship by an agency raises a medical ethics question for the new physician brought into the picture. Such action is occasionally in order however. The counselor contemplating such a move should discuss it thoroughly with his regular medical consultant and carefully follow his detailed advice if this step is decided upon.

This admonition against needlessly switching physicians to provide treatment for the client does not extend to the area of the client evaluation. An agency, like an insurance company or a prospective employer, is at liberty to use its chosen medical examiner to evaluate its client. In the presence of a current doctor-patient relationship the decision to use a different examining physician carries an added responsibility for the agency and its examining physician to not undermine needlessly the existing doctor-patient relationship. Such unwarranted undermining might occur, for example, when the agency suggests a diagnosis or course of treatment different from that of the attending physician even though the opinion of competent members of the medical profession support the methods utilized by the patient's physician.

UTILIZATION OF EXISTING MEDICAL INFORMATION

Many disabled clients have a considerable volume of existing medical information on file with various clinics, hospitals, laboratories and physicians whom they have previously visited. Ideally, all this medical data should be reviewed by the agency and the physician examining this client for additional insights into the client's health and behavior. In actuality a complete review of all this data may not be practical. The press of work on the counselor, the necessity to move the client promptly along in his rehabilitation and, in some cases, the sheer volume and inaccessibility of old medical records dictate a compromise between the ideal and the practical. Judgment must be exercised to select the medical records to request.

With regard to hospitalizations, information on an admission within the last six to eight months should be sought. When admitted to the hospital, a patient almost always is given certain screening-type evaluations; for example, he gets a physical examination, a urinalysis, a blood count, sometimes a chest x-ray and certain blood chemistry. Thus, the admission medical routine is commonly a fairly rich source of information on his current general health status in addition to what it will reveal in regard to the complaint for which he was hospitalized.

Judgment is needed as to whether to ask for old medical records for hospitalizations more than six to eight months ago. Old records are not likely to be of much help if the hospitalization was for a type of disorder or procedure that seldom has residual health problems; for example, appendectomy, herniorrhaphy, hemorrhoidectomy, uncomplicated pneumonia or childbirth. On the other hand, a hospital record may be quite useful to the agency even for hospitalizations as long ago as eight to ten years if the admission was for a disorder commonly of long-range importance; for example, for a nervous breakdown (possibly a clue to a psychotic episode or a fragile psyche) or a colon resection (for a cancer, possibly). For most hospitalizations an intermediate cut-off date for requesting records between these time extremes is appropriate.

Many hospitals prepare a one- to two-page summary for their own use of each patient's most significant findings and events during his hospitalization. The counselor may assume that this document will be adequate for reflecting the level of detail about this hospitalization which he and his agency need.

When the patients are discharged from the hospital, their medical case records are sent for storage to the medical records library. All but the small hospitals employ a medical record librarian. She is the contact point for obtaining medical data. She is thus an important individual for the counselor to get to know since she significantly can influence his success in getting medical data. Her willingness to act promptly upon his authenticated requests for data, to reproduce or facilitate his reproducing parts of records or to track down missing record components make her a key figure to him.

If a hospital regularly does not prepare a discharge summary and the hospital is located in the counselor's community, he may elect to go to the hospital to review the client's old hospital case record and select those items to be duplicated for use by his medical consultant and physicians who will be seeing the client. The following are examples of items to select: the physician's report of the medical history and physical examination obtained upon admission; report of surgery; report of the pathologist's examination of tissue and abnormal laboratory or x-ray finding reports. Hospital records are too bulky and full of information useless to the counselor to warrant the time and expense of duplicating the whole record.

As the counselor grows in his understanding of medicine, he will develop considerable judgment regarding which items to duplicate as he pages through the hospital case record. Before this level of judgment has been reached, he often will be able to get helpful advice from the medical record librarian, an intern or nurse at the hospital.

If the counselor writes the hospital for information rather than visiting it, the medical record librarian, sometimes with the advice of the patient's physician, will give a simple statement about the admission or choose those records to duplicate and send. There may be a charge for this service.

Most hospitals, clinics and physicians will not release any medical information about a patient unless the request is accompanied by a signed authorization by the patient. Therefore, the counselor who realizes as he hears his client's story that he may wish to request existing medical information routinely should explain the need for a signed release to his client and get an authorization from him.

In directing requests for existing medical information to clinics or physicians, it is important that the counselor be as specific as possible as to what he is trying to learn. For example, a request as to whether the patient had a definitely established diagnosis of epilepsy and which drugs had been used with what resulting level of control is preferable to a simple request for medical information. The latter type inquiry might be answered by the physician by his providing data about a recent hernia repair, conceivably not even mentioning the history of seizures which currently were infrequent and not regarded by the physician as particularly important at this time.

In as inexact a science as the practice of medicine, inevitably there will be instances of differences of physician opinion about a given client. In some of these instances, the circumstances will permit the agency's medical consultant to reach a decision as to who is correct. One physician may have had the benefit of knowledge of highly significant developments occurring since the first physician reached his conclusion. A conflict may be about a highly specialized medical problem in a subject area where one is clearly much more knowledgeable than the other.

In those common instances wherein the circumstances do not permit the agency medical consultant to decide with any assurance which opinion is more nearly right, the counselor will arrange for a third physician's opinion. This third examiner should be selected carefully for his competence in the subject area. The counselor should provide him with all available medical information including the differing opinions of the previous examiners.

Competent physicians may reach conflicting opinions; such differences are not necessarily evidence that one or the other is incompetent. Many judgments in medicine must be based on equivocal evidence because the ultimate in conclusive tests for many disorders await future scientific discovery.

THE COUNSELOR-PHYSICIAN RELATIONSHIP

It seems advisable to comment on several matters that currently affect the climate for counselor-physician relationships. The following comments are the writer's opinions, colored by membership in the "fraternity" at former days of clinical practice. They are based on generalizations that will not be true for numerous individual counselor-physician relationships. Considering the above limitations, the question may arise as to why they are being included. I discuss them because I think they often affect how the physician and the counselor will relate to each other and the physician to the vocational rehabilitation program. I think that partial understanding that these factors are operating causes many counselors to be reticent, even apologetic, in portraying to the physician the agency's full requirements on his time and talents. This compromises the effectiveness of both the counselor and the physician and, of course, the program as a consequence.

Generally, physicians are highly supportive of the concept of citizens being self-sufficient and, therefore, embrace vocational rehabilitation program goals. It follows that the counselor should exploit opportunities to make physicians aware that getting persons out of dependency and back to the highest practical level of self-sufficiency is the purpose of this program. Services to his clients are for this objective. This is a powerful force to make vocational rehabilitation attractive to many physicians.

A force exerting an opposite effect stems from the common lack of deep understanding by many physicians of the complexities creating poverty and dependency, even including the effects of physical incapability. In short, many physicians are not well grounded in sociology or the behavioral sciences; these subjects are not prominent in their school curriculum or their subsequent reading.

Realization of the frequency of an attitude by physicians that the poor and the dependent are of limited worth will stand the counselor in good stead. He will anticipate the possibility of some problems in getting certain of his clients established in a solid physician-patient relationship and be resourceful in minimizing these. At the same time, he will not permit this to block up his relationship with such physicians, perceiving it as an area of limited physician's understanding rather than as an expression of mercenary greed or of snobbery.

As this book goes to press we are in a "tight" physician labor market. Exploding medical technology is spawning new treatment methods to offer which take physician time. Rising consumer expectancy, the aging population and other causes for increased demands for health services leave the physician in what may appear to be a desirable situation but is often quite the contrary. He cannot meet the demands for his time. Many, perhaps most, physicians are working much longer hours than they would choose, often 25 to 50 percent longer than the usual counselor.

Many physicians currently view government medical programs with some reservations. Government sponsorship of patients' medical costs seems to many doctors to herald erosion of personal self-responsibility so strongly embraced by them as the basis for a healthy society. Government regulations accompanying cost subsidy to health service consumers grind away at their accustomed patterns of practice and individual decision-making. Is it really progress? They wonder. Many will perceive vocational rehabilitation as another component of government entry into the health care field.

Government fees always have not kept up with rates paid by the private sector. At this writing, rehabilitation agency fees are running well back among government fees. This is occurring at a time when most physicians must turn down some of the work requested of them.

Among the physician's tasks, the performing of physical examinations appears less interesting than most things he does. To do problem-solving for sick patients has considerably more appeal to him. To the extent that the counselor permits the physician to perceive the client's health and desirability evaluation as a perfunctory administrative requirement rather than a key service which will constitute the main basis for several of the major vocational rehabilitation decisions, the counselor can expect these evaluations to have low priority and uninspired execution by the doctor.

Many physicians, like many professionals in various fields, are quite sensitive to any implications that the quality of their practice is questionable. This sensitivity is heightened when such a judgment appears to emanate from a nonphysician or a government agency. This situation creates a need for awareness and careful handling when the agency and the counselor representing it does not follow the physician's recommendations. Of course, the necessity to depart from some or all of a physician's recommendations arises fairly commonly for reasons other than any question of his competence. These include lack of feasibility of the client as a vocational rehabilitation prospect, client refusal, agency policy on subsidizing certain medical procedures and irrelevance to the rehabilitation plan among others. In other instances a question of the wisdom of the medical recommendation is raised by the agency's medical consultant and another opinion is sought.

The physician is a very important man to the patient with a

major illness. He is accorded considerable status by society generally; the counselor knows this. For many counselors, this realization somewhat hampers achieving the most fruitful counselor-physician relationship. The sense of lack of psychological parity between them felt by the counselor tends to undermine the relationship being one between two professionals, each with a contribution to make. The counselor will of course want to afford the doctor the esteem his position deserves but he must not abdicate his own role nor will the well-adjusted physician expect him to.

Perhaps all the potential hazards described above appear to constitute a formidable array of pitfalls awaiting the counselor who ventures into the medical community. How can he hope to effectively harness the potential contribution of the physician if he faces such odds! The answer to this question comes from the actual experience of counselors in dealing with the medical community. The counselor confidently can expect to succeed. The objectives of his program, once understood, are most attractive to physicians. Further, almost all physicians have a strong sense of service which will come into play when the importance of the vocational rehabilitation program is made apparent to them. The dedicated effective counselor attracts the respect of the physician even as he does that of other fellow citizens. The physician's role in rehabilitation can be of absorbing interest to him if the counselor takes that extra step which permits the physician to see his contribution take its place with others in producing successful client outcome.

Thus the competent counselor need feel little anxiety that his relationship with most physicians will be unsatisfactory. However, if he understands something of the larger arena which can influence this relationship, he should fare somewhat better.

ETHICAL CONSIDERATIONS

Physicians have a deeply rooted and rather elaborate code of ethics governing many aspects of how they shall behave professionally. Most physicians take this code seriously and may be offended by actions by their colleagues or outsiders which transgress this code. A few of its tenants will be brought into play as the counselor serves the client who is also the physician's patient. Knowledge by the counselor of several of these points will enable him to avoid inadvertent problems.

Anything told the physician in his professional capacity by his patient is presumed confidential. All medical information about his patient also is held as confidential by the physician. The profession regards the above as within the prerogative of the patient to divulge or conceal regardless of how apparent it may seem to others that the patient would be better served if selected disclosures were made.

Some physicians will presume patient concurrence in sharing patient information with a counselor whose help the patient has voluntarily sought and will tell him what they can which they think will help. Other physicians will ask for a "release of information request" signed by the client before passing on such information. In either case the physician will expect the counselor to observe the same rules of disclosure on information which he has passed. Failure of the counselor to do so will compromise greatly his success in enjoying a free exchange of information and its interpretation with the physician thereafter.

Use of medical information in administrative reporting, research and placement of it on file in the counselor's office, thus available to secretaries and associates, is not regarded as a transgression. However, associates are expected to read this information only on a bona fide "need-to-know" basis and must observe the same security against use other than in the client's service.

Ethics constrain physicians' criticizing each other's competence except in accordance with prescribed rules designed to protect physicians from ill-informed and unwarranted judgments by colleagues. The consideration here is that patient confidence is a vital ingredient in the physician's successful handling of many disorders, and this is not to be undermined without adequate cause.

The counselor is well advised to adopt this ethic as his own in his relationship with the medical community and his clients. If he must guide clients away from agency-sponsored medical services by a given physician or resolve a conflict of medical opinion, his explanation to his client should be made with this consideration in mind.

A third consideration in ethics of occasional importance to the counselor is that a physician is not to undertake management of a patient who is still under the care of another physician. The consideration here, of course, is that the simultaneous and uncoodinated management of a patient by two or more physicians is fraught with possibilities for adverse consequences for the patient such as drug overdose, incompatible treatment regimens and so forth.

This principle will be a consideration in those very occasional instances wherein very competent examiners and the agency medical consultant are in agreement that if a given physical restoration regimen is to be purchased by the agency it should be provided by a different physician than the one currently treating the impairment. The handling of this situation should be by the agency medical consultant.

More commonly this principle becomes a consideration for the counselor due to an oversight by him. He has had the client examined by a generalist or a specialist other than the treating physician and has received recommendations for a medical treatment program. The counselor proceeds to authorize and arrange for this treatment. The existence of a current medical treatment program by another physician is overlooked.

A situation arises somewhat related to the last two ethics principles described above when the counselor exercises insufficient discretion in reviewing with and interpreting medical data to his client. It is very easy in interpreting this technical data to a client, who may have little background to facilitate understanding, to appear to be saying something quite different from what was said by the treating physician. This admonition is included here not to suggest that the counselor never amplify or reinforce physician explanations to the patient but rather to sensitize him to remain alert that he and the physician do not pull in opposite directions either in fact or as perceived by the client because of the use of different terms, different analogies, et cetera.

THE PHYSICIAN AS A SOURCE OF REFERRALS AND AS A REFERRAL SOURCE

The counselor will find in the physician more than a needed service resource; the physician is also a potentially rich source for good referrals. Commonly the physician is the first to know when disability strikes since one of the victim's first actions is to seek medical care.

At this early time the disabled person may have numerous resources to facilitate rehabilitation which will fade by a later date. He may have tenure on his job and an employer expectation that he will return. He may still have the psychological posture of self-sufficiency and a like expectation of him by his family as well as some economic resources, insurance, work skills and so forth.

Thus, the counselor will want to actively cultivate the physician as a referral source. He will be able to reciprocate for such referrals by assisting the physician in his role through occasional agency sponsorship of medical evaluation, treatment or hospitalization of client patients. Additionally, the counselor's capability to assist the patient generally will be most welcome by the physician.

The counselor should try to assure that physicians in his area know the basic elements of the vocational rehabilitation program and how to get their patients served. The heavy work schedule of most physicians complicates the counselor's efforts to get these points across. Written descriptions of the program often go unread in the avalanche of the physician's mail. Personal calls by the counselor to the physician at his office to explain vocational rehabilitation and invite his referrals will reach most physicians. The counselor skilled in public speaking may gain considerable understanding of his program by giving a concise, brief and hard-hitting presentation before the hospital staff meeting or the county medical society.

When a physician first opens his office in a community, he is less busy than most will be later. He also is then striving to identify with his new community. This is a particularly appropriate time for the counselor to meet with him, perhaps more than once, to build understanding and a relationship that will last after the busier days arrive. This underoccupied physician may particularly welcome referrals at this time and unattached patients may be properly referred to him by the counselor if the new physician is qualified. His accessibility for prompt appointments may be a welcome change from what the counselor has been experiencing heretofore in trying to get client appointments in the tight medical labor market.

In the course of conducting business concerning clients, the counselor should watch for opportunities to help each physician to better understand the vocational rehabilitation program through submitting notes, letters, follow-up reports and so forth to him.

A particularly fruitful opportunity arises whenever the counselor is serving a client in whom the physician has an interest, a patient the physician has referred or for whom he has performed a service at vocational rehabilitation's request sufficient to have an interest in the outcome.

The counselor should acknowledge referrals promptly and drop additional notes to the physician when he accepts or rejects the client for service (stating why in the latter instance). Additionally, he should let the physician know rather promptly when there is a major development in the case, such as when the client is sponsored for college, employed, closed unrehabilitated or if he drops out.

Over a period of time, the physician receiving this kind of feedback from the counselor will develop fairly accurate understanding as to what services vocational rehabilitation offers and what types of cases constitute good referrals.

THE MEDICAL CONSULTANT IN REHABILITATION

There is one physician with whom the counselor has a special relationship which warrants special comment. This is the agency's regular medical consultant. This physician is usually a part-time employee of the agency who meets periodically with the counselor to consider with him the client's medical factors in the counselor's case load. He assists in interpreting the medical reports and their rehabilitation implications, in planning for client evaluation or treatment and in evaluating the quality and adequacy of the medical services provided the agency's clients.

The consultative session will be much more fruitful if the counselor carefully prepares for it each time. The ingredients of his preparation include reviewing the cases to be discussed so that the facts are fresh in his mind. He should assure that the medical and other reports of work which have been completed are in the case file for ready reference. He must have thought out what his specific questions for the consultant are about each client. He will want to know the aspects of agency policy which may bear on the discussions. He should have thought through to the extent that available information permits what the rehabilitation plan and the vocational objective for each client are likely to be.

This quality of preparation by the counselor will save much valuable time for both men, assure that the dialogue takes advantage of all the evidence available and help assure that significant points which should have been the subject of discussion are not recognized only after the session has terminated. The counselor will commonly open the discussion on each case to be examined with a concise review of key points concluding with his questions.

The roles suggested for the counselor and for the physician earlier in this chapter also pertain here, although as the consultant becomes increasingly knowledgeable about the whole rehabilitation process and the counselor gains experience in medical factors, the dividing line between roles becomes less distinct.

In the continuing relationship between the counselor and his physician-consultant, the counselor should aim to continually upgrade his colleague's understanding of the total rehabilitation process, the counselor's role and those portions of agency policy which potentiate the consultant's performance.

The consultant should, in addition to assisting with the medical factors of individual cases, give conscious attention to the continued growth of the counselor in understanding the common medical factors relating to his operation and their effective application in rehabilitation. The counselor should encourage the physician to serve as teacher as well as case consultant.

The counselor also should recognize the value which the consultant can be to the agency in providing liaison and building rapport with the medical community, resolving points of friction, interpreting each to the other and personally handling sensitive points in counselor-physician relationships.

Much of the content of this chapter is little more than common sense which the astute counselor will himself recognize as he gains experience. Perhaps the preceding remarks, however, can hasten his acquisition of understanding of these issues and advance the date when his clients will be reaping the full benefit of an effective counselor-physician relationship.

25

The Psychologist and Rehabilitation

Wayne S. Gill

The Psychologist as a Rehabilitation Specialist
The Traditional Role of the Psychologist in the Rehabilitation Program
Contents of the Psychological Evaluation
Making Referrals for Psychological Testing
How Testing Services Are Provided
Vocational Evaluation and the Psychologist
Innovations in Rehabilitation and Psychology
Group Treatment/Training Approaches
Summary
References

WHILE IT IS TRUE that "Psychology is as old as the inquiring, self-concious mind of man"[15] psychology as a profession is of rather recent vintage. The American Psychological Association, for example, grew from a membership of only 893 in 1929 to a present membership of over 30,000.

Psychology is at one time a scholarly discipline, a scientific field and a professional activity. Its overall function is the scientific study of human behavior and related mental processes. As a scholarly discipline, it represents a major field of study in academic institutions. As a science, its focus is on research through which investigators collect, quantify, analyze and interpret data describing human and animal behavior. As a profession, psychology involves the practical application of knowledge, skills and techniques to the solution of human problems. This professional role provides an opportunity to enhance the dignity and worth of the individual human being, increases man's understanding of himself and others and thereby contributes to the human welfare.[4]

Many people erroneously believe that psychologists work primarily in the field of mental illness and deviant behavior, often confusing psychology with psychiatry, a medical specialty. While some psychologists, particularly clinical psychologists, deal with abnormal behavior, the concerns of psychology are considerably more diverse.

Historically, psychology began in the classroom as a philosophical approach to understanding behavior and in the laboratory as a scientific approach. Now psychologists work in various social, institutional and industrial settings, as well as schools, community agencies, mental health clinics and private industries. Some psychologists function primarily as scientists and scholars; they may function in academic and research areas. Other psychologists work in the applied specialties and may function as clinical psychologists, counseling psychologists or in such areas as industrial psychology, consumer psychology or related areas.

Statistically, about 30 percent of psychologists listed with the APA consider themselves as clinical, 20 percent as school psychologists, 15 percent in other categories. Forty percent are employed mainly by colleges and universities, 12 percent by other schools, 11 percent by clinics, hospitals and medical schools, and others by government agencies and private industry. About 6 percent of psychologists are self-employed, however, less than 3 percent of all psychologists work in the area of mental deficiency and only 2.5 percent are engaged in programs for the physically handicapped.[2] The psychologists most often associated with vocational rehabilitation work are counseling or clinical psychologists.[4]

To insure that the psychologists who perform public services are adequately trained, most states have restricted the use of the title "psychologists" by those in independent practice to individuals whose training and experience have met certain standards as prescribed by law. There are now laws to license or certify psychologists in forty-two states and six provinces. Eight states, the District of Columbia and the Province of British Columbia have nonstatutory certification programs.

Standards set by the profession and by most state laws define the qualified professional psychologist as one with a doctoral degree in psychology and at least one year of supervised experience in the practice of psychology.

THE PSYCHOLOGIST AS A REHABILITATION SPECIALIST

There is a rapidly expanding field of common concern between rehabilitation workers and psychologists who have special interest and training in dealing with handicapped workers. These common concerns have developed with the increasing complexity of society and the world of work along with increased philosophical attention to the person as a biopsychosocial being.

Not to be ignored in these changes is the influence of significant legislation. The 1943 Amendments to the Vocational Rehabilitation Act broadened the scope of the rehabilitation program and, for the first time, extended services to the mentally ill and mentally retarded as well as to the physically handicapped. While having the salutary effect of opening the door of rehabilitation to thousands of incarcerated mental patients and mentally retarded individuals, the broadened scope of rehabilitation carried with it the "medical model" concept originally designed for persons with physical handicaps. The medical model concept implies that the etiology of the deviant behavior is to be found within or inside the individual. The unusual or strange behavior is regarded as a symptom of illness or disease which the person has and for which he should be treated by a medical doctor.

Treatment in the medical ideology consists of various types of therapies. Many advances have been made over the years and such approaches as psychosurgery, insulin coma therapy and incarceration have been replaced by other approaches. Now the psychotropic drugs, electroconvulsive therapy and various forms of psychotherapy are all that remain of traditional treatment. A variety of activity therapies have been introduced, which reflect the thinking of the "sociopsychological model."

Albee[1] charges that the illness explanation of psychopathology supports the forces of reaction and delays necessary social changes that would prevent emotional distress. He argues that if mentally disturbed persons suffer from unknown and undiscovered illness, then the strategy for action is to discover the cause of the disease. If on the other hand, as he contends, they have been damaged by hostile and evil social environments, then we must change the "dehumanizing forces of society." Szasz[13] calls mental illness a myth and states that mental symptoms refer to a patient's communication about himself, others and the world about him. Mowrer[11] insists that "the primary, basic cause of psychopathology is deliberate, choice mediated behavior of a socially disapproved, reprehensible nature which results in emotional disturbance and insecurity." Albee[1] supports this view by contending that emotional disorders are acquired defects in social interaction and social participation. Evidence continues to accumulate from the laboratory, from psychoanalysis and from psychotherapy that conditions influencing the stability and strength of the child's social world "have profound effects on the rate and kind of subsequent emotional disorder."

The sociopsychological model conceives of abnormal phenomena as coming from the outside. A basic concept is that the person and his current environment are interdependent. The axiom is that the individual responds to his environment and when emotional disturbance results, they are not due to internal illness but to inability to cope with the stresses and strains of living. Furthermore, "problems" with people or the demands of one's responsibilities should not be labeled "Diseases."

In the midst of this raging controversy, there have developed some rather innovative programs which have won at least temporary acceptance in rehabilitation circles. In fact, subsequent amendments of the Vocational Rehabilitation Act of 1954 have reflected the efficacy of the sociopsychological approach through research and demonstration programs and the institution of graduate training programs for psychologists with emphasis in rehabilitation.

The 1968 Amendments to the Vocational Rehabilitation Act have continued to underscore the validity of this interactional concept of mental disorders by broadening the definition of eligibility for vocational rehabilitation services to include behavioral disorders. The definition of behavioral disorders for purposes of the act is based upon descriptions of faulty interaction between the individual and his environment.

The implication of this trend in both rehabilitation and psychology for the professionals in these two fields lies in the orientation of the communication between counselor and psychologist. Under the medical model approach to consultation it was valid for the psychologist to be primarily interested in categorizing behavior. As we have moved from the medical model to the sociopsychological model, the role of the psychologist in the rehabilitation setting has changed to a primary concern for describing behavior in the context of the individual's environment.

THE TRADITIONAL ROLE OF THE PSYCHOLOGIST IN THE REHABILITATION PROGRAM

Perhaps the most traditional role of the applied psychologist is that of the "tester." Certainly, in rehabilitation circles, the psychologist has been mostly as someone who gives tests and writes reports on his findings. This, still, is a legitimate, though certainly not exclusive, role of the rehabilitation psychologist.

The psychological evaluation should serve at least three purposes: (a) to help the client learn about his own assets and liabilities, his interests and his capacities; (b) to help the counselor "tune in" on the specific individuality of his client, to understand him sufficiently to be able to plan intelligently with him in his efforts to move toward rehabilitation and independent living, and (c) to establish eligibility in specific disability groups such as mental retardation or behavior disorder.

Psychological testing services are definitely needed when (a) mental retardation is suspected, (b) behavioral disorders are suspected, (c) serious emotional problems such as anxiety or depression are thought to be present, (d) when the vocational goal selected by the client seems unrealistic and efforts at modifying the goal through counseling are unsuccessful, (e) when long-range training such as a college or university program is involved, or (f) when the rehabilitation plan calls for a relatively large expenditure of funds.

It should be added parenthetically that in many states the counselor himself is expected to administer and evaluate certain tests of mental capacity and personality traits within the normal range. The amount of testing that an individual counselor does will depend upon his training and experience, the amount of time he has available for testing and the policy of the rehabilitation agency with whom he is employed. However, according to Hardy and Cull[7] whether or not the counselor is doing psychological evaluation, he should be familiar with the instruments being used.

CONTENTS OF THE PSYCHOLOGICAL EVALUATION

The fact that most clinical psychologists have traditionally received their training in mental hospitals and clinics working in treatment programs primarily associated with psychiatry often makes them ill-equipped to produce an adequate evaluation for a rehabilitation agency. Understanding, however, the purpose of the evaluation in a rehabilitation framework, the psychologist can more adequately concentrate on those areas of primary interest to the rehabilitation counselor. The counselor generally has little interest in psychoanalytic concepts such as "libidinal forces" or "intrapsychic conflicts"; he is obviously most interested in the client's interpersonal skills, his ability to learn new jobs, his emotional stability and his motivation to follow-through on a vocational plan.

Channels of communication must first be opened between the counselor and the psychologist; the formal report of findings should routinely be supplemented with person-to-person conferences.

The psychological report should usually deal with the ten areas described below; it follows that interviews and testing must be sufficiently comprehensive to allow the report to deal in detail with each area.

1. *Review of Background Data.* This review should include information on the client's family history, age, physical limitations (if any) and reason for referral to the psychologist.

2. *Educational History.* This history should include not only

how many years the client attended school but should reflect the seriousness of his efforts, his attendance record and any additional vocational training which he may have gained.

3. *Work History*. This section should include the types of jobs he has had; the seriousness of his work efforts and any part-time work or hobbies which may be pertinent to present vocational goals.

4. *Intellectual Ability*. This should be measured by appropriate tests (individual and group) with both verbal and performance areas being reported. In instances where the subject is bilingual or has a language barrier (such as deafness) care must be exercised that the subject is not unduly penalized. It is obvious, though not always recognized, that inability to speak or write English is a function which may be entirely independent from general intelligence. A comparison of verbal and performance scores may give valuable data which may affect job training and placement decisions of the counselor.

5. *Educational Assessment*. Some standard measure of literacy skills (if not already available to the counselor) should be used to make predictions regarding readiness for entrance into various programs. An individual with a low reading level would not usually be recommended for college training and persons with low scores in reading and spelling would not usually qualify for secretarial occupations.

6. *Perceptual-Motor Functioning*. This is an area which is often omitted from an otherwise adequate psychological report. Performance on visual-motor tests often gives clues to neurological impairments as well as fine and gross motor dexterity and efficiency.

7. *Specific Aptitude Tests*. Such tests are applicable for various job families and vary widely depending on vocational goals being considered.

8. *Personality Factors*. Here the examiner attempts to rule out the presence of interfering personality factors which might predispose the client to failure in one or more occupational pursuits. Factors like emotional control, interpersonal skill, frustration tolerance and so forth should be considered. The presence of

anxiety, depressive trends or significant personal and social maladjustment should be studied.

9. *Synthesis and Summary.* In order to make the report comprehensive, an attempt should be made to synthesize and summarize the salient factors pertinent to the vocational rehabilitation of the client to help both client and counselor to "clue-in" on what job families and/or training opportunities would likely be most profitable for the client.

10. *Diagnosis.* Finally, a psychological diagnosis or classification based on the evidence just presented should be given along with recommendations.

MAKING REFERRALS FOR PSYCHOLOGICAL TESTING

Often there is some initial resistance on the part of a client when it is suggested that he should take some psychological tests. Such resistance may indicate that adequate trust has not developed between the client and his counselor or that the counselor has not properly gauged the client's "fear of the unknown." The attitude and approach of the counselor in making the referral is of utmost importance; he must be able to explain to the client the positive results which can accrue as a result of the information which will be obtained. While he should not attempt to "sell" the client, he should present the material realistically and in such a manner that the client himself can see the value of the testing procedure.[10] In addition, the counselor should provide thorough feedback to the client so that he is able to share in each step of the planning process in a meaningful way.

After discussing the rationale of referral for psychological evaluation with the client, the counselor's responsibility relative to referral then shifts to discussing the referral with the psychologist. All too often the counselor refers a client with no more specificity than merely requesting a "psychological evaluation." An intelligent referral to a psychologist should provide him with adequate information to determine the reason for referral and the use to which the data will be put. For example, if the vocational goal selected by the client seems unrealistic and efforts at modifying the goal through counseling are unsuccessful, this should be communicated in the referral to the psychologist. His evaluation report would be considerably different than one on a client referred because of the suspected presence of emotional problems such as anxiety or depression which the counselor feels would interfere with the successful completion of a vocational plan.

HOW TESTING SERVICES ARE PROVIDED

In some rehabilitation agencies psychological evaluations are provided by consulting psychologists on the local or state staff or by outside psychologists who have special training in the area of rehabilitation. In some instances where the counselor must purchase these services, he may be reluctant to do so, perhaps believing that he may save money thereby. According to Cull and Wright[5] the counselor should not avoid securing psychological testing, for it is his responsibility to see that all clients receive those necessary services which will insure satisfactory vocational, social and economic adjustment. Failure to secure adequate psychological information is no less grave an omission than that of failing to make a thorough investigation of a physical abnormality. Neglecting important psychological data can easily result in accentuating adjustment problems of the client and continued repetition of abortive rehabilitation efforts.

VOCATIONAL EVALUATION AND THE PSYCHOLOGIST

An extension of the traditional psychological evaluation into the actual work experience has brought a new role to the rehabilitation psychologist. This new facet added to the traditional role of the psychologist is that of vocational evaluation. A vocational evaluation not only attempts to be more comprehensive in scope than the routine psychological evaluation but also combines the benefits of various disciplines as well as using the work-trial or job sample techniques. There are various models in this area and new ones are still developing.

Essentially, the comprehensive vocational evaluation attempts to combine three basic components: the physical, psychosocial and the vocational. The physical component represents the medical or paramedical personnel; the psychosocial represents social work and psychological personnel; and the vocational component represents personnel essential to the vocational assessment. The vocational assessment may involve standardized work samples or the evaluation of a worker in a job station, performing certain specified tasks. While these components may be identified as distinct aspects, there is an inseparable interrelation geared toward the common objectives of assessment and rehabilitation.[6]

Pruit[12] claims the following advantages for work samples over the usual psychological tests: (a) the client sees himself as performing a work task rather than taking a test, (b) taking a test has a strong negative connotation while working has a positive connotation and (c) a more realistic picture of work potential is obtained from work sample evaluation than from psychological testing.

It seems important that all aspects of the evaluation procedure should be combined and interchanged for the sake of variety in the use of the client time as well as to provide for more honest sharing of evaluation data among the professional staff. It is also recommended that the client be involved in each step of the evaluation so that the material can have constant relevance as well as to provide consensual validation.

INNOVATIONS IN REHABILITATION AND PSYCHOLOGY

Many psychologists and rehabilitation workers have not been content to maintain the *status quo* and as a result many innovative programs have developed. It is interesting by way of example that many psychologists are employed in social and rehabilitation service to review and process R & D proposals in Washington. Others serve on study groups which review and comment on proposals. Many state agencies now employ psychologists to head-up research units or to serve as consultants in research utilization.

One of the most interesting innovations in rehabilitation which highlights the role of the psychologist has been the halfway house movement whose real impetus was the Vocational Rehabilitation Administration. Although halfway houses are not new, going back in history at least to 1781 in England, they are relatively new in the United States; a 1960 survey made by the Joint Commission on Mental Illness and Health disclosed that seven of the nine existing halfway houses had been founded since 1952. Since 1960, there have been numerous new programs established for disability groups ranging for drug addicts to individuals with superficial adjustment problems. Essentially a transitional residence, the halfway house program integrates personal, social and vocational services into a program of community adaptation. The program varies from facility to facility, some programs emphasizing one aspect of rehabilitation and others emphasizing quite a different aspect of the resocialization process.

There are, however, common elements which all or most halfway houses seem to share: (a) The house is usually located in a residential section in a large, private dwelling with sufficient bedrooms to accommodate the residents. Each house has between seven and twenty-five residents; housing is temporary in nature though this may vary from one year to less than three months. (b) Each program provides socialization and/or resocialization in a sheltered setting where there is greater tolerance for deviant behavior and freedom from the usual stresses of community life. (c) Each provides some vocational assistance which may be given through the vocational rehabilitation agency or more informally by hospital staff or halfway house staff.[14]

Residents for the most part share a common experience of previous institutionalization. They are selected as eligible because they are unable to go directly from the hospital to independent community living. A study conducted at Brentwood Veterans Administration Hospital regarding persons who would be eligible for residence at Portals (Los Angeles) found 15 to 20 percent of the patients would be eligible. Patients were not considered eligible if they had behavior patterns which might be disruptive to group situations. Residents tended to be young to middle age (20 to 40); this may be attributed to the fact that residents were required to find and maintain jobs in the community.

The staff usually included at least one staff member in residence, such as a house director, housemother or housekeeper.

Residents usually had access to assistance from social workers, psychiatrists or psychologists.

Halfway house routine usually involved only a part of the life space of the individual resident inasmuch as most residents work at jobs outside the home and are free to seek recreation in the community. Group activities usually included both formal and informal situations; there was usually freedom of choice regarding participation. Responsibilities of the resident usually included cleaning his own room and sharing in some light housekeeping chores.

In some houses this responsibility included occasionally preparing meals. Decisions about readiness for leaving the halfway house were usually made in conjunction with a consultant or staff member.[14]

The growth of halfway houses in the last decade has been so rapid that individual enthusiasm and personal dedication no longer suffice. The ideal halfway house program is a community effort, well led and with a broad base of community support.

GROUP TREATMENT/TRAINING APPROACHES

Several innovations have been forthcoming in group treatment and training; these approaches range from behavior modification techniques, carried on in a closed social system whereby reward–no-reward alternatives are highly structured and carried out in a systematic fashion, to formal programs of instruction about personal and social behavior. Modified group counseling programs have also met with success. Keller and Alper[8] describe three basic group treatment approaches: group counseling, psychoanalytic group psychotherapy and guided group interaction. Group counseling is the least demanding in frequency, depth and training; whereas, the other two group approaches, by contrast, involve relatively frequent meetings which aim to probe rather deeply. In group discussion, the participant begins to realize that others have problems similar to his own, that their suggestions may help him solve some of his difficulties as well as making him aware that others are interested in him. As he, in turn, attempts to assist others, he gains confidence and self-respect; he begins to behave in helpful rather than hurtful fashion.

The guided group interaction approach stresses the group as a distinct entity; with group culture being evident and participants developing a strong "we" feeling, newfound ease of communication leads to increased independence, cooperation and commonality of interests in sharing of norms and values.

Group psychotherapy tends to emphasize the individual within the group situation; it maintains that problems are best solved by not rational deduction but rather through exploration of unconscious materials. Traditional group psychotherapy holds that the person must relive the traumatic episodes of earliest childhood, thereafter transferring the re-experience emotions of love and hate to other group members.

Although professionally trained staff members may conduct a group session, these discussions may be conducted by persons who have received only the briefest instruction. Guided group interactions maintain that an intelligent and sensitive person can be trained to be a competent leader within a matter of weeks or months. Few universities offer such instruction and leave persons interested in them no choice but to intern at guided group centers in order to develop competence. In contrast, group psychotherapy holds to the view that leaders should undergo years of training, even to the inclusion of medical degree and extensive clinical experience in individual psychotherapy.[8]

A more direct, instructional approach to changing behavior is illustrated by Kraus,[9] who developed a simple series of lesson plans on subjects ranging from the use of employment agencies, tips on shopping for a car or a place to live, getting a bank loan, advice on use of leisure time and restaurant etiquette.

SUMMARY

While the psychologist's most traditional contribution to vocational rehabilitation has been in the area of mental testing, psychological research has contributed to the most encompassing changes in vocational rehabilitation techniques and programs. The change in emphasis from a limited physical restoration program to a comprehensive network of rehabilitation services as reflected in the rehabilitation amendments of 1943, 1954 and 1968 is itself a reflection of a way of thinking about health and "wholeness." It carries with it an implicit recognition of man as a biopsychosocial being as well as concern for the quality of the human condition. In this recognition and this concern, psychology plays a unique role.

REFERENCES

1. Albee, G.W.: The short, unhappy life of clinical psychology. *Psychology Today*, September 1970.
2. Allen, W.S.: *Rehabilitation: A Community Challenge.* New York, John Wiley & Sons, May 1967.
3. American Association of State Psychology Boards: *Newsletter*, Vol. 6, August 1970.
4. American Psychological Association: *A Career in Psychology*, 1970.
5. Cull, J.G., and Wright, K.C.: Psychological testing in the rehabilitation setting. *Insight*, 1970.
6. DiMichael, S. G.: *Psychological Services in Vocational Rehabilitation.* Washington, D.C., U.S. Department of Health, Education and Welfare, Office of Vocational Rehabilitation, 1959.
7. Hardy, R.E., and Cull, J.G.: Standards in evaluation, *Vocational Evaluation and Work Adjustment Bulletin*, Vol. 2, No. 1, January 1969.
8. Keller, O.J., and Alper, B.S.: *Halfway Houses: Community Centered Correction and Treatment*, Lexington (Mass.), D.C. Heath & Company, 1970.
9. Kraus, E.A.: *Pathways Back to the Community*, New York, Spring Publishing Company, 1970.
10. McGowan, J.F., and Porter, T.L.: *An Introduction of the Vocational Rehabilitation Process.* Washington, D.C., Department of Health, Education and Welfare, Office of Vocational Rehabilitation, 1967.
11. Mowrer, O.H.: Learning theory and behavior therapy. In Wolman, B.B. (Ed.): *Handbook of Clinical Psychology.* New York, McGraw-Hill, 1965.
12. Pruit, W.A.: Basic assumptions underlying work sample theory. *J Rehab*, January 1970.
13. Szasz, T.S.: The myth of mental illiness. *American Psychologist*, 1960, pp. 15, 113-118.
14. Wechsler, H.: Transitional residences for former mental patients: A survey of halfway houses and related rehabilitation facilities. *Mental Hygiene*, 45:65-76, 1961.
15. Woodworth, R.S.: *Contemporary Schools of Psychology*, 3rd ed., New York, Ronald Press, 1964.

26

Planning for Psychological Services in Vocational Rehabilitation: A Priority Consideration

Richard E. Hardy and John G. Cull

Developing and Using Psychological and Related Services.
Indications for Psychological Evaluations
Contraindication for Psychological Evaluation
Referral for Psychological Services
Selection of a Psychologist
The Psychologist's Report
Use of Psychological Evaluation
Cautions in Using Psychological Test Scores
Developing Models of Psychological Services for State Rehabilitation Agencies
Description of Models
References

DEVELOPING AND USING PSYCHOLOGICAL AND RELATED SERVICES

THE REHABILITATION counselor has been called the key to effective rehabilitation work and rightly so since he is the center of activity, the coordinator and often the developer of services to his clients. The responsibility for the success of various steps in the rehabilitation process rests upon the counselor's shoulders—psychological and related services are no exception.

Psychologists are engaged in a wide variety of activities, many of which relate directly to the goals of the vocational rehabilitation program. The rehabilitation counselor must develop professional psychological resources in much the same way that he de-

---

Note: A resource for this paper was Dr. DiMichael's Book listed in the references.

Planning for Psychological Services

velops community resources. Of the wide array of services offered by psychologists, three which the rehabilitation counselor will be particularly interested in include the following:

1. General psychological evaluations—relatively superficial but broad spectrum screening evaluation.

2. Speciality psychological evaluations—narrow in-depth evaluations (diagnosis of learning disabilities, determination of abilities, aptitudes and interests, and description of personality patterns of handicapped clients).

3. Individual and group adjustment counseling.

Rehabilitation counselors are becoming increasingly aware of the need for making the most effective use of psychological services during the counseling process. Therefore the new rehabilitation counselor should acquaint himself thoroughly with the services provided by the psychologist and the role each of these services ploys in the rehabilitation process. He can then provide the most needed services to his client at the appropriate time in the professionally appropriate manner.

INDICATIONS FOR PSYCHOLOGICAL EVALUATIONS

Quite often the new rehabilitation counselor is in a quandary concerning when he should obtain additional psychological data. He feels, as a counselor, it is his responsibility to evaluate his client in order to counsel him. While he can agree on the necessity for psychological evaluation in the rehabilitation process, he needs some rather specific guidelines relative to securing such evaluation. The most obvious response to this question is, "The counselor should secure a psychological evaluation when he has a specific question regarding his client's personality or personal attributes." More specifically, the counselor should obtain a psychological evaluation when he is developing a rehabilitation plan which will be of long-term. If a long-term plan is developed, some basic assumptions are made relative to mental ability, interests, aptitudes and emotional stability. These assumptions should be checked out early in order to help insure the ultimate success of the plan. If the assumptions are not verified by means of a psychological evaluation but are found erroneous, a great deal of the client's time and energies can be wasted. Similarly, if an expensive rehabilitation plan is being developed, a psychological evaluation should be obtained for almost the same reasons.

Many psychological evaluations are obtained at the beginning of the rehabilitation process during the diagnostic phase when the individual's eligibility is being established. A psychological evaluation should be made in cases in which eligibility is based upon mental retardation, functional retardation and behavioral disorders.

In developing the rehabilitation plan the counselor needs to have a fairly complete understanding of the client's functional educational level, mental ability, aptitudes and interests. If this needed information is missing, it should be obtained. If part of the information the counselor has is unclear, ambiguous or contradictory the counselor should clear up the confusion with a psychological evaluation. For example, if the client has a reported educational achievement level or reported level of intellectual ability substantially lower than that required on a job the client performed successfully, the counselor should clarify the obvious contradictions by psychological testing.

If the counselor suspects important talents, capacities, abilities or disabilities which are unreported but have a bearing on the probable vocational objective, a psychological evaluation should be purchased to delineate these attributes. Also an evaluation should be obtained if the client has certain disabilities which later on materially affect his capacities, abilities, skills or personality. For example, a client who is experiencing mild anaesthesia in his hands and fingers should be tested for manual dexterity prior to settling on a vocational objective calling for a manipulative ability. A client interested in electronics assembly work should be tested for color blindness.

Lastly, a psychological evaluation should be obtained if the client is exhibiting or has exhibited behavior the counselor does not understand. If the client's current behavior patterns are not predictable and are difficult to understand, the counselor should enlist the aid of the psychologist to explain the client's personality

Planning for Psychological Services

structure. If the client's past history is filled with events or actions the counselor can not reconcile, such as unexplained job changes, frequent moves from one community to another, a lack of organization to the client's vocational history and so forth, a psychological evaluation is in order to describe the client's personality structure in an effort to explain his behavior patterns.

CONTRAINDICATION FOR PSYCHOLOGICAL EVALUATION

Perhaps looking at cases when psychological evaluation is unnecessary would be meaningful. An obvious case in which a psychological evaluation is unnecessary is when the client recently has been successfully employed and intends to return to his particular vocation following the physical restoration and other rehabilitation services he will receive.

If the client has been successfully employed but is now unable to find similar work because of employer prejudice toward the handicapped, it is necessary for the counselor to use his counseling and vocational placement skills to convince the employers of the client's ability. In this case it would not be appropriate to obtain a psychological evaluation in an effort to change the client's vocational objective.

Psychological testing is not needed when a client has been successfully employed and the new vocational objective constitutes only a minor shift or the new job is directly related to his prior work. There is no need for testing when the client has developed a long and rich background of information regarding a particular industry or job family and his new vocational objective, though not previously performed by him, is sufficiently related for the counselor and client to be safe in assuming he can meet the demands of the job. A separate but related case concerns the client having a long and rich background of educational information and experience, and the client plans to study or work in areas related to his background. Evaluation is not needed in this case.

In essence, a psychological evaluation is needed when the client's behavior is to be predicted over a long period or his behavior is difficult to predict over a short period of time. An evaluation is not needed when the client's behavior is understandable and predictable or if he has established a related pattern of vocational growth over an extended period of time.

At times, counselors will threaten to deny rehabilitation services if a client refuses to submit to the testing and interviewing of a psychologist. In many instances, if the client continues to refuse, the case is closed—"The client is not motivated." Even though this occurs much less frequently than it has in the past, it is appropriate to discuss. As rehabilitation counselors become more professional and more aware of the needs of clients, they will be more attuned to the motivating factors operating in the client. If the client refuses services which the counselor offers, the counselor should seek to understand and modify behavior through counseling rather than being threatened and defensive himself and reacting in a punitive manner toward the client.

REFERRAL FOR PSYCHOLOGICAL SERVICES

When securing psychological services, the counselor should ask himself some basic questions: What specific knowledge can be obtained from the psychologist which will be of value in the rehabilitation counseling process? What data can he (the counselor) obtain and what data should he request from the psychologist? When these questions have been asked and answered, the counselor is better prepared to make an intelligent referral to the psychologist. As mentioned above there are numerous types of psychological evaluations; therefore, it is inadequate for a counselor to merely refer a client for a "psychological evaluation." If he is expecting highly specific definitive information from the psychologist, the rehabilitation counselor must set definite limits for the psychologist and provide him with the appropriate background information. Gandy's referral form which, if used, will tend to increase materially the quality of psychological reports the counselor receives. This referral form should constitute the minimum information forwarded to the psychologist; however, generally little more than a request for an evaluation is sent.

REFERRAL FOR PSYCHOLOGICAL-VOCATIONAL EVALUATION

FROM:_____ DATE:_____

TO: _____

IDENTIFICATION:

Name of Client_____

Social Security No._____

Address_____

Sex_____ Age_____ Race_____ Marital Status_____

No. Dependents_____

SOCIAL-VOCATIONAL-MEDICAL:

Economic Stratum_____

Family Environment_____

Formal Education_____

Usual Occupation_____

Vocational Success_____

Leisure Activities_____

Physical or Mental Impairments_____

General Health_____

BEHAVIORAL OBSERVATIONS:

General Observations (appearance, mannerisms, communication, attitude, motivation) :

_____
_____
_____

REASON FOR REFERRAL:

Statement of Problem_____

_____

Specific Questions_____

_____
_____

Enclosures:_____

Note: This form was taken from Gandy, J.: The Psychological-Vocational Referral in Vocational Rehabilitation. Unpublished Master's Thesis, University of South Carolina, 1968.

Much of the information called for on the form is already in the case folder so it is easily accessible to the counselor. In order to select the appropriate instruments and interpret them, the psychologist needs the social-vocational-medical background information. Therefore, to facilitate the work of the psychologist and relieve the client of having to answer the same questions repeatedly and to increase the effectiveness of the psychological interview, the counselor should make a concerted effort to supply the psychologist all pertinent information.

An individual's economic status, home situation, the degree of vocational success he has experienced and the physical or mental impairments he has will have a direct and major bearing on his behavior and personality. Test responses and results have to be evaluated in comparison with the above factors. If this information is not provided to the psychologist, he will have to interview the client at some length. The more time he spends in this duplicative effort, the less time he has to evaluate the client.

The counselor generally has had several contacts with the client before the client is referred to the psychologist. Also, the counselor is a professional who is skilled in observations; therefore, it is of particular value to the psychologist to have access to the observations the counselor has made. These observations can be quite meaningful since the counselor sees the client under a variety of conditions and the psychologist sees the client only in the testing and interview situation on one occasion.

Perhaps the most important information the psychologist should receive is usually not given to him. This is a statement of the problem which prompted the counselor to refer the client to the psychologist. In order to specifically meet the needs of the counselor, the psychologist should have this statement since it will, in many cases, determine the particular instruments the psychologist will use. In conjunction with this statement of the problem, the counselor should outline the specific questions he wants answered by the psychologist. By considering these questions, the psychologist can further tailor his evaluation to the specific needs of the counselor.

Lastly, a good referral should include other reports, evaluations and examinations which have a direct bearing upon the psychological evaluation. These would include other psychological evaluations, social evaluations and reports, psychiatric data, the general medical examination report and some medical examinations by specialists.

SELECTION OF A PSYCHOLOGIST

After deciding upon what information the counselor himself will obtain and what information will be expected from the psychologist, the counselor has to select a psychologist. The counselor can obtain psychological data himself or he may rely upon a psychometrist (an individual skilled in the administration and interpretation of psychological, vocational and educational tests; an individual trained at a lower level than that of a psychologist), a psychologist in private practice outside the agency, a staff psychologist or a consulting psychologist (these latter two will be discussed later). Generally, if he selects either the psychometrist, the staff psychologist, or the consulting psychologist, the agency will describe the mechanics of referral in a policy manual or procedure manual. Therefore, here we will concern ourselves only with using the psychologist in private practice.

When the counselor is attempting to do part of the psychological study himself, it is very important for him to recognize his limitations in the field of evaluation. Certainly few counselors are skilled in psychological evaluation to the degree that they are able to use a wide variety of instruments. All counselors, however, should be able to use skillfully a small number of tests comprising a specific battery. When the counselor is inexperienced in the type of testing which he feels should be done, he must be able to secure the services of a qualified psychologist.

When obtaining the services of a psychologist in private practice, the counselor should have at hand a list of psychologists who are well known for their competency and who are experienced in working with handicapped persons. It is generally felt that psychologists who belong to the division of clinical psychology, the division of counseling psychology or the division of psychological aspects of disability of the American Psychological Association will be interested in the field of rehabilitation and will be most helpful to the counselor. However, the counselor must recognize that psychologists, like other professionals, have areas of special interest. A psychologist who is knowledgeable concerning the emotionally disturbed or the mentally retarded may be relatively inexperienced in testing the physically handicapped.

When the client is sent to the psychologist he is referred on an individual basis just as he is for a general or speciality medical examination. The payment is made according to a fee schedule developed by the agency and usually the state or local psychological associations. As with a new physician, a psychologist in private practice who is being utilized for the first time should be contacted. The counselor should discuss the vocational rehabilitation program, its goals, its procedures for referral, reporting, payment and the agency's fee schedule.

THE PSYCHOLOGIST'S REPORT

After the referral of the client the counselor has every reason to expect and should demand speedy service for his client. This speedy service entails both a prompt appointment to see the client and a written report of the finding submitted. While the report should be received within ten days of the client's appointment quite often it takes longer; however, if it routinely takes longer and at times exceeds three weeks, the counselor should discuss the problem with the psychologist so that he may receive better service or change psychologists. When the counselor receives the psychological report, it should cover five basic areas:

1. Clinical observations of the psychologist
2. Tests administered
3. Results and interpretation of results
4. Specific recommendations
5. Summary

The observations of the psychologist are important since they provide the flavor of the evaluation and, without them the evaluation would be quite sterile. These observations will comment on the client's emotional behavior, appearance, motivation, reaction to the testing and so forth.

The tests which were administered should be spelled out for two reasons; first, most fee schedules are based upon the number and type of tests administered; but, more importantly, the counselor needs to know upon what data the psychologist is basing assumptions and making recommendations. In the reporting and interpreting of results, the counselor should find the results of all the tests given with an explanation of their importance. This section is highly technical, however, it should be very logical since this is where the psychologist builds his case. If some of the test results are not noteworthy or are not used in the diagnosis and recommendations, this fact should be mentioned and explained in the interpretation section. Essentially this is where the psychologist logically bridges the gap between his clinical observations, the test results, the diagnosis and recommendations he will make. Above all the sections should be very sensible and understandable.

In the recommendations section the psychologist should make a number of suggestions which are addressed to the specific referral problem and the questions the counselor asked on referral of the client. Recommendations should be stated clearly and concisely. If the counselor does not understand them he should never hesitate to call the psychologist for clarification. The summary is a short, clear summation of the evaluation stated in nontechnical terms.

USE OF PSYCHOLOGICAL EVALUATION

After receiving the report the counselor is confronted with how to use the evaluation. The use of the data will be easier if psychological evaluations are viewed as an integral part of counseling and closely related to all other rehabilitation services and not as an isolated event or service. The evaluation can be used in counseling sessions to aid the client in better understanding himself and in identifying his major problem areas. Additionally the counselor can use the psychological evaluation as a counseling tool to aid the client in developing insights specifically related to his relative strengths and limitations and in helping him in making reasonable plans and decisions.

In interpreting the test results to the client, the counselor should develop short, clear, concise methods of describing to the client the purpose of the tests he took and the meaning of the results; but, by all means, the counselor should communicate only on the level at which the client is fully "with" the counselor. A most effective means of interpreting test results is relating test data in meaningful terms to the client's behavior. A trap to avoid is becoming overly identified with the client's test scores. They should be presented in a manner that will allow him to question, reject, accept or modify the presentation and interpretation without having to reject the counselor. The counselor should not project his own subjective feelings into the results he is using.

CAUTIONS IN USING PSYCHOLOGICAL TEST SCORES

While psychological testing plays a vital role in the rehabilitation process, there are some cautions which need to be exercised in their use. It should be remembered that test scores are just that—only test scores. The indications are a product of the interpretation of the scores. Tests are only an *aid* to the counselor; they should never become the prime reason for a program of action in a client's rehabilitation. They are too fallible. They are too susceptible to human error to be relied upon completely. While scores are valuable in indicating vocational areas which merit consideration, the counselor should remember that tests are rather weak in industrial validation. But most importantly, it should be remembered that the individual can adjust to several occupations. Inherent in testing philosophy is the concept that an individual is "predestined" to only one occupation.

DEVELOPING MODELS OF PSYCHOLOGICAL SERVICES FOR STATE REHABILITATION AGENCIES

As the scope and commitment of vocational rehabilitation has expanded to include services to the culturally disadvantaged and those with behavioral disorders, so has the reliance on and need for psychologists in rehabilitation work. Psychologists who are trained at the doctoral level and who are aware of rehabilitation objectives and procedures are needed urgently.

The number of psychologists employed in vocational rehabilitation is limited. In order to obtain psychological services on a statewide basis, many vocational rehabilitation departments have generally taken one of three approaches in developing models of psychological services. The approaches might be labeled as (a) the consultation model, (b) the strict panel model and (c) the supervising psychologist model.

DESCRIPTION OF MODELS

The *consultation model* is relatively simple in structure. The department of rehabilitation must develop cooperative relationships with psychologists who are employed by institutions or who are in private practice. Usually rehabilitation area office supervisors contact these individuals and ask that they serve as consultants in psychology to the vocational rehabilitation program.

There are some problems with this approach. Many rehabilitation workers are not knowledgeable about the selection of qualified psychologists, and many psychologists are unaware of the objectives of rehabilitation. Unless there is considerable effort on the part of rehabilitation personnel and psychologists to develop understanding, the relationship between the rehabilitation department and consulting psychologists can be strained. This type of working relationship results in complaints from rehabilitation personnel that they are not getting the type of information they really need from psychologists. In addition, psychologists may not become fully involved and committed to the objectives of the rehabilitation programs. In addition, there is often confusion about fees and the selection of psychologists for various types of work such as psychotherapy and psychological evaluation of clients with catastrophic disabilities.

The *strict panel model* is the second approach which is used by some departments of rehabilitation. In this model, a part-time state consultant in psychology is usually hired. The state consultant in psychology and the rehabilitation department, in cooperation with the state psychological association, selects a panel of psychologists who represent various phases of professional psychology. The panel rules on the qualifications of psychologists who apply to perform various service functions for the vocational rehabilitation department and specifies areas of competency of individual psychologists. The state psychological consultant for the vocational rehabilitation department usually chairs the panel. Panel members develop a list of psychologists and describe services psychologists are qualified to offer to the vocational rehabilitation department.

This approach can be criticized as duplicated effort if the state has a certification or licensing board. Such boards examine the credentials of psychologists and determine areas of competency. The state licensing or certification board also is concerned with violations of ethical standards. The strict panel model can be very useful in states where no state board of examiners has been appointed.

The *supervising psychologist model* is a third approach which is used by departments of vocational rehabilitation. This model requires the employment of a full-time psychologist who serves as state supervisor of psychological services. The supervising psychologist has statewide responsibility for developing effective working relationships with other psychologists employed on either a full-time or part-time basis. He recommends psychologists for work with the rehabilitation department. He may also act as chairman of a panel of psychologists which meets to consider special psychological problems in vocational rehabilitation. The panel can also help in developing cooperative relationships between the rehabilitation department and consulting psychologists.

The supervising psychologist helps rehabilitation staff members develop understanding of concepts that will be of value to them in their work in vocational rehabilitation. He should participate actively in in-service training activities for professional rehabilitation staff members. He visits area offices and facilities in order to work with consulting psychologists and rehabilitation personnel.

In addition, the supervising psychologist assures that psychologists working for the rehabilitation department maintain standards of practice in accordance with the laws of the state and with standards established by the American Psychological Association.

He may also plan training programs for them in order that they may develop improved understanding of the complexities of vocational rehabilitation work.

These models and general variations of them have been used by most state rehabilitation departments, although some departments have not yet developed psychological services on a statewide basis.

Of the three described models, the supervising psychologist approach seems most effective, mainly because it allows an individual who is a psychologist to devote a substantial portion of his time to psychological services within the department of rehabilitation. A supervising psychologist should hold a doctoral degree in psychology or a closely related field. He must be carefully selected. He has crucial responsibility for the effectiveness of psychological services in an important statewide social service program.

Effective rehabilitation work requires comprehensive evaluation of clients. Psychologists offer invaluable information to the total vocational evaluation effort. The fullest and most effective use of their services by state rehabilitation departments is of high priority.

REFERENCES

1. Cull, J. G., and Hardy, R. E.: State agency administrator's views of psychological testing. *Rehab Lit,* 1970.
2. Cull, J. G., and Wright, K. C.: Psychological testing in the rehabilitation setting. *Insight,* 1970.
3. DiMichael, G.: *Psychological Services in Vocational Rehabilitation.* Washington, D. C., U.S. Government Printing Office.
4. Hardy, R. E., and Cull, J. G.: Standards in evaluation. *Vocational Evaluation and Work Adjustment Bulletin,* Vol. 2, No. 1, January 1969.
5. Lerner, J.: The role of the psychologist in the disability evaluation of emotional and intellectual impairments under the Social Security Act. *American Psychologist,* Vol. 18, No. 5, 1963.

27

State Rehabilitation Administrators' Views on Psychological Evaluation

John G. Cull and Richard E. Hardy

Considerations in Obtainig Psychological Evaluations
Administrators Sampled
Results
References

THE REHABILITATION process relies, of course, upon a thorough understanding of the rehabilitated client. Counselors develop this understanding by careful evaluation and study of medical, social psychological and vocational components.

According to Hardy and Cull[3] the widening range of vocational rehabilitation services, along with the increasing complexity of disabilities with which rehabilitation has become involved heightens the need for more comprehensive evaluation services in the rehabilitation process. Even though a high level of evaluation is essential to providing adequate services to the rehabilitation client, obtaining pertinent and topical psychological information has been a continued source of frustration to the rehabilitation counselor. Not only does obtaining psychological information present a problem to counselors who have difficulty locating psychologists to evaluate their clients, but the psychological evaluation of clients presents a challenge to the rehabilitation administrator who must plan budgetarily for the provision of psychological evaluation.

Note: See *Rehabilitation Literature*, Vol. 32, No. 3, March, 1971.

CONSIDERATIONS IN OBTAINING PSYCHOLOGICAL EVALUATIONS

The dilemma of handling psychological evaluations is a topic of frequent discussion by counselors and administrators. A basic question seems to be how the rehabilitation counselor can obtain an adequate psychological evaluation of his client without paying prohibitively large amounts in psychological fees for the increasing numbers of clients who need this type of evaluation.

Rehabilitation counselors and administrators generally acknowledge that from their experience, psychological examinations are extremely important in overall planning in the rehabilitation process. A study by Sindberg, Roberts and Pfeifer[4] has confirmed this acknowledgment by indicating that, in terms of the usage of recommendations of psychologists, reports are definitely useful in the rehabilitation process. More than half of the recommendations of psychologists were followed completely or were followed to a large extent by rehabilitation counselors involved with the cases in the rehabilitation process.

ADMINISTRATORS SAMPLED

This current study is concerned with reactions of state rehabilitation agency directors relative to satisfaction with psychological services obtained from psychologists in private practice and the use of rehabilitation counselors in obtaining psychological information. All state vocational rehabilitation agencies were surveyed during the summer of 1969; of the ninety-one questionnaires sent out, fifty-five or approximately 60 percent were returned. Thirty-two of the fifty-five questionnaires which were returned indicated that state agency administrators do not believe that rehabilitation counselors should be prepared to administer a basic battery of psychological tests. Of the administrators responding to the questionnaire, 49 percent (or twenty-seven) did believe that rehabilitation counselors should be trained to administer interest tests, 47 percent (or twenty-six) felt they should learn to give aptitude tests, and 44 percent (or twenty-four) believed that they could administer intelligence tests with training.

RESULTS

All fifty-five administrators who participated in this study stated that private psychologists are their primary source of psychological evaluations. Almost half of those persons returning questionnaires indicated that their state agency had hired psychologists on a full-time basis. Forty-three of the fifty-five agency administrators indicated that they were generally satisfied with the adequacy of reporting and professional services offered by outside psychologists. The most often expressed reasons for dissatisfaction by the twelve agency administrators who were not satisfied with outside consulting psychologists were (a) reporting was not sufficient for rehabilitation purposes and (b) there was an unacceptable time lag in getting material from the psychologists. Agency administrators concerned with programs serving blind individuals stated that psychologists in private practice often were not trained to evaluate blind persons. This observation apparently supports Allen's[1] statement that less than 3 percent of all psychologists work in the area of mental deficiency and only 2.5 percent are engaged in programs for the physically handicapped.

A majority of the administrators (58 percent) indicated that rehabilitation counselors should not attempt to administer a basic battery of tests because counselors lack an understanding of the principles of testing and evaluation. Additionally, thirty stated that in their opinion counselors lacked the time necessary to achieve effective testing and evaluation.

In states that recommend that the counselor have a counselor's test kit for his personal use in evaluation of clients, the following tests were most often recommended:

1. *Tests of Intellectual Functioning*
   Peabody Picture Vocabulary Tests
   Wechsler Adult Intelligent Scale
2. *Tests of Academic Achievement*
   Wide Range Achievement Tests
3. *Tests of Vocational Interest*
   Kuder Performance Record-Vocational
4. *Tests of Motor Dexterity*
   Purdue Peg Board

5. *Tests of Vocational Aptitude*
   General Clerical Tests
   Mechanical Comprehension Tests

In some states, the Otis Self-Administering Tests of Mental Ability and the Revised Beta Examination are being used in lieu of the Wechsler Adult Intelligence Scale and the Wechsler Intelligence Scale for Children. The following comment from a state director on the Eastern Seaboard indicates the general thinking of state administrators concerning the use of a counselor test kit, "We feel very strongly that counselors should be able to administer basic pencil-and-paper tests requiring level B^2 competency and preparation. We strongly urge that they not become involved with projective techniques and complex personality inventories."

Results of this survey seem to indicate that about 42 percent of the state agencies are moving toward having counselors use tests to make initial screening judgments of their clients relative to some of his basic needs and toward gaining an understanding of the client. Also, it appears that these screening procedures being utilized by rehabilitation counselors are helpful to them in making decisions which concern whether the client should have further evaluation by psychologists or should be involved in extended evaluation. Since fees for psychological services represent a substantial portion of the case service budget in the state agencies' overall budget, it seems practical to screen many of these clients through the use of a counselor's testing kit along with evaluating other data from the social and medical areas which may be available in order to make basic decisions regarding the rehabilitation process for individual clients. After such screening, the number of clients referred to psychologists for in-depth psychological testing and evaluation can be substantially reduced. This procedure would seem to allow for improved services to all clients since much of the money expended for psychological evaluation could be spent on other case services and comprehensive psychological testing could be completed only when, in the counselor's opinion, it would be necessary for the rehabilitation of the client. As a result of this study, it is the opinion of the authors that agency administrators have confidence in their counselors and generally believe that they can depend upon them to make the complex decisions which are required regarding the variety of types of psychological evaluation needed.

In summary, it was found that almost half of the state agency administrators felt counselors should be equipped to administer interest tests, aptitude tests and intelligence tests; however, a majority felt administration time requirements precluded counselors' routine administration of a basic battery of tests. While over half of the agencies have employed full-time psychologists the major source of psychological evaluations in all cases was from psychologists in private practice. Although a large majority of state directors were satisfied with this arrangement, the main dissatisfactions concerned the relevancy of evaluations to vocational rehabilitation and the time lag in getting reports from psychologists.

REFERENCES

1. Allan, W. S.: *Rehabilitation: A Community Challenge.* New York, John Wiley & Sons, 1958.
2. American Psychological Association: *Ethical Standards of Psychologists.* Washington, 1953.
3. Hardy, R. E., and Cull, J. G.: Standards in evaluation. *Vocational Evaluation and Work Adjustment Bulletin,* Vol. 2, No. 1, January 1969.
4. Sindberg, R. M., Roberts, A., and Pfeifer, E. J.: The usefulness of psychological evaluations to vocational rehabilitation counselors. *Rehab Lit,* Vol. 29, No. 10, October 1968.
5. University of Arkansas: *Psychological Evaluation in the Vocational Process,* Fayetteville, Arkansas, In-service counselor training project for vocational rehabilitation counselors in Arkansas, 1957, Monograph 3.

28

Working with the Rehabilitation Facility

Harry W. Troop

Types of Workshops
Goals and Objectives of Sheltered Workshops
What a Sheltered Workshop Can Accomplish
Type of Clients to Be Referred to a Sheltered Workshop
What a Counselor Can Expect from a Sheltered Workshop
What the Sheltered Workshop Can Expect from the Rehabilitation Counselor

THE NEED to clarify the nature, makeup and value of workshops has long been apparent. New counselors (or for that matter, more experienced counselors) have very few guidelines to help them fully utilize the workshops in their geographic areas. Questions such as Which clients should or should not be referred to a workshop? What services does a workshop offer? How good is a service of a particular workshop? What responsibility does the workshop have to me? need to be answered. It is the hope of the author that this chapter will supply some of these answers.

One generally accepted definition of a sheltered workshop, which has been adopted by the National Association of Sheltered Workshops and Homebound Programs (1966), is as follows: "A sheltered workshop is a work-oriented rehabilitation facility with a controlled working environment and individual vocational goals which utilize work experience and related services for assisting the handicapped person to progress toward normal living and productive vocational status." Within this definition the concepts of "work-oriented rehabilitation facility" and "individual goal" are of prime importance. In the past two decades the sheltered workshop has changed greatly from the early concept of a custodial care institution.

The workshop is now seen as a unique type of rehabilitation facility which affords an individual an opportunity to develop his assets within the framework of a remunerative work setting. Thus, the individual is not only pointing toward competitive employment and a regular, earned wage but is able to do this within an environment that enables him to experience the dignity and self-respect that comes with being a productive individual.

TYPES OF WORKSHOPS

A work activity center is viewed by the Department of Labor and is described in part 25 of the Federal Register, July 23, 1968, as a ". . . workshop or physically separated department of a workshop having an identifiable program . . . planned and designed exclusively to provide therapeutic activity for handicapped workers whose physical or mental impairment is so severe as to make their productive capacity inconsequential. . . ." The Federal Register goes on to state that this is determined on a basis of whether the average productivity per handicapped worker is less than $850.00 per year as measured by dividing the total annual earned income of the work activity center work program, less the cost of purchasing materials used; in the case of a work activity center paying at piece rates where the average annual labor rate per client is less than $600.00 as measured by dividing the total annual wages of the client by the average number of clients in the work program.

The term *transitional* reflects emphasis on the development of an individual to a higher level of functioning with the primary emphasis being on moving the person toward employment in the regular labor market. In certain instances, however, the individual may not possess the potential need to function on a job in a regular labor market. In such instances, the goal may be modified to prepare the person for placement in extended employment (in a long-term workshop), additional education or further supportive services. The transitional workshop is a work setting, not a school, not a hospital, not a clinic, not an activity center.

Working with the Rehabilitation Facility

Each of the other facilities has distinct programs geared toward meeting specific needs of the clients. The transitional workshop offers a work experience, an opportunity to identify with the role of a worker (with the resulting dignity that comes from being a productive individual), an environment ideal for evaluation of functioning ability and a setting for work adjustment training (training in self-control, self-discipline, work tolerances, work habits, work performance, work attitudes and knowledge of the world of work itself).

Within a transitional workshop, a client is referred for a specific purpose and for a specific period of time. It is the responsibility of a workshop to document that goals have been established for the client, that they are realistic and that there is movement toward these goals throughout the client's program in the workshop. If the movement toward these goals does not take place, then either the goal has been unrealistic, the workshop has not done everything it can to help that person reach the goal or the client has reached the point where no more movement is possible. If the goal has been unrealistic, an attempt should be made to correct the goal and bring it within the line of reasonable expectation. If the workshop has not done everything possible, this should be corrected. If the person has reached a plateau and is no longer "moving," the client should be terminated or referred to another more appropriate agency (such as a long-term workshop) if additional movement cannot be forecast within a reasonable period of time.

It is extremely important to keep in mind that there are too few agencies offering services to the handicapped in the community. When a person is maintained in a program longer than is necessary, another individual in that community is, in effect, denied service. If, on the other hand, there is movement but it is slow, consideration should be given to allowing this individual additional time to "grow" at the rate that he is capable. It should not be forgotten that in many cases a person has been disabled all of his life and this has left tremendous "damage." These elements cannot be eliminated in a short period of time. Nevertheless, movement toward a goal is essential within a transitional workshop.

Since the goal of a transitional workshop is to develop a person to his highest level of functioning and to move that person out to the regular labor market, emphasis must be on placement. To prepare a person for work but to deny him the opportunity to get a job is folly. Regardless of who does the actual placement, the workshop should have the responsibility either for doing the placement work itself or for following up on the referral to the appropriate agency that will handle the placement activities. Follow-up is a major segment of the workshop program and should not be taken lightly. Too often, people go through a program and are able to function on a job, but since there is no follow-up, the chances of that person's maintaining a job and succeeding are diminished. Much too often minor difficulties arise once the person is out of the workshop, and these difficulties cannot be worked through unless the workshop is in touch with the former client and the employer, and the counselor has established some system whereby the client feels free to contact the workshop if a difficulty arises. Needless to say, follow-up services are expensive and quite often handled when "there is time to handle this type of thing." However, unless the workshop develops a meaningful follow-up program, much of the value that it accomplishes will be lost in the long run. In keeping with this, it is important for the workshop to include follow-up services in its entire funding process so that it has sufficient funds to handle this very important segment of its program.

The evaluation and work adjustment center is a highly professional service that falls within the scope of a transitional workshop. Since all transitional workshops make some attempt to evaluate and train clients, transitional workshops that offer evaluation and work adjustment training services must be classified by the type of evaluation and training services they offer.

The *long-term, or extended, workshop* denotes a continuation of services for individuals who, while in the transitional workshop, have mastered the ability of handling themselves within a sheltered work setting but, upon completion of the transitional program, are unable to meet or to sustain the demands of competitive employment. By moving these individuals into extended employment workshops, they are able to function at their maximum level and are able to achieve success and a level of productivity that is in keeping with their capabilities.

There has been considerable discussion about the advisability of the extended employment workshop being separated from the transitional program when both services are being offered by the same center. The argument that is offered in favor of a separation is based on the desire to provide the person moving into the long-term workshop with a sense of "change." Also, it is felt that it is advisable, by the people who argue for a separation, to remove the person who will be functioning in a long-term workshop from the competition and the possibility of not being able to keep up with more competent individuals who are within the transitional workshop program.

The argument in favor of the two programs being together is based on the value of having each group of clients benefit from the stimulation of the other group. While there will always be exceptions to any general rule, most people coming into the transitional workshop may well establish a pattern of competitiveness that would be beneficial for a client in the long-term program. On the other hand, clients in long-term programs will most likely have acquired the discipline, self-control and good work habits that many of the people coming into the transitional program have not yet learned to adopt.

Regardless of whether the two facilities are separated physically, it is important to remember that movement from the transitional to the extended program should not be considered a failure or "terminal" for this disabled person. Many people in industry reach a level of their capacities and spend their working lives at benches, machines or assembly lines. For them, this is terminal employment for which they need not apologize. There should be a similar understanding of the disabled individual who reaches his potential by functioning successfully within a long-term workshop setting.

What is even more important is the need for periodic reevaluation of the client's place in the extended employment. Disabilities change, human beings continue to grow, the labor market regularly changes and over a period of time these individuals may be able to move from a sheltered environment into regular employment.

GOALS AND OBJECTIVES OF SHELTERED WORKSHOPS

To ascertain the goals and objectives of a particular workshop, one must examine the stated services offered by the center and then seek clarification of exactly how these services are rendered. It should be clear that not all workshops can offer all services and, indeed, not all workshops should attempt to meet all the needs of all clients. The important thing is that the workshop does, in fact, offer the services it describes in its literature and that it can show evidence that these services are carried out.

Organizational Structure—Staff

A workshop should have adequate staff to carry out its stated goals. To assess the services that an agency offers, it is necessary to identify who is responsible for each service and how the service is carried out. An example of a basic method of assessing a service, such as counseling, is to find out who does the counseling, what the background of this individual is, how this background prepares this person to provide this service and how much time during the week this person devotes strictly to counseling.

Programs of Service

Intake

While each workshop will follow its own general procedure for preparing intake reports, it is recommended that a written intake report be prepared after the initial intake interview and that this report be sent to the rehabilitation counselor. Items that should be covered in such a report would include the reason for referral, the intake interviewer's impressions of the applicant, the family background, past educational experiences, test material received, medical information, past employment history and vocational goals. The end of the report should include some type of summary that would generally review the material covered in the intake report and would make recommendation as to the acceptability by the workshop of the applicant. If the applicant is an acceptable candidate for the program, suggestions concerning services should be written detailing the significant points that the workshop staff should be aware of in dealing with the client, the general goals for the client and how the workshop can go about providing a program that will help the person reach those goals.

Evaluation

In addition to the admission evaluation, which every workshop must offer, there are many types of evaluations that can take place within a facility. The five areas, beyond admission's evaluation, described below may or may not be offered by any one center; however, the rehabilitation counselor should be aware of what type of specific evaluations can be provided by workshops and where they can obtain the type of evaluation they need for a particular client.

The purpose of the admission's evaluation is to assess, immediately after a person has entered a workshop, his personal and social characteristics and his present level of functioning; to identify vocational disadvantage (s) (when applicable) and/or limitations; to formulate an appropriate vocational goal; and to determine the services the individual needs and, if the services are offered, whether the individual is able to utilize these services.

Upon completion of the admission's evaluation, a person in a workshop program must be classified as (a) a person not suitable for additional services within the scope of the workshop; (b) a person who can reasonably be expected to become employable after a program of service; or (c) a person in need of a longer period of extended evaluation (rehabilitation determination program). This procedure clarifies whether or not he could be reasonably expected to become employable after a program of service.

As mentioned earlier, the workshop is not a medical setting geared to evaluating a person medically. What the workshop can do is to evaluate the client's functioning ability in regard to what he can and cannot do, from a medical point of view.

As a person proceeds through the program, keen attention

should be directed to any possible areas of medical limitations which were not originally noted in the medical information. If such evidence does develop, then additional medical consultation is in order. It should be kept in mind at all times that the person is an individual with a specific medical or mental problem—not a diagnostic label without individual identity. Much too often, areas of employment or areas of training are arbitrarily put off because the person is "an amputee who could not handle such a job." Anyone who has been involved with workshops for even a short period of time will bear witness to the fact that many people can accomplish many things that, on pure medical grounds, are not indicated. While this does not mean that chances should be taken with a person's medical health just to see how far he can go, it does mean that two individuals with the same diagnostic label function in different fashions. The workshop can be the setting to test a person's functioning and train him to develop as far as he is capable of developing.

A workshop can offer psychological evaluation, either through its regular staff members or by obtaining these services on a consultative basis. Most likely the evaluation will take place prior to the applicant's entering the workshop (rehabilitation counselors customarily refer their clients for psychological evaluation prior to referring them to a workshop); however, additional testing may be indicated during and at the conclusion of the workshop program, which will assist the staff and the client in planning for the future.

In addition to specific tests, the individual overall functioning within the workshop tells quite a story about a person's makeup. Many times an individual can function at a much higher level than his IQ, or level of academic achievement, would suggest. In other instances, a person with an average, or better than average, IQ score cannot effectively use his potentials and may be, in fact, functioning much less effectively than a person with a significantly lower test score. In addition, a person's ability to handle pressure, deal with supervisors and co-workers, handle failure, peer pressure and a host of other elements related to day-to-day activity of a workshop may be extremely revealing as to the person's psychological composition.

Working with the Rehabilitation Facility

More and more social and cultural elements loom bigger and bigger as obstacles that hamper the individual's ability to utilize his potentials and to function successfully within the community. Individuals who fall into this category need rehabilitation services just as much as a person with any other type of disability that hampers his ability to function as a productive and useful individual.

A review of the individual's educational experiences may reveal areas of strength, weaknesses, interests, level of academic achievement and potential for additional training. Likewise, his learning ability within the workshop itself will point up significant information as to how he learns best, how well he retains information, whether he can transfer learning and in what areas he exhibits the best potentials.

Within the workshop, vocational evaluation takes place as the client is tested in various work situations. Obviously, some workshops will be much more capable of testing people in a variety of work settings than will others. However, most workshops will be able to test people on office assignments (duplicating, collating, stapling, sorting, addressing, et cetera), quality inspection (visual or mechanical), service functioning (cafeteria work, messenger work, laundry work, maintenance work), bench work (wrapping, packing, assembling), machine operation and, possibly, outside or greenhouse type of work that may be available.

Observation of the client will point up information relating to his ability to follow, retain and carry out directions in a systematic way; capabilities in regard to eye-hand and eye-foot coordination; and skills related to depth perception, color blindness and overall visual ability. Also, information can be obtained in regard to the person's physical strength, fatigue level (physical, mental and emotional) and level of efficiency, organization and consistency of performance. Additional points would include quality and quantity of work under various conditions, personal and social adjustment in regard to co-workers and supervisors, tolerances for routine and monotonous tasks, realistic level of aspiration, level of motivation and drive, habits related to motivation, punctuality and dependability and ability to handle criticism, correction and a variety of assignments.

Training

The term *work adjustment training* is used to cover a variety of experiences geared toward assisting the person who, by virtue of his handicap, does not possess the attitudes and skills needed to succeed within the regular labor market. Work adjustment training is *not* trade training. Rather, its goal is to help the individual to develop self-confidence, self-control, work tolerances, ability to handle interpersonal relationships, an understanding of the world of work and a "work personality" that will enable him to handle the day-to-day demands of a work situation in the labor market.

Work conditioning involves numerous items, starting with how to punch in on a time clock all the way through to how to handle the receiving of a paycheck in a sophisticated manner. Areas that fall within the scope of work conditioning also include the development of various work tolerances. A few of the work tolerances needed by an employee include the ability to sustain a work effort for a prolonged period of time, maintain a steady flow of production at an acceptable pace and at an acceptable level of quality, handle a certain amount of pressure, get along with all types of co-workers and do the unsavory aspects of the job.

It should be remembered that the goal of work conditioning is to help the person acquire as many skills and tolerances as possible. No one person will necessarily achieve all the tolerances that are "desirable"; however, in most cases, work conditioning training can result in the individual's being able to function at a level commensurate with his potential.

Areas that fall within the scope of attitude modification are the development of motivation to work, the desire to give one's best effort to the job at hand, the characteristic of taking pride in what one does, the ability to gain gratification from being productive, the ability to follow the rules and regulations, to do a job one does not like and to accept correction. The desire to maintain as perfect an attendance record as possible, and the acquisition of a sufficiently high level of self-confidence and self-esteem will enable the person to see himself as an individual worthy of respect because of what he can accomplish. When such an attitude is acquired, the person will most likely be able to handle the day-to-day pressures imposed by a job and to handle himself in a mature, self-controlled fashion.

In order to help the client in learning about the world of work, various techniques such as group meetings can be used. Individual counseling, field trips and experiences within the workshop regarding the various areas of the world of work that are discussed can also be helpful. Emerging from these will be concepts such as why do people work, why does an employer hire a person, and what does the employer expect, plus numerous items concerning earning and spending of money, unions, insurance, vacation, fringe benefits, taxes and so forth. Suffice it to say that most individuals within a workshop do not have a good understanding about the world of work and most likely have learned to bluff quite well when asked questions about their knowledge of the work world. By concentrating on helping the person to acquire knowledge about the world of work in a concentrated fashion, the individual can slowly acquire details regarding these matters.

When follow-up takes place for individuals who have been placed by a workshop, a pattern often appears of a person who can make an adjustment to work but who has difficulty handling the personal and social adjustments necessary to function as an independent person. While many of the elements tied into personal and social adjustment should be learned within the home situation, the fact remains that if a person does not achieve this training when he is in the workshop, he may not achieve it at all. In line with this, it is generally felt that some type of personal and social adjustment training is a necessary adjunct to work adjustment training. Areas that fall under the area of personal adjustment training include self-care, grooming and the ability to manage one's life outside a work situation.

A clear distinction should be kept in mind in regard to the difference between vocational training and work adjustment training. Work adjustment training, which has been described earlier, is basically the satisfying of an individual's needs prior to being ready for specific vocational training (that is, training in auto mechanics, motor winding, et cetera). In many cases, dealing with the more severely handicapped person and the mentally retarded, vocational training may not be indicated as much as an entrance type of job that a person may enter after acquiring the skills stressed in work adjustment training. Nevertheless, for an individual who is capable of mastering a particular vocational field that requires specific training, vocational training may well be in order. In certain instances, a workshop may be well equipped to test a person in regard to a specific vocational training. For example, the workshop may well test a person in regard to an interest in clerical work. However, unless they have a specialized department that is geared to prepare people for the clerical field, it may be much more appropriate to refer this individual to a specialized vocational training program dealing with clerical work, once the person has mastered the items stressed within the work adjustment program.

On-the-job training is often an ideal type of situation for an individual who may not fit into a specific, formalized program of vocational training but who can learn the specifics of a particular job outside a workshop. In cases such as these, the employer might be willing to train a person, providing the workshop can establish that the individual has demonstrated the maturity, attitudes and potentials to benefit from a specific program of on-the-job training.

Rehabilitation Potential Determination

The purpose of a rehabilitation determination program is to determine whether or not there is a reasonable expectation that additional rehabilitation services might render the client fit to engage in a gainful occupation. It is the rehabilitation counselor's responsibility and prerogative to determine whether or not a client is in need of this type of service.

Under the law, services can be provided within this program for a period from six to eighteen months. However, it should be clearly understood that these are maximum allowable periods of time for the establishment of the state agency's third condition of eligibility. During the extended evaluation period, staffings should be held regularly by the workshop and counselor, and justification for remaining in the program should be established.

This justification would be derived from reports received from the facility and the staffing sessions that are held prior to the preparation of these reports. It is extremely important that the rehabilitation counselors attend these staffings.

In every workshop there is an admission's evaluation program. This initial evaluation ranges from four to eight weeks depending on the nature of the program and the makeup of the client served. The focus of this initial evaluation is to clarify the individual's level of functioning, appropriate vocational goals and the services needed to reach these goals. When working with the more severely or multiple handicapped, it is often virtually impossible to make this determination during the initial evaluation period; thus, the determination of the rehabilitation potential (extended evaluation) program provides from six to eighteen months of additional time to determine that there is a reasonable expectation that additional rehabilitation services might render the client fit to engage in a gainful occupation.

The extended evaluation program is not a means to keep a person in a workshop for a prolonged period of time just for the sake of keeping him in the program. The extended evaluation period is for evaluation; however, this does not mean to imply that growth and development do not take place during this time. In fact, considerable training goes on during the evaluation period, and it is this program that brings the person to a point where a judgment can be made as to his future employability. In a case where a person is able to grow and to develop during the extended evaluation program, he can reach a point where it can be reasonably expected that he could be moved on to gainful employment after a period of additional services are provided.

Education

Remedial education may or may not be part of a typical workshop program. Much could be said about the value of offering clients in workshops additional remedial education to help elevate and develop their potentials to make them better equipped to function in the world of work and in the community at large. However, this type of education can often be found in the community, either through regular classroom work or through individual, tutorial work. In workshops that do provide this type of experience, the rehabilitation counselor should give attention to examining the nature of the program and the background of the individual providing this training.

Counseling

Psychiatric counseling is needed when a person's disturbances are rather severe and hamper his ability to function effectively. Obviously, psychotic individuals need psychiatric counseling. Likewise, neurotic individuals and people with other disabling emotional difficulties can benefit from psychiatric services. Quite often in a workshop, psychiatric consultation is available to assist the staff in being better able to understand and work with their clients. In general, this seems to be a very advisable way to utilize psychiatric services and when an individual who is within a workshop program seems to be so disturbed that he does need psychiatric assistance, a referral to an appropriate clinic or therapist is indicated.

Some form of psychological counseling seems indicated when an individual has a handicap that necessitates his being in a workshop program. The trauma of being handicapped, or just being different, often injures a person much more than one would believe on casual contact. The stigma of not being able to perform at an acceptable level, of always being less than adequate, of never being able to live up to one's own, or to others' expectations leaves a tremendous mark on an individual. Only through some type of psychological counseling, be it intensive or casual, can an individual hope to work through some of his trauma to the point where he can utilize his potentials. In certain instances, this psychological counseling need only be supportive in nature. In other instances, it can become intensive to the point that it verges on services better described under psychiatric counseling.

Vocational counseling is geared toward helping the person establish an appropriate vocational goal and moving toward that goal. Within this area, many issues regarding preparation for employment are covered. Testing can be administered and general guidance provided to help the individual arrive at an appropriate vocational goal.

In most workshop settings, a rehabilitation counselor is responsible for the counseling program of the clients. While emphasis will be placed on helping the client establish and prepare for a realistic vocational goal, many of the points mentioned under the section dealing with psychological counseling become an integral part of what is often labeled "vocational counseling," and effective vocational planning cannot be achieved unless the client enters into some type of counseling relationship.

In addition to providing individual counseling by rehabilitation counselors, a social worker can be extremely valuable as an individual who is able to handle intakes, work with the client and the client's family. Anyone who has worked within a workshop is well aware of the individual who does not make it because of lack of family cooperation. While getting the families involved with the workshop may be an extremely difficult task, every effort should be made to involve the parents of the client so that everybody is working towards the same goal and so that lines of communication are kept open.

Medical Services

Depending upon the facility, medical services can be a major area of service offered to the client. In workshops that are associated with medical facilities, these medical services can greatly enhance the services that can be offered by the workshop. In cases where medical services are not extensive in nature, the workshop should have access to medical consultation. Prior to entering the workshop, a general medical is obtained by the rehabilitation counselor and, in certain instances, specialized medical information is obtained. This information is important in planning for the program of the client. Much can be said about involving a medical specialist in helping to develop a person's vocational goal in keeping with his medical and physical condition. Likewise, the question of endurance and physical ability to handle a particular goal is extremely valuable. Consultation services or additional specialized medical evaluation may be indicated as a person proceeds within the workshop program.

Recreational Services

On casual contact with a workshop, recreational services may appear to be a nice addition to a regular program but not necessarily significant in achieving the desired change in the clients. However, as one looks into the background of a typical client in the workshop, it becomes rather apparent that the stigma and deprivation associated with being handicapped affects an individual in many dimensions. One of the major areas in which the person experiences a void is social and recreational experiences associated with the growth patterns of a normal youngster. Clients in the workshop, especially the mentally retarded, are often quite deprived in regard to recreational experiences that are so important in developing coordination, self-confidence, the ability to participate as a team member, physical well-being and a sense of adequacy. Within the workshop, the client acquires a sense of self-worth and in being able to acquire the role of a productive individual. If a person can go beyond this role and acquire the additional sense of being competent within other dimensions of life, such as social or recreational areas, his total growth will be enchanced.

Job Placement

All counselors who deal with workshops are well aware of the time, energy, creativity and hard work involved in placing a handicapped person in a job situation that is in keeping with that individual's interests and capabilities. While there are a number of resources in the community for securing jobs for handicapped people (state employment service, vocational rehabilitation, etcetera), no one can argue that the more resources a person has in terms of seeking job opportunities, the better the chances of finding an adequate position. In addition, a placement person who is in the employ of a workshop has a much better opportunity to be completely familiar with an individual's assets, liabilities, interests and overall functioning than a placement person in another agency. By being aware of these factors, that placement person can take the time necessary to develop an individualized program of placement, prepare the person for the interview, take the person for the interview and follow-up to see that everything runs smoothly. The workshop cannot expect another agency to take on all these responsibilities and to do them with as much detail and time-consuming effort that a regular staff member in the workshop can.

Follow-up

Experience indicates that most individuals who complete the workshop program will need some type of supportive assistance during their initial experience on the job and will have a greater chance of success if they know there is someone to turn to if they run into difficulty, even though they are no longer in the workshop. A placement person or a counselor should be available to the individual when needed. Often, minor difficulties that arise on a job can be cleared up without a great deal of effort by a staff member who is able to provide follow-up services. If this minor event is left unattended, the entire job situation may fall apart. Likewise, the workshop has a responsibility to follow up, at regular intervals, all people who move out of the workshop in order to insure that they are progressing satisfactorily.

WHAT A SHELTERED WORKSHOP CAN ACCOMPLISH

A sheltered workshop can provide an environment that is conducive to the modification of a client's overall functioning. It can also offer a setting in which an individual can experience success as a productive human being. The makeup of the center can be adapted to meet certain needs of the client through individual programming. A sheltered workshop can develop a work and counseling milieu that enables a person to develop his potentials and to plan realistically for the future.

In certain instances, where the workshop is a long-term facility, the center can provide a work situation that enables a person to function effectively even though he does not have the capabilities to handle a job in the regular labor market.

A workshop is not the answer to every client's problems. If an individual is emotionally disturbed to the point that he needs intensive therapy, he will not magically get well in a workshop.

Only when psychiatric services can enable the person to work through his difficulties can he effectively utilize his potentials. Likewise, if a person possesses good work attitudes and basic work discipline, he may need selective placement, special trade or academic training rather than workshop services which are generally geared to the work adjustment approach.

In effect, what services does a client need and does a workshop specifically provide these needed services?

TYPE OF CLIENTS TO BE REFERRED TO A SHELTERED WORKSHOP

In referring a client to a workshop, the counselor should have in mind specific questions that he wants answered. By posing these questions to workshop personnel, both the staff of the workshop and the counselor can focus on finding answers to the specific elements of the client's makeup that appear to make him unemployable. For example, if a client has had several jobs but has been unable to retain these jobs, the question that can be asked the workshop is, What is the cause of this job failure? Has it been that the client has been pushed into jobs that he was unable to handle? Is it the client's inability to cope with supervision? Is it the client's lack of speed or versatility? Does the job lack interest? Does the client lack the ability to do things that he doesn't like?

A counselor may unintentionally view the individual client as a "disability" rather than as a person who has a disability. While the difference may seem subtle, it is quite real when a person is viewed as a "retardate." Certain generalizations are made about that person that may not be valid. On the other hand, if a person is viewed as an individual who tested out as a retarded individual, then much more emphasis is placed on how the person differs from other people who have a similar disability.

A good example of the need to examine a person as an individual rather than as a disability lies in the generalization often made about retardates being good on boring, repetitious tasks. While it is quite true that many individuals who are retarded do function quite well on repetitious and somewhat boring tasks, it is also quite true that just as many individuals who are retarded become bored and disenchanted with repetitious tasks. One of the nicest statements that has ever been made regarding characteristics of mental retardation is a statement made by a teacher when asked to sum up the characteristics of a retardate. The answer to the question was that "mentally retarded people are . . . people."

In extending this concept of looking at the person as an individual, it becomes quite apparent that while some individuals who are retarded may need a program whereby they can mature, other individuals who have the same label may well be able to move on to a job without a long period of maturation. When people are viewed as individuals and not as disabilities, they are often given an opportunity to try out something; whereas, if all emphasis is placed on a disabling condition, the door to imagination might well be closed. This closing of the door is an unfortunate situation. A discussion with any staff member of a workshop will indicate that in many instances a client in the program has greatly outdistanced the original opinion as to how far he could develop and to the extent of growth he could achieve.

WHAT A COUNSELOR CAN EXPECT FROM A SHELTERED WORKSHOP

Workshops have a responsibility to make known to the community the role of the vocational rehabilitation agency and to clarify the nature of their services, misunderstandings and misconceptions about handicapped people. In doing this public relations work, referrals are received by the workshop. These referrals should be referred, in turn, to the vocational rehabilitation agency so that eligibility for services can be determined. The workshop has a responsibility to contact other agencies within the community to make them aware of the type of services the workshop provides and the relationship that the workshop has with the vocational rehabilitation agency.

When a referral comes to a workshop, regardless of how it does come in, an interview should be set up with the intake person to explain the program to the referred person and to establish, as much as possible, the appropriateness of that person's making application to the center. In addition, the individual should be informed of the services offered by the agency and if the person has not already become a client of the agency, he should be referred to the local office. The intake procedure of a workshop is quite significant and should be done by a professionally competent person. The exact details of what an intake report should contain and how it should be used are described earlier in this chapter.

The workshop should accept the responsibility of handling all necessary intake procedures of referring the client to the vocational rehabilitation agency (if this has not already been done) and of keeping in touch with the agency to ascertain if the applicant is acceptable by them for sponsorship in the workshop. If the applicant is an acceptable vocational rehabilitation agency client, the workshop should notify the rehabilitation counselor when an opening in a workshop is available and when it could accept that particular client.

Throughout the program, the workshop should keep in contact with the rehabilitation counselor, set up staffings and invite the rehabilitation counselor to such staffings and notify him of any significant changes in the client or his program.

The vocational rehabilitation agency is purchasing a specific program for a specific client. It is the responsibility of the workshop to see that this service is provided and to document that the stated program is, in fact, provided to the referred client.

The workshop has the responsibility of preparing the necessary evaluation reports and of sending copies to the counselor. These reports not only document what has happened to the client, but they also point out the nature of the program that will be provided for the next given period of time.

Workshops have been very greatly misunderstood by many people and by other agencies within the community. It is the workshop's responsibility to correct these misunderstandings and to establish a positive program whereby it tells its story to the community and obtains its fair share of recognition and support. By so doing, the needs of handicapped persons can be more adequately met and the workshop can achieve more favorable funding support. If the workshop movement is not understood correctly by the people in the community, it is the fault of the workshop

—it has not given enough attention to the public relation needs of a service agency.

WHAT THE SHELTERED WORKSHOP CAN EXPECT FROM THE REHABILITATION COUNSELOR

Attention was given above to methods by which a counselor could assess a given workshop. It is the responsibility of the counselor to follow this process and to become familiar with what the workshop offers and how a counselor might use the services of a workshop for a given client. As mentioned earlier, this can best be achieved by visiting the workshop and meeting with staff personnel. It should be remembered that workshop programs are changing at a very rapid pace and the counselor who may not have had occasion to visit a given workshop for a year or so should, by all means, attempt to revisit and refamiliarize himself with that center.

The rehabilitation counselor has the responsibility to review his client case load and to assess the possibilities of referring appropriate clients to a given workshop for a given service. In certain instances, it might be very clear that a particular client could be served effectively within a workshop program. In other cases the question of the appropriateness of referral may not be clear. It is in these situations that the rehabilitation counselor should speak with the intake worker of a particular workshop to discuss the appropriateness of a referral.

The rehabilitation counselor should assume responsibility for gathering sufficient case material to evaluate fully the client's handicap, previous contact with other agencies and present status. Too often, only sketchy material is available on the client and this lack of information hampers the rehabilitation counselor, as well as the workshop intake worker, in accurately ascertaining the client's status and the appropriateness of the referral to the rehabilitation facility.

When it is deemed appropriate for a client to be referred to a workshop and the workshop has agreed that the client is an appropriate applicant, then the rehabilitation counselor should begin processing the case. This involves a medical examination and psychological testing. In many instances, it may be very necessary to obtain other evaluations to clarify further the appropriateness of the client's being referred and the type of service he may need in addition to the workshop program. The necessary authorizations must be sent to the workshop in accord with the working agreement with the vocational rehabilitation agency. As the client proceeds through the workshop program, it may become necessary to have additional evaluation of services. It is at these times that the rehabilitation counselor should discuss with the staff of the workshop the need for these services and the most appropriate method of obtaining them.

There is no question that the rehabilitation counselor's schedule is quite full and that time to attend meetings at various workshops is demanding. Nevertheless, it is his responsibility to attend and to participate in these staffings, if the client is to receive the best service possible. By attending and by participating in the staffings, the rehabilitation counselor is kept informed of the program that the person is receiving and can offer his expertise in developing plans with the staff of the workshop. If additional services are needed, the rehabilitation counselor is involved in the initial discussion and decision-making.

One additional fact that should not be taken lightly is that when the workshop staff knows that the rehabilitation counselor is truly involved in the program offered his client, the facility is going to make a special effort to provide the best program possible and to work closely with the counselor. Few things stimulate workshop staff more than having outside people ask questions. Often, the workshop may be so "wrapped up" in its own program that it has difficulty seeing things from an outside perspective. The rehabilitation counselor, by asking these questions, can provide this stimulation.

The report that the workshop sends to the counselor should be reviewed and, when necessary, clarified by asking questions. Too often, reports are briefly scanned without giving attention to the details that tell the total story. Thus, a clear picture is often not obtained and the client may well suffer.

Each workshop has an agreement with the vocational rehabilitation agency which spells out in detail the exact relationship between the center and the agency. By being familiar with this agreement, the counselor is aware of what services the workshop offers, how these services are provided and what he can expect from the center. From the workshop's point of view, by having the counselor familiar with the working agreement, there is less chance for misunderstandings and confusion.

The rehabilitation counselor has the responsibility to be familiar with workshops and their operation. This can be accomplished by becoming familiar with the working agreement between the state agency and workshops in his area; by exchanging information with workshop staff members; by attending professional meetings and by keeping up on professional literature regarding the field. With this type of information, the rehabilitation counselor can better utilize the facilities in his area and can make a contribution to the overall movement of workshops in general.

In the preceding sections, an attempt has been made to describe the responsibilities of the workshop and of the vocational rehabilitation agency. In reference to mutual responsibilities, the most significant element is to work together as a team. A workshop's only purpose for existence is to provide meaningful programming for handicapped individuals. The state agency's only purpose for existence is to provide services to these same handicapped individuals. Much too often communication breaks down between agencies and misunderstandings develop. Both the workshop and the rehabilitation counselors have a responsibility to maintain close and open communication, to raise issues that are not clear and to resolve these issues as they occur. By maintaining this type of cooperative arrangement, the client obtains the best possible services as quickly and as effectively as possible.

29

Working with the Community

Keith C. Wright

Shortcomings of Traditional Delivery Systems
Historical Review
Need for Changes in Manpower Utilization
Orientation to the Community.
Some Selected Community Resources for the Rehabilitation Counselor
References

MOST COMMUNITIES in this country are either organized, in some fashion, to help the handicapped or are disorganized in this effort. Our national government, with its state and local counterparts—citizen groups and voluntary agencies and organizations—have developed a very complex system of helping individuals and families to solve their problems. We have created scores of agencies which, in turn, have developed hundreds of programs aimed toward meeting the needs of people.

We have devised systems to deal with major groupings of the problems of people. Welfare and social security programs deal with income maintenance; Medicare, Medicaid and other medical programs deal with health problems; educational systems deal with the provisions of educational training and opportunities for various other types of training; while other systems deal with evaluation, counseling or employment; other systems are concerned with various combinations of these groupings.

SHORTCOMINGS OF TRADITIONAL DELIVERY SYSTEMS

It is evident that all of the problems of one individual—or family—cannot be dealt with within one system, one agency, or one professional discipline. Leaders in planning for services for people have recognized the inadequacies of systems in helping needy individuals—and the problems accompanying the interrelatedness of systems, organizations and disciplines. One of the major emphases we will surely work on during the next decade will be to either break down the systems of delivery of services to people as we have practiced them or to bring these systems into effective relationships with each other. With the proliferation of agencies and services that now exists in most communities, it is imperative that we develop more effective delivery systems. To say that delivery systems are well thought out, well organized and well developed, with clear-cut lines of responsibilities and with congruent goals by all concerned, would be untruthful. There is much indecision, confusion and differences of opinion and emphasis in the teamwork approach to rehabilitation as it is practiced today. Some of this is caused by the variance in training programs (college and in-service) for the various rehabilitation disciplines; some of it is caused by vested interest problems of the agencies; some of it is caused by the mere fact that we have a proliferation of professional disciplines, volunteer personnel and agencies serving the handicapped; some of it is caused by inadequate administrative standards. There are probably many more valid reasons why our delivery systems are under pressure and challenge today as never before.

However proficient an institution or agency may be in fulfilling its special purpose, it cannot meet all human needs—or serve all human beings equally well—even within the universe it is designed to cover. The needs of people are too many and diverse. There must be recognition of the multiple problems of people and recognition of the interrelationships of these problems and then an understanding of the need for coordinated and cooperative efforts to solve them.

Studies of social pathology have clearly demonstrated the "clustering principle"—the clustering of such problems as poverty, unemployment, undereducation, residentital mobility, inadequate housing, delinquency and crime, marital incompatability, divorce, alcoholism, mental illness and poor health. Within families, a serious illness or behavioral problem in one member invariably is reflected in the health and well-being of the entire family unit. A growing recognition of the clustering principle by those responsible for formulating public policy, designing programs of social welfare and implementing different kinds of rehabilitation can have a significant impact on the nature of rehabilitation programs and their response to conditions of social change.[4]

HISTORICAL REVIEW

A brief historical review of rehabilitation counselor assignment over the years reveals that the old-time counselor was a "field" counselor, with a large case load, usually including hundreds of clients (with all types of disabilities and handicapping conditions) and a large territorial assignment often including several counties. There was little specialization and few rehabilitation facilities. In the early years, the rehabilitation counselor tried to be all things to all people—a one-man operator, a jack-of-all trades. How he worked and functioned, how he selected his clients and his services, and the criteria he used in all aspects of his work was more or less known only by him and his supervisor. In effect, he had his own little bag of tricks which were often not shared with others. This so-called professional bag-of-tricks or mysticism is probably not unique to the rehabilitation counselor. This professional isolationism is no longer adequate as a system of delivery of services to clients.

NEED FOR CHANGES IN MANPOWER UTILIZATION

The smooth merging of many professional skills is needed more and more, as programs are called on to deal with an ever-widening range of disabilities and with ever more severe and complicated problems of disability and dependence. No one professional worker can do the job. Neither can a whole series of professionals, working one at a time. They must work together, all at once, if they are to come up with the best answers for their handicapped clients.[5] Mary Switzer[6] stated "There is only one alternative to coordination in the field of human services—and that is chaos." She also stated, "Coordination cannot simply be achieved, in principle, at the federal level. The efforts that really count, those that will pay dividends, begin where the service is, where the need for it exists, and where a willingness to organize to improve services is essential—in the community."

Interagency cooperation, interdisciplinary teamwork and effective community resource utilization are recognized by the Federal Government as necessary attributes for effective helping programs.

Organization of CAMPS (Cooperative Area Manpower Planning System) is evidence of the government's concern. The proliferation of agencies, programs and services—all designed to aid the disadvantaged-were operating under authority from different legislation, with each imposing its own conditions for the use of funds. Gaps and duplications resulted. Some needy people were left out because they did not fit readily into existing programs. Others needed several types of help (the clustering principle). Often they did not know where to find help to their problems.

CAMPS, therefore, came into existence as a cooperative planning and action system for effective utilization of manpower. It encompasses many of the manpower and related programs of eight federal agencies. It recognizes that the focal point for joint action is the local area (the rehabilitation counselor's area) where services and clients come together. Counselors may obtain more information on CAMPS by contacting the local office of their state employment service.[1]

Dr. Edward Newman, Commissioner, Rehabilitation Services Administration, has also emphasized the importance of interagency and community resource relationships in his discussion and review of the 1968 Amendments to the Vocational Rehabilitation Act relating to vocational evaluation and work adjustment.

Dr. Newman[2] states that Section 15 of the Act provides for rehabilitation services to support "all manpower and manpower-related programs in a community. Manpower programs—such as the Concentrated Employment Program and the Work Incentive Program as well as other programs of the Department of Labor." He further states that this section of the act authorizes for disadvantaged individuals, among other services, those of outreach, referral and advocacy. These three important services cannot be administered effectively without counselor knowledge and understanding of his community.

Services for the disadvantaged are being performed by a number of different agencies which are often competing with each other to assist the same client or to enlist the cooperation of the same employer. The client who needs several types of service often finds himself bounced around from one agency to another with little or no information sharing on the part of these agencies concerning the needs and with too little support from the referring agency to ensure that the referral results in effective services.[3]

Another major problem in effecting better utilization of community resources is the fact that certain professional disciplines become associated with various systems and then become defenders of these systems; for example, the teacher in education, the social worker in welfare and the counselor in rehabilitation agencies. In addition to this vested interest problem is the fact that very few people really know their community, really understand the requirements, functions and charges of the various agencies, organizations and disciplines. Turnover of staff serves to enlarge this problem.

Training programs for the helping professions also must share a large part of the blame for inadequate community organization and poor community resource utilization. In too many universities, health care training programs develop without ever talking to each other. Each specialty stakes its claim to space and program and then proceeds to build its own little empire. According to Wright and Hardy[7] duplication is rampant and an excellent opportunity for cross-fertilization is lost. This is true of many programs in the helping professions. Teamwork is preached by all faculty members—but not practiced by all. The professionals who must practice teamwork and who must work together following graduation unfortunately do not study together while matriculating at the university. Teamwork becomes either effective or ineffective through trial and error on the job. There is need for some interdepartmental and interdisciplinary programs in the universities. There are, certainly, many areas of common concern for all disciplines. The clustering principle certainly shows some relationships. The client presents the same problems to all of us. There must be some justification for one or more interdepartmental, interdisciplinary classes on campus; for instance, Interdisciplinary Relationships, Rehabilitation Concepts and Principles or Community Resources. We should at least question the necessity for a proliferation of seemingly identical courses on campus such as Psychiatric Information for Rehabilitation Counselors —then one for psychologists, another for social workers, and so forth.

ORIENTATION TO THE COMMUNITY

The newly employed rehabilitation counselor will require a considerable amount of time getting acquainted with the available resources in the community. It takes time to establish effective working relationships with the variety of resources and persons in any community. It becomes imperative therefore that the counselor prepare an ongoing itinerary which will afford him the opportunity to develop the necessary contacts needed in order to do his job.

The counselor should set aside a specified amount of time each week for community relations and community contact work. Perhaps this should amount to one day per week. His itinerary for that time should be specific. Much of the itinerary should be scheduled with appointments.

There is much more to effective community organization and community resource utilization than referral. The rehabilitation program must be interpreted to the community. Relationships between rehabilitation and other community services must be pointed out. Working relationships must be established. Knowledge of community service programs and services must be learned. All of this takes time.

Many communities have directories of social services and most rehabilitation offices have available directories of organizations most used, yet, it must be realized that these directories serve as the starting point for personal involvement. Effective working relationships are based on personal contact. It is necessary that the counselor know people. It is necessary that he know them well.

Effective personal relationships increase as we move from letter correspondence to phone contact to personal visit. People work more effectively together when they know each other.

Getting acquainted is the first step in establishing effective community resource utilization. Once the formalities of introduction are achieved, we then move into exchanging information and in this exchange of information we can establish the relationship between the community resource and the rehabilitation program. At that point we might move into the establishment of referral activities to be followed by joint planning and coordination with concurrent cooperative services.

There are several problems inherent when we are concerned with effective community resource utilization. Perhaps one of the major areas in which we recognize problems is the lack of knowledge about each other. Another would be personnel turnover. This fact, incidentally, indicates that maintenance of effective community relationships is an ongoing activity.

Other barriers to effective teamwork would be "agency mindedness" whereby we become so involved in our own little world, our own agency, that we fail to establish relationships outside the agency bounds. It is necessary to keep in mind that rehabilitation and the rehabilitation counselor supplement community services to the disabled and that the counselor many times must coordinate the community services for an effective rehabilitation plan for his client. Another barrier to teamwork is the age-old stereotyping of other professionals and agencies. We could of course add the problems of vested interest, personality complex and professional jealousies. There is certainly a real need for us to understand and accept differences among ourselves as professional persons to the same extent that we try to do this with our clients.

The counselor should recognize the fact that a scheduled itinerary each week for the purpose of working in the community and establishing working relationships in essence helps him to serve more people. This itinerary does not detract from his production in serving as many people as possible. This itinerary emphasizes the fact that rehabilitation is a concern of many people. It emphasizes that rehabilitation is a community concern. It eventually

Working with the Community

results in more clients receiving more services at one time than would otherwise be possible.

One of the primary problems encountered when counselors are transferred from one territory to another, when they are promoted to administrative and supervisory positions or when they resign is that the new counselor coming into the community must begin to establish effective relationships with the community all over again. This is the principle reason why the newly employed counselor usually is not expected to achieve the same number of rehabilitated clients during the first year as the counselor who has already established himself in the community.

A typical day's itinerary for community services development might include one or two regularly scheduled weekly meetings with the counselors' counterpart in the welfare office and the employment service office. It might include one or two visits to local physicians, a scheduled visit for a plant or job survey and then some visits for follow-up purposes to employers who have employed rehabilitation clients. It would be appropriate for this weekly itinerary to always include at least one new employer or business, one or more employers for follow-up and one or more visits to cooperating agencies who serve people in the community. The wide variety of community resources available in most communities would assure that this one-day itinerary would not be static. It could offer a variety of changing visits each week. It would provide the opportunity to meet with clients who have been placed in the community and in addition the opportunity to find new clients within the community.

The newly employed rehabilitation counselor might utilize the statistics available from sources of referral when planning his community resource itinerary. For instance, he might prepare a table which shows all sources of referral to his case load for the past year. From this compilation he might be able to determine which referral sources need special emphasis and he could plan his itinerary accordingly.

The rehabilitation counselor also could identify the source of referral for all clients rehabilitated during the prior year. When combined with the new referral statistic, the counselor might be able to determine to some degree the effectiveness of referral by some of the referral sources. This could also help him in planning a more effective community resource itinerary. Incidentally, it should be mentioned that reporting back to referral source at closure and at other times during the rehabilitation process might also serve as an effective case finding tool for the rehabilitation counselor. Referrals are more apt to be made when the referring agency and referring persons know what has happened to their referrals.

SOME SELECTED COMMUNITY RESOURCES FOR THE REHABILITATION COUNSELOR

The State Employment Service

The local state employment service can help the rehabilitation counselor in a number of ways. This agency can provide for employment counseling for job choice, job change and job adjustment. The agency also administers the GATB for use by the agency and the counselor in arriving at a suitable job objective. The employment service can help the rehabilitation counselor in selection and referral to job openings. It provides for selective placement and individualized job development. In addition, this agency prepares labor market information for employers and for applicants and rehabilitation counselors. Generally, the employment service has entered into a written agreement with the state vocational rehabilitation agency which recognizes the common goal of each—namely, employment. The employment service should serve as a good source of referral for rehabilitation and the rehabilitation counselor should recognize the employment service for its special abilities in placement and should think seriously about referring all rehabilitation clients who become ready for employment. Each employment service office has designated a person to serve as a counselor for the disabled. The rehabilitation counselor should know this person in his own locality.

State Welfare Department

State welfare departments provide a variety of services which can be of help to the rehabilitation counselor. For instance, it is possible for the welfare department to provide assistance to family members when the rehabilitation counselor has entered into a rehabilitation program with the family breadwinner. Perhaps the rehabilitation counselor has developed a program at a rehabilitation center which necessitates an absence from home by the breadwinner. The family assistance by the welfare department during this time would enhance the rehabilitation plan of the client. Most welfare programs have also entered into work incentive programs for their clients and these should enhance the relationships between the two agencies. Welfare departments should serve as a good source of referral for rehabilitation and a source for cooperative programming. Most state welfare departments have entered into written agreements with the state vocational agencies and have described what the contributions of each should be in a cooperative program. Generally speaking the goal of vocational rehabilitation is independence and in this instance would include removal from welfare rolls. This is not always possible but vocational rehabilitation can result in a substantial reduction of welfare payments and this in itself is a worthwhile rehabilitation goal.

Family and Children's Service

Most communities have a family and children's service which provides a series of services which might be of help to the rehabilitation counselor when working with his client. This agency generally provides for marital counseling and in many instances it can arrange for, in cooperation with the local bar association, a legal aid type of assistance to provide legal counsel to persons in need. In many instances the family service society can provide short-term financial assistance to meet emergency needs, usually when such help is not available through other sources such as the Department of Public Welfare. This organization often provides for budget counseling for families on limited income and in some instances provides for homemaker service. This service would provide trained and supervised household workers daytime coverage to families faced with emergency for such help but unable to secure it through usual resources. It generally provides a variety of services concerning various types of family and individual social and emotional problems.

Sheltered Workshops

Many communities have sheltered workshops which can serve the rehabilitation counselor in a number of ways. Many workshops can provide for prevocational evaluation, training for various type jobs, development of work tolerance, development of work habits, personal adjustment and job tryout, and many will provide for interim employment and employment. In addition, many workshops have developed work evaluation units whereby the counselor can evaluate a rehabilitation client through reality testing. Here the unit often provides for actual job samples and real work under real work conditions. The client is evaluated not only according to his aptitudes and performance but also in order to obtain information on work habits, work tolerance, ability to take supervision, ability to follow instructions and the ability to get along with his fellowman. He can actually be evaluated along those lines in which employers are really interested. Since many persons, disabled or not disabled, are poor employees not on the basis of their ability to perform a job but on their inability to profit from supervision, get along with others and for personality reasons, this kind of evaluation can actually help the counselor to know his client better as a person and be better able to represent his client and employer. Utilization of sheltered workshops can often provide for prescription services from the counselor.

Medical and/or Dental Schools

The rehabilitation counselor often has available at the medical and/or dental schools a variety of services which might help him in serving his client. Many of these schools operate a wide variety of clinics which offer more extensive evaluation than may be available elsewhere. Many of them offer a number of special clinics which the counselor might use; for instance, prosthetic clinics, seizure control clinics or diabetic control clinics. Since many rehabilitation agencies frown somewhat upon the purchase of dentures or tooth extraction and fillings, the dental school can provide these services for the rehabilitation counselor without the necessity of extensive use of his case service funds.

Voluntary Organizations and Agencies

There are a large number of voluntary agencies which provide a wide variety of services which might help the counselor. Many of these agencies are concerned with specific disabilities. In such instances these agencies might provide counsel to the client and to the counselor concerning the specific problem. Many of these agencies have literature which can aid the counselor in understanding the specific problem and help him in his counseling with the client. In addition, many of these agencies have literature which is available to the rehabilitation client which can help him in understanding his condition and how to live with it. There are other voluntary organizations that operate or conduct loan closets. In such instances the counselor might secure a wheel chair, crutches and other equipment which might be necessary on a temporary basis. Some voluntary organizations provide for transportation services and homemaker services. Others such as the YMCA, Salvation Army, American Red Cross, et cetera, might provide for temporary lodging, meals and emergency assistance. Many times these types of services are necessary immediately and they can serve until the client overcomes the emergency or is accepted into an ongoing program in one of the public agencies.

Training Facilities

Most communities offer a wide range of training resources which rehabilitation counselors might use effectively when developing training plans with their clients. We have already mentioned a sheltered workshop as a training resource. To this we might add several other types of training resources such as business schools, technical schools, colleges and universities and other institutional-type training programs. The counselors should also be aware of employment or on-the-job training with employers in his community. At times there would be a need also for correspondence training and tutorial training.

REFERENCES

1. U.S. Department of Labor: *Cooperative Area Manpower Planning System, Concentrating Manpower Services Against Poverty.* Washington, D.C., Manpower Administration, U. S. Government Printing Office, 1970.
2. Newman, E.: Vocational evaluation and work adjustment: A future thrust of the rehabilitation movement. *Rehab Rec,* January-February 1971.
3. Odel, C. E.: Improving opportunities through coordination. *J Rehab,* March-April 1969.
4. Straus, R.: Social change and the concept of rehabilitation. *Rehab Rec,* May-June 1965.
5. Straus, R.: Teamwork. *Rehab Rec,* March-April 1969.
6. Switzer, M. E.: Coordination: A problem and a promise. *J Rehab,* March-April 1969.
7. Wright, K. C., and Hardy, R. E.: An alternative to duplication. *J Rehab,* November-December 1970.

Index

A

Acceptance, 212
Accountability, 305, 306
Acculturation, 157
Accuracy of information, 218
Actual body image, *see* Body image
Addams, Jane, 20
Addictive disabilities, 112
Adjustment to disability, 421ff
Administration on Aging, 49
Advisory committee, 300
Air Force Classification Test Battery, 190
"Agency mindedness," 532
Aging, 437
 employment needs, 442
 psychological aspects, 438
 social needs, 443
Albee, G. W., 472, 483
Allan, W. S., 483, 502
Alper, B. S., 481, 483
American Association of Industrial Physicians and Surgeons, 15
American Association of Work Evaluators, 193
American Association of Workers for the Blind, 414
American Board, 455
American Federation of Labor, 9
American Journal of Psychology, 16
American Mutual Insurance Alliance, 240, 242
American Personnel and Guidance Association, 24, 141
American Psychological Association, 141, 470, 491
American Red Cross, 20, 537
American Rehabilitation Counseling Association, 141, 171, 173
Anderson, R. P., 64, 127
Annual Institute for Rehabilitation Personnel, 128
Anthony, Susan B., 12, 69
Anthony, W. A., 174
Appropriation Act, 278
Archambault, R. D., 54
Army Alpha, 25
Army Beta, 25
Assurance of the counselor, 216
Axelrad, L., 60, 64

B

Baccalaureate degree, 120
Background data, 475
Baker, H. J., 54
Barber, B., 141, 148
Barden-La Follette Act, 43
 see also Public Law, 1943
Barillas, M., 149
Baron, S. W., 54
Barrett, A. M., 187, 255
Bauman, M. K., 254, 402, 405
Baxt, R., 187
Beck, R. H., 54
Beecher, Henry Ward, 18
Beers, Clifford, 17, 20, 54
Behavioral disorders, 473, 474
Behaviorally disabled, 111
Bender-Gestalt Test, 368
Binet, Alfred, 16
Binet-Simon IQ Test, 16
Blicksler, Paul, 416, 420
Blind, 90, 242
Blindness, 401
Blum, J. M., 53, 54
B'nai B'rith, 19
Board-certified physician, 455
Board eligible physician, 455
Body image, 422
Borow, H., 64
Bregman, M. H., 190, 210
Brewer, J. M., 16, 54

539

Bridgeport Project, 293
Bridges, C. C., 247, 254
Brill, A. A., 64
Buck, D. P., 350
Bureaucratization, 157, 158

C

CAMPS, 529
Career opportunities, 74
Careers (new), 71
Carkhuff, R. R., 169, 174, 405
Carnegie Corporation, 19
Carroll, T. J., 401, 405
Case finding techniques, 135, 185
Case supervision, 263
Case planning and management, 288
Case supervision, 263
Center for Study of the Unemployed, 7
Character disorders, 270
Children's Bureau, 49
Citizen Groups, 526
Classification committees, 364
Client, 409
Client-centered placement, 237
Client responsibility, 263
Clinical psychologists, 471, 475
Closure, 263, 268
"Clustering principle," 527
Cogan, M. L., 152, 166, 174
"Comeback," 186
Committee on Employment of the Physically Handicapped, 240
Committee to Promote the Employment of the Handicapped, 184
Community, 341ff, 373, 375, 526
Compensation, 432
Compensatory Skill Training, 230, 231
Confidentiality, 464
Consultation model, 495
Contemporary poor, 114
Control, 285
Conversion reactions, 421
Coolidge, Calvin, 36
Cooperative Area Manpower Planning System, 529
Cooperative programming, 275ff, 294ff, 304ff, 326ff, 346
Cooperative public school-vocational rehabilitation programs, 280ff
Coordinator, 127
Correctional institution, 351ff
Correctional setting, 357ff, 381
Counseling the blind, 396ff
Counseling session
   anatomy of, 212
   development of, 214
   greeting, 214
Counseling techniques, 212
Counselor, 449ff
Counselor-physician relationship, 460
Counselor trainees, 119
Crippled Children's Service, 290
Cull, J. G., 445, 478, 483, 497, 502
Cummings, H. B., 153, 154
Cybernation, 63

D

Davis, R. V., 237, 254, 255
Day-Care Facilities and Services, 290
Defense mechanisms, 426
Denial, 427
Dental schools, 536
Detroit Day School for the Deaf, 23
Dewey, John, 20, 21, 22
Diagnosis (psychological), 477
Dickson, W. J., 64
Dictionary of Occupational Titles, 249
Di Michael, S. G., 483, 497
Disability, economics of, 79
Disadvantaged, 6
Discovery method, 332
Division 22, 141
Dix, Dorothea, 17
Documentation, 267
Dumas, N. S.,
"Dynamic conservatism," 45

E

Easter Seal Society, 20
Eclectic, 397
Economics of disability, 79
Educational assessment, 476
Educational history, 475
Effective counseling, 134
Egerman, Karl, 198, 210
Egerton, A. H., 36, 154

Index 541

Eisenhower, Dwight D., 44, 82
Eligibility, 88, 135
Emotional problems, 270
Empathy, 354
Employability factors, 203
Employment
　getting client ready, 246
　needs of the aging, 442
　opportunities, 244
Employment Security Commission, 43
England, G. W., 255
English, A. C., 422, 434
English, O. S., 335
Ethical conduct, 262
Ethical considerations, 464ff
Evaluation, 316, 509
Existentialism, 195
Exploratory occupational experiences, 319
Extended evaluation, 514
Extended workshop, 506

F

Family and Children's Service, 535
Fantasy, 430
Farwell, G. F., 54
Faulkes, W. F., 26, 150
Federal Board for Vocational Education, 26, 27, 28, 30, 35, 38, 153, 155
Federal Emergency Relief Administration, 38
Federal Rehabilitation Agency, 116
Federal Security Agency, 41ff
Fine, S. A., 335
Fiske, D. W., 194, 210
Follow-up, 263, 323, 324, 512, 519
Formal training methods, 232
Forster, W. O., 53
Foster, Terry, 39
Free-standing rehabilitation center, 104
Freud, Sigmund, 16
Fulton, W. S., 379

G

Galbraith, J. K., 64
Galludet, Thomas, 22
Galston, Iago, 53
Galton, F., 445

Gardner, John W., 6, 49, 51, 52, 75, 117
GATB, 534
Gellman, William, 194, 210
General Aptitude Test Battery, 225
General clerical tests, 501
Gibbons, James, 18
Gilbert, J. L., 210
Ginsburg, S. W., 60, 64
Ginzberg, E., 60, 64
Glanz, E. C., 54
Gompers, Samuel, 9, 10
Goldstein, Sidney E., 19, 54
Goodwill Industries, 19
Governor's Committee to Promote Employment of the Handicapped, 184
Greeks, 61
Greeting, *see* Interview
Greenwood, Ernest, 166, 167, 174
Griswold, P., 148
Gross, E., 165, 174
Group counseling, 331
Group psychotherapy, 482
Group treatment, 481
Guidance Testing Class, 191
Gustad, J. W., 396, 405

H

Halfway houses, 374, 393, 479ff
Hall, G. S., 15, 21
Hall, J. H., 128, 148
Hamilton, K. W., 235
Handlin, O., 53
Hanlon, J. J., 53
Harding, Warren, 36
Hardy, R. E., 254, 405, 483, 497, 502, 538
Harrington, Michael, 114
Hatt, P. K., 53
Haug, M. R., 124, 144, 149, 350
Helms, Edgar, 19
Henry Street Settlement, 20
Hensley, G., 350
Herma, J. L., 60, 64
Hill, David S., 24, 25
Hobby, Oveta Culp, 44, 45
Hoffman, P. R., 210
Hofstadter, R., 53
Holbert, W. M., 137, 148

Holland, J. L., 64
Hoover, Herbert, 36
Horace, H. B., 422, 434
House Ways and Means Committee, 39
Hull House, 20
Hylbert, K. W., 71, 148

I

Ideal body image, *see* Body image
Identification, 431
Income maintenance, 79
Industrial gerontology, 436
Industrial Revolution, 8, 9
Industrialization, 20
In-hospital services, 391ff
In-service training, 268
Institute for the Crippled and Disabled, 191, 192
Institute for Crippled and Disabled Men, 37, 90
Institutionalization, 363
Intake, 508
Intellectual ability, 476
Interview, 214, 224
 acceptance, 216
 closing, 224
 development, 214
 greeting, 213
 opening, 214
Intrapsychic conflicts, 475
IQ, 435, 510

J

Jacques, M. E., 142, 143, 148
James, William, 15, 16
Jeffrey, D. L., 254
Jeffrey, R. P., 254
Jewish Employment and Vocational Service, 196, 208
Job analysis, 199, 248, 249
Job Placement, 238, 312, 323, 388, 518
Job training, 312
 advanced, 322
 community, 321
 on-campus, 320
Job tryout, 202
Joint Committee on Mental Illness and Health, 480

Joint Liaison Committee, 126
Johndrow, R. F., 445
Johnson, D. E., 174
Johnson, F. E., 18, 54
Johnson, L. T., 127, 148, 254
Jordan, J. E., 405
Joynes, V. A., 124, 144, 149, 350

K

Kaplan, Max, 64
Keller, O. J., 481, 483
Kessler, Henry H., 33
Krantz, Gordon, 194, 195, 210
Krantzler, M., 140, 142, 143, 148
Kratz, John, 40
Kraus, E. A., 482, 483
Kuder Preference Record, 368, 500

L

Laird Amendments, 278, 279
Laird, Melvin, 278
Landis, P. H., 53
Lane, P. A., 235, 335
Larson, K., 379
Lasch, C., 54
Lerner, J., 497
Lewin, K., 193, 210
Liberty Mutual Insurance Company, 164
Libidinal forces, 475
Lincoln, J. T., 415, 420
Little, R. M., 15, 26
Locating employment opportunities, *see* Employment opportunities
Lofquist, L. H., 237, 254, 255
London, Jack, 13
Long-term workshop, 506
Lorge, I., 445

M

Maas, M. J., 91
Mager, R. F., 335
Maisel, A. Q., 53, 54
Manpower, 74
Manpower Development and Training Programs, 208, 290
Manpower utilization, 63, 528
Margolin, R. J., 379

Marshall, H. E., 54
Martin, S. P., 132, 133, 148
Marx, Karl, 60
Maslow, A. H., 251, 254
Massachusetts School for the Blind, 22
Mayer, G. H., 53
McAlees, D. C., 124, 125, 136, 137, 148
McCauley, W. A., 174
McGowan, J. F., 52, 187, 254, 483
McMurtie, Douglas C., 27
McNamee, H. T., 254
Medicaid, 109, 113, 290, 526
Medical consultant, 467
Medical evaluation, 451
Medical Facilities Survey and Construction Act, 83
Medical history, 453
Medical model, 472
Medical referral, 134
Medical schools, 536
Medical services, 364, 517
Medical Services Administration (Medicaid), 49
Medicare
Mental Health Association, 309
Mental illness, 386ff
 see also Mentally ill
Mentally ill, services for, 391
Miller, J. H., 137, 148
Miller, L. A., 149
Mills, D. L., 151, 174
Milwaukee Conference on Rehabilitation, 154
Mink, D. G., 55
Minnesota Multiphasic Personality Inventory, 368
Mobility, 109
Morgan, C. A., 405, 414, 420
Moriarty, E. J., 126, 127, 148
Morrill Act of 1862, 21
Morrison, S. E., 53
Morrow, J. C., 335
Moser, L. E., 55
Moser, R. S., 55
Mowrer, O. H., 473, 483
Munsterberg, Hugo, 16
Murray, H. A., 64, 194, 210
Muthurd, J. E., 70, 149

N

Nadolsky, J. M., 195, 210
National Association of Mental Health, 20
National Association for Retarded Children, 309
National Association of Sheltered Workshops and Homebound Programs, 503
National Citizens Advisory Committee on Vocational Rehabilitation, 67
National Conference of Charities and Corrections, 20
National Conference of Social Welfare, 20
National Conference on Vocational Rehabilitation, 153
National Easter Seal Society for Crippled Children and Adults, 20
National Employ the Physically Handicapped Week, 44
National Rehabilitation Association, 37, 39, 69, 173, 193, 198, 237
National Rehabilitation Counseling Association, 124, 141, 171, 173
National Society for Vocational Education, 34
National Tuberculosis Association, 20
National Vocational Guidance Association, 24
Neff, W. S., 64, 192, 199, 210
New careers, 71
New Deal, 38
Newman, Edward, 144, 145, 149, 529, 538
Nixon, R. A., 7, 53, 71, 124, 138, 149
Nonverbal communication, 219
Nursing services, 98

O

Obermann, C. E., 34, 35, 42, 48, 50, 53, 54, 139, 149, 150, 153, 154, 174
Odel, C. E., 538
Office of Economic Opportunity, 113
Office of Education, 38, 39, 41, 153
Office of Vocational Rehabilitation, 42, 43, 44, 83
On-the-job training, 514
Orientation, 259

Otis Self-Administering Tests of Mental Ability, 501

P

Parents, 339
Parsons, Frank, 23, 25, 55
Parsons, Talcott, 167, 174
Patterson, C. H., 127, 130, 131, 149
Peabody Picture Vocabulary Tests, 500
Pearson, G. H. J., 335
Pencil and paper tests, 501
Perceptual-motor functioning, 476
Perkins Institution, 22
Personal Adjustment Training, 229, 230
Personality factors, 476
Personnel and Guidance Journal, 199
Peters, H. J., 54
Pfeifer, E. J., 502
Physical restoration services, 266
Physician, 449ff
Placement, 134, 263
  see also Vocational placement
Plan development, 134, 267
Plunkett, George Washington, 11
Pneumoconiosis, 275
Populist-Progressive political movement, 12
Portals (Los Angeles), 480
Porter, T. L., 52, 187, 254, 483
Portvillez School, 190
Poulke, R. M., 64
President's Committee on Employment of the Handicapped, 44, 91, 186, 240
Prevocational evaluation, 188, 189
Prevocational training, 230, 317
Prison staff, 362, 367
Probation and parole, 372
Professional bearing, 217
Professional placement, 245
Professionalism, 139
Program coordination, 328, 349
Projection, 431
Prossner, C. A., 27
Protestant Ethics, 61
Pruit, W. A., 479, 483
Psychiatric counseling, 389, 516
  professional preparation for, 394
Psychological counseling, 516, 517
Psychological evaluation (use of), 493
Psychological report, 475, 492
Psychological services, 484ff, 499
Psychological testing, 474, 487
Psychological test scores, 494
Psychologist, 491
Psychologist and rehabilitation, 470
Psychology, 15
Psychology as a profession, 470ff
Psychometric testing, 200
Psychosomatic medicine, 421
Public Health and Marine Hospital Service, 13
Public Law
  1917 Smith Hughes Act, 22, 25, 27
  1918 P. L. 65-178, 26
  1920 P. L. 66-235, 8, 25, 81
  1943 P. L. 78-113, 42, 43, 82, 153, 155, 308, 386, 388, 472, 482
  1954 P. L. 83-565, 44, 45, 46, 82, 83, 159, 191, 242, 291, 292, 309, 356, 388, 473, 482
  1965 P. L. 89-333, 85, 177, 178, 206, 227, 278, 356
  1968 P. L. 90-391, 473, 482, 529
Public schools, 280ff
Purdue Peg Board, 368, 500
Puth, A. D., 161, 174

R

Rationalization, 430
Reaction formation, 429
Reality-oriented therapy, 382
Recreational services, 518
Redkey, Henry, 192, 210
Referral source, 466
Referrals, 263, 477
  psychological services, 488
Rehabilitation, 80
  centers, 93, 95, 97
  facilities, 93, 99, 102, 503
  new services, 285
  plan, 227
  potential determination, 514
  process, 95
  system, 85
Rehabilitation counseling, 118, 398
Rehabilitation Counseling Bulletin, 70

Rehabilitation Counselor, 161
  administrative role, 300
Rehabilitation Counselor's Association, 141
Rehabilitation Generalist, 67
Rehabilitation Literature, 192
Rehabilitation Movement, 11
Rehabilitation Services Administration, 49, 208, 264
Regression, 428
Relief fund, 38
Religion, 17
Remedial education, 515
Reporting, 267
Repression, 429
Rerum Novarum, 18
Revised Beta Examination, 501
Rights to rehabilitation, 110
Roberts, A., 502
Rockefeller Foundation, 19
Rockefeller, Nelson, 45
Roe, Anne, 60, 64
Roethlisberger, F. J., 60, 64
Rogers, C. R., 50, 335
Roles, 127
Romans, 61
Roosevelt, F. D., 38
Rugg, H., 54
Rusalim, H., 187

S

Salomone, P. R., 70, 149
Salvation Army, 18, 537
Samler, J., 137, 149
School unit, 295ff, 302, 310ff, 315, 327, 336ff
School unit counselor, 336ff
  functions of, 343
SCORE, 443, 445
Scott, W. Richard, 158, 159
Screening committee, 299
Secondary sources, 183
Section 2, 277, 279, 282
Selective Service Agency, 43
Self-care, 90, 98, 109
Service Corps of Retired Executives, 443, 445
Severely disabled, 95, 97

Shay, H. F., 350
Sheltered workshops, 347, 435, 504ff, 519ff, 536
Shryock, R. H., 53
Silverstone, L. S., 235, 335
Sinclair, Upton, 13
Sindberg, R. M., 502
Sinick, D., 254
Situation approach, 201
Skilled manpower, 79
Smith, C. E., 55
Smith, D. R., 149
Smith-Hughes Act, 22, 25, 27
  see also Public Law, 1917
Smith, J., 149
Smith, R. L., 110
Smith-Sears Veteran's Rehabilitation Act, 26
  see also Public Law, 1918
Soares, L. M., 235, 335
Social Darwinism, 18
Social reform, 20
Social and Rehabilitation Service, 6, 49, 193
Social Security Act, 39, 81, 113
Socialization, 157
Socially and culturally handicapped, 112
Sociopsychological model, 472ff
Soldier Rehabilitation Act, 26
  see also Public Law, 1918
Somatopsychology, 422
Special education, 280ff, 344
Specific aptitude tests, 476
Sprague, Norman, 436, 445
Staff development, 73, 120
Staffing committee, 299
Staffing pattern, 71
Staffings, 514
Stalnaker, W. O., 254
Stanford-Binet Test, 16
Stanton, Homer L., 32
State Employment Service, 534
State-Federal Program, 99
State Welfare Department, 534
State Council of Rehabilitation Administrators, 85
Straus, R., 538
Strauss, George, 174

Strict panel model, 495
Stussman, M. B., 350
Suinn, R. M., 65
Super, D. E., 60, 64, 149
Supervising psychologist model, 496
Supportive counseling, 332, 334
Sussman, M. E., 124, 144, 149
Switzer, Mary, 6, 44, 45, 49, 147, 149, 528, 538
Synthesis and summary, 477
Szasz, T. S., 473, 483

T

"Target" groups, 275, 289
Taylor, F. W., 16, 64
Techniques of counseling, 212
Terman, Louis, 16
Tertiary sources, 183
Tessler, B., 379
Test Administration, 135
"Tester", 474
Testing services, 478
Tests of mechanical comprehension, 501
Therapeutic efforts of medicine, 95
Therapeutic workshops, 103
Third-party funds, 279ff
Thomason, B., 187, 255
Thompson, A. S., 149
Thompson, R. C., 37
Tilgher, Adriano, 64
Total client evaluation, 301
TOWER, 192
Towle, C., 132, 149
Training, 228, 229, 247, 267
Transitional, 504, 505
Treatment team, 388
Truax, C. B., 133, 149

U

United Cerebral Palsy Association, 191
United Mine Workers of America, 164
U. S. Department of Health, Education and Welfare, 45
U. S. Department of the Interior, 38, 39, 41
U. S. Department of Labor, 133, 208
U. S. Public Health Service, 14

V

Verbal communication, 218
Vernile, R. T., Jr., 379
Veterans Administration, 160
Vocational
 adjustment, 323
 behavior, science of, 237
 counseling, 134, 325ff, 331
 education, 22, 23, 270
 evaluation, 188, 189, 190, 478, 511
 guidance, 23, 325ff, 331
 placement, 236, 250, 248
 rehabilitation, 6, 38
 schools, 103
 training, 230, 231
Vocational Bureau, 23
Vocational Evaluation and Work Adjustment Association, 193, 237
Vocational Evaluation and Work Adjustment Bulletin, 237
Vocational Guidance Association, 265
Vocational Rehabilitation Act, 23, 25, 27, 177, 277, 279
Vocational Rehabilitation Agency, 191, 333
Vollmer, H. M., 151, 174
Voluntary agencies, 526
Voluntary organizations, 537

W

Wald, Lillian, 20
Walk-ins, 180
War Manpower Office, 43
Warren, S. L., 128, 148
Watson, R. I., 53
Weaver, E. W., 24
Wechsler Adult Intelligence Scale, 368, 500
Wechsler, H., 483
Wechsler Intelligence Scale for Children, 501
Weiss, D. J., 255
West, J. A., 350
White, Barbara, 210
White, T. K., 149
Wide Range Achievement Test, 204, 500
Wilson, Woodrow, 12, 26
Withdrawal, 427

Withers, W. M., 54
Woodworth, R. S., 483
Work
 activity center, 504
 adjustment, 188, 189, 512
 evaluation, 188, 190, 202ff
 evaluator, 206, 207
 history, 476
 "personality," 237
 release, 373
 samples, 200, 479
 tolerances, 512
 world of, 513
Workmen's Compensation, 14
Workshops, *see* Sheltered workshops
Wright, K. C., 254, 478, 483, 497, 538

Y

Yoder, N. M., 254, 402, 405
Younie, W. J., 350

Z

Zytowski, D. G., 228, 235